The Future of Medicine: Frontiers in Integrative Health and Medicine

Editors

Robert H. Schneider
Mahadevan Seetharaman

MDPI • Basel • Beijing • Wuhan • Barcelona • Belgrade • Manchester • Tokyo • Cluj • Tianjin

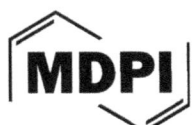

Editors
Robert H. Schneider
College of Integrative Medicine
Maharishi International University
Institute for Prevention Research
USA

Mahadevan Seetharaman
Institute of Transdisciplinary Health Sciences and Technology
India
AYUSH Global
USA

Editorial Office
MDPI
St. Alban-Anlage 66
4052 Basel, Switzerland

This is a reprint of articles from the Special Issue published online in the open access journal *Medicina* (ISSN 1010-660X) (available at: https://www.mdpi.com/journal/medicina/special_issues/Integrative_Medicine).

For citation purposes, cite each article independently as indicated on the article page online and as indicated below:

LastName, A.A.; LastName, B.B.; LastName, C.C. Article Title. *Journal Name* **Year**, *Volume Number*, Page Range.

ISBN 978-3-0365-3202-8 (Hbk)
ISBN 978-3-0365-3203-5 (PDF)

Cover image courtesy of Shutterstock.

© 2022 by the authors. Articles in this book are Open Access and distributed under the Creative Commons Attribution (CC BY) license, which allows users to download, copy and build upon published articles, as long as the author and publisher are properly credited, which ensures maximum dissemination and a wider impact of our publications.

The book as a whole is distributed by MDPI under the terms and conditions of the Creative Commons license CC BY-NC-ND.

Contents

About the Editors vii

Mahadevan Seetharaman, Geetha Krishnan and Robert H. Schneider
The Future of Medicine: Frontiers in Integrative Health and Medicine
Reprinted from: *Medicina* **2021**, *57*, 1303, doi:10.3390/medicina57121303 1

Wayne B. Jonas and Elena Rosenbaum
The Case for Whole-Person Integrative Care
Reprinted from: *Medicina* **2021**, *57*, 677, doi:10.3390/medicina57070677 9

Robert Keith Wallace
The Microbiome in Health and Disease from the Perspective of Modern Medicine and Ayurveda
Reprinted from: *Medicina* **2020**, *56*, 462, doi:10.3390/medicina56090462 21

Hari Sharma and Robert Keith Wallace
Ayurveda and Epigenetics
Reprinted from: *Medicina* **2020**, *56*, 687, doi:10.3390/medicina56120687 33

Supaya Wenuganen, Kenneth G. Walton, Shilpa Katta, Clifton L. Dalgard, Gauthaman Sukumar, Joshua Starr, Frederick T. Travis, Robert Keith Wallace, Paul Morehead, Nancy K. Lonsdorf, Meera Srivastava and John Fagan
Transcriptomics of Long-Term Meditation Practice: Evidence for Prevention or Reversal of Stress Effects Harmful to Health
Reprinted from: *Medicina* **2021**, *57*, 218, doi:10.3390/medicina57030218 41

Frederick Travis
On the Neurobiology of Meditation: Comparison of Three Organizing Strategies to Investigate Brain Patterns during Meditation Practice
Reprinted from: *Medicina* **2020**, *56*, 712, doi:10.3390/medicina56120712 59

Robert Keith Wallace
Ayurgenomics and Modern Medicine
Reprinted from: *Medicina* **2020**, *56*, 661, doi:10.3390/medicina56120661 75

Dinesh Gyawali, Rini Vohra, David Orme-Johnson, Sridharan Ramaratnam and Robert H. Schneider
A Systematic Review and Meta-Analysis of Ayurvedic Herbal Preparations for Hypercholesterolemia
Reprinted from: *Medicina* **2021**, *57*, 546, doi:10.3390/medicina57060546 83

Archana Purushotham and Alex Hankey
Vegetarian Diets, Ayurveda, and the Case for an Integrative Nutrition Science
Reprinted from: *Medicina* **2021**, *57*, 858, doi:10.3390/medicina57090858 107

Suzanne Steinbaum
The Future of Women and Heart Disease in a Pandemic Era: Let's Learn from the Past
Reprinted from: *Medicina* **2021**, *57*, 467, doi:10.3390/medicina57050467 113

Syed Ghazanfar Ali, Mohammad Azam Ansari, Mohammad A. Alzohairy, Ahmad Almatroudi, Mohammad N. Alomary, Saad Alghamdi, Suriya Rehman and Haris M. Khan
Natural Products and Nutrients against Different Viral Diseases: Prospects in Prevention and Treatment of SARS-CoV-2
Reprinted from: *Medicina* **2021**, *57*, 169, doi:10.3390/medicina57020169 . . . . **119**

Suhas G. Kshirsagar and Rammohan V. Rao
Antiviral and Immunomodulation Effects of Artemisia
Reprinted from: *Medicina* **2021**, *57*, 217, doi:10.3390/medicina57030217 . . . . **131**

Ioannis-Fivos Megas, Dascha Sophie Tolzmann, Jacqueline Bastiaanse, Paul Christian Fuchs, Bong-Sung Kim, Matthias Kröz, Friedemann Schad, Harald Matthes and Gerrit Grieb
Integrative Medicine and Plastic Surgery: A Synergy—Not an Antonym
Reprinted from: *Medicina* **2021**, *57*, 326, doi:10.3390/medicina57040326 . . . . **143**

Diego A. Arteaga-Badillo, Jacqueline Portillo-Reyes, Nancy Vargas-Mendoza, José A. Morales-González, Jeannett A. Izquierdo-Vega, Manuel Sánchez-Gutiérrez, Isela Álvarez-González, Ángel Morales-González, Eduardo Madrigal-Bujaidar and Eduardo Madrigal-Santillán
Asthma: New Integrative Treatment Strategies for the Next Decades
Reprinted from: *Medicina* **2020**, *56*, 438, doi:10.3390/medicina56090438 . . . . **151**

About the Editors

Robert H. Schneider, MD, FACC, is an internationally renowned physician scientist and leader in evidence-based integrative medicine. He is currently Dean and Professor of the College of Integrative Medicine at Maharishi International University, as well as director of the NIH-funded Institute for Prevention Research. Dr. Schneider is a specialist in preventive and integrative medicine, and has been elected as Fellow of the American College of Cardiology. For over 30 years, Dr. Schneider has directed or co-directed a series of pioneering clinical trials in integrative preventive medicine from the US National Institutes of Health and Department of Defense. Among these awards was a center of excellence for research in complementary and integrative health award, sponsored by the NIH. The results of these studies have been published in more than 150 peer-reviewed articles, chapters and abstracts. Based on his groundbreaking research and clinical experience, Dr. Schneider authored the popular book *Total Heart Health: How to Prevent and Reverse Heart Disease with the Maharishi Vedic Approach to Health*. He is currently editing a textbook on integrative medicine for physicians and health professionals.

Mahadevan Seetharaman, PhD is a Duke Integrative Healthcare Leader and Founder of AYUSH Living. He is Visiting Professor at the Institute of Transdisciplinary Health Sciences and Technology, India and guest faculty at the Hindu University of America. As an Ayurveda Diet & Nutrition Consultant and Yoga Teacher, he provides Ayurveda/Yoga related health and wellness information, directory, research, news, and reviews through his website, AYUSH Living. Dr. Mahadevan serves on the Boards of the Council for Ayurveda Research (CAR), the American Academy of Yoga and Meditation (AAYM), American Association of Ayurvedic Professionals (AAAP) and co-founded the Texas Ayurveda Professionals Association (TAPAS). He was previously the CEO and Managing Director at one of the largest integrative research university hospitals in India—the Institute of Ayurveda & Integrative Medicine (I-AIM). During this time, he served as Professor & Dean, School of Health Sciences, Transdisciplinary University. As COO, he has also helped set up an Integrative Healthcare Centre for the Isha Arogya Research Foundation.

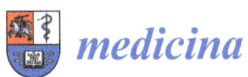

Editorial

The Future of Medicine: Frontiers in Integrative Health and Medicine

Mahadevan Seetharaman [1,2,*], Geetha Krishnan [3] and Robert H. Schneider [4,*]

1. School of Health Sciences, Institute of Transdisciplinary Health Sciences and Technology, Bengaluru 560064, India
2. AYUSH Global, Sugar Land, TX 77479, USA
3. Traditional, Complementary and Integrative Medicine Unit, Service Delivery and Safety Department, World Health Organization, 1211 Geneva, Switzerland; drgk2000@gmail.com
4. College of Integrative Medicine, Maharishi International University, Fairfield, IA 52556, USA
* Correspondence: mahadevan.seetharaman@gmail.com (M.S.); rschneider@miu.edu (R.H.S.)

1. Background

Despite advances in modern medicine, contemporary society has experienced a series of epidemics and pandemics of noncommunicable, chronic diseases and communicable, infectious diseases [1,2]. These public health crises are related, at least in part, to behavior and lifestyle [3]. There is increasing interest and growing evidence that the integration of conventional medicine with traditional, complementary, and alternative medicine (TCAM) may be useful for the prevention and treatment of communicable and chronic diseases related to behavior and lifestyle [4–6]. The World Health Organization (WHO) has been developing standards and documentation for the state and practice of TCAM [7]. The aim of this special issue of *Medicina* on "The Future of Medicine: Frontiers in Integrative Health and Medicine" was to explore the scientific evidence for these approaches of integrative medicine, which hold promise for the future of healthcare and medicine.

According to the Consortium of Academic Health Centers for Integrative Medicine and Health, integrative medicine is defined as the practice of medicine that reaffirms the importance of the relationship between practitioner and patient, focuses on the whole person, is supported by evidence, utilized all appropriate therapeutic and lifestyle approaches, healthcare professionals and disciplines to achieve optimal health and healing [8–10]. TCAM includes modalities such as Ayurveda, Yoga, traditional Chinese medicine, other traditional systems of medicine, meditation, herbal medicines, nutritional supplements, movement therapies, and other mind-body practices. The World Health Organization (WHO) now refers to this set as Traditional, Complementary and Integrative Medicine (TCIM) [11].

There has been a surge in the public interest and the use of TCIM globally. Nearly 50% of the population in developed nations (United States, 42%; Australia, 48%; France, 49%; Canada, 70%), and similar or greater numbers in developing countries (India, 70%; China, 40%; Chile, 71%; Colombia, 40%; up to 80% in Africa) use some form of TCIM [12]. The World Health Organization and governments of several countries have established agencies to support research and practical utilization of TCIM [13].

The trends driving integration of TCIM in contemporary healthcare are presented in Figure 1. According to the WHO, non-communicable or chronic diseases continue to rise globally [14,15]. These diseases are not adequately prevented or treated by modern medicine and are often accompanied by high rates of adverse side effects. With an ageing population using polypharmacy, adverse events are also increasing [16] The costs of modern healthcare are high [17], with chronic disease accounting for approximately 75% of the US aggregate health care spending according to the Centers for Disease Control and Prevention (CDC) [18–21]. The trends also show high utilization of complementary and alternative medicine (CAM) amongst the public with most patients using CAM in conjunction with modern medical care and majority of them do not inform their primary care physicians about the use of CAM modalities [4]. There is inadequate education of physicians and other health professionals about CAM methods, and high interest amongst medical professionals in CAM education according to the Academic Consortium for Integrative Medicine and Health [22]. New clinical practice guidelines from conventional medical organizations are starting to include considerations of CAM practices, e.g., in cardiovascular health [23], cancer [24], pain [25] and mental health [26].

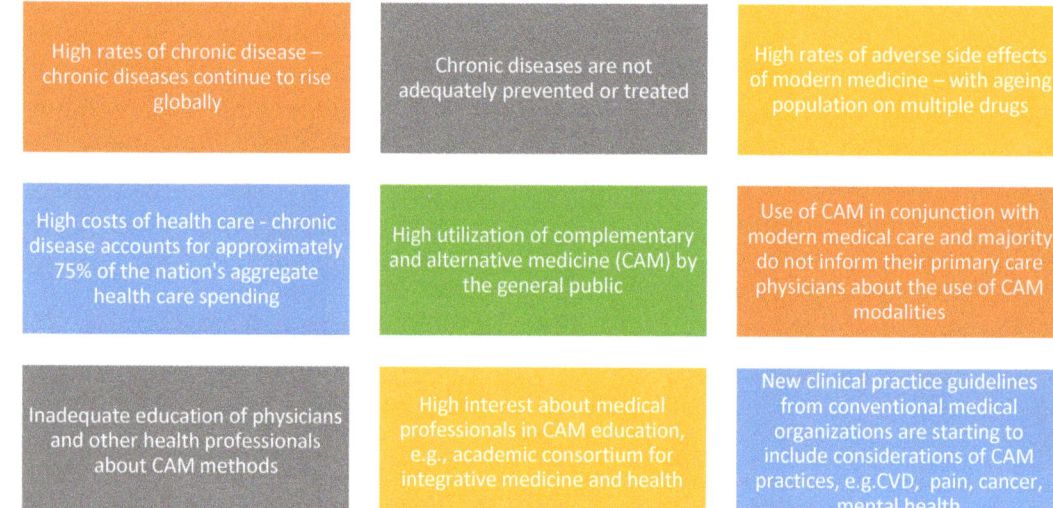

Figure 1. Trends driving integration of TCIM in contemporary healthcare. TCIM: Traditional, Complementary and Integrative Medicine; CVD: cardiovascular disease.

At present, the growing use of integrative medicine has stimulated the scientific community, national and global policy organizations to investigate the clinical efficacy, mechanisms of action, healthcare costs, standards, protocols and policy implications of these therapies [27–29]. However, with notable exceptions, much of this effort has been on quality, safety, and efficacy of TCIM products mainly due to the potential for exploitation in drug discovery and development [30].

2. Current Contributions

The goal of this special issue of *Medicina* was to address these gaps in collective understanding and to promote the integration of TCIM into contemporary medicine and public health. This collection of articles will stimulate further research and support healthcare professionals, consumers, and policy makers to make informed decisions about the utilization of evidence-based integrative medicine for the future of healthcare.

There are several critical observations and implications on the management of communicable and non-communicable diseases based on this series of papers. Using microarray experiments, Wenuganen et al. studied the effects of Transcendental Meditation (TM) practice on the expression of 200 genes [31]. Compared to control group, 49 inflammation related genes were downregulated, while genes associated with antiviral and antibody components of the defense response were upregulated. Meditation might have an important role to play in the management of chronic diseases, including anxiety, post-traumatic stress disorder (PTSD), cardiovascular disease (CVD) and communicable diseases. As meditation practices have become more common place, Travis presents three strategies to organize and study brain patterns during meditation practice [32].

We are still in the midst of the SARS-CoV-2 pandemic and the scientific and medical community is looking for novel therapeutic and preventive anti-viral candidates. Ali et al.

(2021) highlight natural medicines that could be used against SARS-CoV-2 including plants like *Glycyrrhiza glabra (licorice), Alnus japonica (alder), Allium sativum (garlic), Houttuynia cordata, Lycoris radiata, Tinospora cordifolia (guduchi)* and *Vitex trifolia (nirgundi)* [33]. Vitamins such as A, B2, B3, B-12, C, D and E, and minerals such as Zinc may have a possible role in SARS-CoV-2 prevention by enhancing immunity.

Kshirsagar and Rao (2021) present recent studies that have investigated derivatives from the plant Artemesia that is widely used in Ayurveda and traditional Chinese medicine (TCM) for its antiviral, antifungal, antimicrobial, insecticidal, hepatoprotective and neuroprotective properties [34]. The notable phytochemical Artimesinin from Artemesia has shown not only to have potent antiviral actions but also utility against the severe acute respiratory syndrome coronavirus 2 (SARS-CoV-2). Youyou Tu was awarded the Nobel Prize in 2015 for the discovery of antimalarial properties of Artemisinin [35], which holds promise for anti-viral and anti-inflammatory drug discovery from traditional plant sources.

The traditional healthcare system of India, Ayurveda typically recommends changes in diet, lifestyle, behavior, digestion, stress, and environmental factors for prevention and treatment. These are factors that cause epigenetic changes and affect gene expression. Sharma and Wallace propose that epigenetics is an important mechanism of Ayurveda and studying the effects of Ayurveda-based modalities on gene expression will increase understanding between Ayurveda and modern medical science [36]. Wallace reviews and provides an update on the developments in Ayurgenomics, the field that integrates concepts in Ayurveda, such as Prakriti, with modern genetics research. He suggests that the *Tridhosha* theory of Ayurveda (the combination of three physiological modulators—Vata, Pitta and Kapha) correlates with the expression of specific genes and physiological characteristics [37].

According to Ayurveda, the gut has an important link to the health of an individual. Diet and digestion influence the composition of the gut microbiome. Ayurveda has been focusing on the role of digestion in health and disease for millennia. The author presents the connection between the gut microbiome and various prevention and therapeutic approaches of Ayurveda [38]. This has major implications in the field of integrative Ayurveda that combines the best practices of Ayurveda with modern medicine.

Arteaga-Badillo et al. (2021) present new integrative treatment strategies for the management of asthma [39]. Scientific evidence suggests that diet including fruits, vegetables, seeds, whole cereals, consumption of vitamins A, C, and E and the use of plants and natural extracts (phytotherapy) may help relieve symptoms of asthma. In particular, plants such as *Glycyrrhiza uralensis, Angelica sinensis, Pinellia ternata, Astragalus membranaceus, Helichrysum stoechas, Eucalyptus globulus, Rosmarinus officinalis, Zingiber officinale, Inula helenium* and *Allium sativum* L., have shown significant benefits.

A systematic review and meta-analysis of Ayurveda based herbal preparations for hypercholesterolemia is presented by Gyawali et al. (2021). These authors found that three Ayurvedic herbs—garlic, guggul and black cumin, were safe and effective in reducing cholesterol biomarkers. Several other Ayurvedic interventions that include the herbs, holy basil, ginger, fenugreek, arjuna and Indian gooseberry may also ameliorate hypercholesterolemia [40].

Megas et al. hypothesize that conventional therapy integrated with Anthroposophic therapies may be potent and beneficial for plastic surgery patients. In this approach, not only functional and physical approaches are stressed, but also mental state, creativity, and self-determination. Complementary approaches include Anthroposophical massage (rhythmical massage and streaming massage), breathing therapy, ergotherapy, eurythmy therapy, hyperthermia, painting therapy, clay modelling therapy, music therapy, physiotherapy, and psychotherapy. Along with these mind body practices; natural products are incorporated [41].

Steinbaum argues in her perspective article that women have been proportionately affected by the COVID-19 pandemic. Of the 5 million women-run businesses, 25% of them closed within two months of the pandemic outbreak. These stressors impact psychological and physical health. Stress and lack of self-care increases chances of heart disease, the number one killer in women. Stress impacts behavior, resulting in overeating, sedentary behavior, poor diets, increased alcohol intake and lifestyle, all preventable risk factors for heart disease [42].

Jonas and Rosenbaum shared their perspective on the need for standardization of whole-person models and research using whole systems approaches [43]. Whole person medicine includes dimensions of health that consider behavior and lifestyle, social and emotional dimensions, and an individual's mental and spiritual dimensions. The authors present the status of current evidence on holistic models for improved health outcomes, patient satisfaction, health care costs and clinical experience.

Purushotham and Hankey [44] conducted a detailed comparison of the dietary intake of food groups in two cohort studies of diet and stroke that had disparate results. They applied the nutritional principles of Ayurveda to suggest how these apparently contradictory results may be explained. The authors propose that traditional systems of medicine, such as Ayurveda possess clinically relevant knowledge of the effects of food on physiology and health.

The TCIM modalities reported in this special issue may be applied to the COVID-19 pandemic, prevention of future pandemics, and to address the on-going epidemic of non-communicable, lifestyle-related diseases. This collection of articles stimulates further research in integrative medicine and supports healthcare professionals to make informed decisions about the practice of evidence-based integrative medicine in contemporary healthcare settings around the world.

3. Post-COVID-19 Era: An Integrative Vision of Healthcare—Public Health and Policy Recommendations

At the time of writing, COVID-19 infections and death continue in pandemic proportions [45]. Clinical management, research and therapeutic strategies for COVID-19 have focused on either tackling the virus directly or immunize against it. Over the past century, society experienced a series of pandemics or epidemics, notably polio, smallpox, cholera, plague, dengue, AIDS, West Nile, tuberculosis, severe acute respiratory syndrome (SARS) and now COVID-19 [1,46]. On the contrary, Ayurveda, amongst the oldest and most widely practiced traditional healthcare systems, recommends preventive measures for improving immunity through healthy lifestyle in addition to acute therapy when indicated. Ancient Ayurveda texts, notably *Charaka Samhita* discuss epidemic management and immunity enhancement to prevent disease, arrest its progression and to maintain health on the individual and public health scales [47]. The Ayurvedic texts explains the onset of pandemics when there is collective human stress the disrupts endogenous preventive capacities. The concept of building and maintaining balanced functioning of the mind and body to cope with internal and external stressors, including infectious microorganisms, is the fundamental strategy of Ayurveda [48]. Many of these preventive principles have garnered modern scientific evidence which then supports the proposal that they are physiologically applicable across cultures and geography [48–50].

An integrative approach to healthcare that focuses on prevention and immunity building is imperative to preventive future pandemics. Such an approach to healthcare would involve modern medicine education and practice incorporating traditional, complementary, and alternative medical approaches including Ayurveda, Yoga, Chinese medicine, and other traditional systems of medicine. The development of an integrative curriculum will lead to a more complete understanding of optimal health and wellness. In modern scientific language this is termed, systems medicine which encompasses the individual, family, community, and the environment [51,52]. Ayurveda describes this systems approach to health care in the concept of '*Swasthya*' or wholeness. That is, optimal health and well-being are based on inner wholeness together with a balance of mind, body, social and physical environments [49,52,53]. This would require a revision of health care for the 21st century that shifts the paradigm from a standardized approach to personalized prevention and treatment, from a short-term to long-term sustainable intervention, from single molecular targets to an integrated system of networks and, from treatment with adverse effects to prevention and holistic health promotion.

In a way, the COVID-19 pandemic has been an eye opener for the scientific community and policymakers alike. It has shown to us that the resources and knowledge, the skills and human capital, the medicines, and the infrastructure, all fall behind expectations when faced with a pandemic of this stature [54]. It calls out at us that the current preparedness to achieve the sustainable development goals (SDG) of the United Nations is a mirage and unachievable, unless deliberate drastic, and systemic changes are brought about in their approach by communities and nations, in its pursuit [55]. It is evident that unless all resources available to human societies are utilised in the most effective an appropriate manner, we might be found formulating an SDG 2050, in the year 2030 without much change of its expected outcomes. Integrative medicine therefore is not a possibility but and a necessity. Human societies, whether technologically and financially advanced or deprived, will have to find their own integrative models in public health to achieve their expectations in health outcomes by 2030. In Africa, for example, an integrative model might look at skilling traditional practitioners to identify diseases, create knowledge base of available medicinal interventions, support evidence generation, provide guidelines for specific clinical interventions which are safe and effective, and develop and establish clear referral models [56–59]. In India, the home of Ayurveda, the contemporary health care system might utilize the country's range of traditional modalities (AYUSH) in prevention and early management of diseases, and health management of categorised population groups such as the aged, women and children, healthy adults, palliative care etc [60]. In the United States, Germany, or Canada it might evolve to support specific public health initiatives in cancer care, pain management, palliative care etc. It could also extend to clinical conditions such as sleep medicine and support specific neurodegenerative conditions. Emerging areas such as wellness or mental health promotion, will progress faster, when TCIM knowledge gets integrated into research, practice, education, and policy. Whichever may be the course taken by contemporary society, integrative medicine is here to stay and nations who ignore its precious resources would do so at their own economic and health costs.

Funding: No external funding was provided for this manuscript.

Institutional Review Board Statement: Not applicable.

Informed Consent Statement: Not applicable.

Data Availability Statement: Not applicable.

Acknowledgments: The Editors would like to thank Rammohan Rao for valuable discussions.

Conflicts of Interest: Where authors are identified as personnel of the World Health Organization, the authors alone are responsible for the views expressed in this article and they do not necessarily represent the decisions, policy, or views of the International Agency for Research on Cancer/World Health Organization

References

1. Huremović, D. Brief History of Pandemics (Pandemics Throughout History). In *Psychiatry of Pandemics*; Huremović, D., Ed.; Springer: Cham, Switzerland, 2019; pp. 7–35.
2. Jamison, D.T.; Gelband, H.; Horton, S.; Jha, P.; Laxminarayan, R.; Mock, C.N.; Nugent, R. (Eds.) *Disease Control Priorities: Improving Health and Reducing Poverty*, 3rd ed.; The International Bank for Reconstruction and Development; The World Bank: Washington, DC, USA, 2017.
3. Noce, A.; Romani, A.; Bernini, R. Dietary Intake and Chronic Disease Prevention. *Nutrients* **2021**, *13*, 1358. [CrossRef] [PubMed]
4. Eisenberg, D.M.; Kessler, R.C.; Foster, C.; Norlock, F.E.; Calkins, D.R.; Delbanco, T.L. Unconventional Medicine in the United States—Prevalence, Costs, and Patterns of Use. *N. Engl. J. Med.* **1993**, *328*, 246–252. [CrossRef] [PubMed]
5. Complementary, Alternative, or Integrative Health: What's In a Name? Available online: https://www.nccih.nih.gov/health/complementary-alternative-or-integrative-health-whats-in-a-name (accessed on 1 October 2021).
6. Frass, M.; Strassl, R.P.; Friehs, H.; Müllner, M.; Kundi, M.; Kaye, A.D. Use and acceptance of complementary and alternative medicine among the general population and medical personnel: A systematic review. *Ochsner J.* **2012**, *12*, 45–56. [PubMed]
7. Ong, C.K.; Bodeker, G.; World Health Organization. *WHO Global Atlas of Traditional, Complementary, and Alternative Medicine*; World Health Organization, Centre for Health Development: Kobe, Japan, 2005.

8. Witt, C.M.; Chiaramonte, D.; Berman, S.; Chesney, M.A.; Kaplan, G.A.; Stange, K.C.; Woolf, S.H.; Berman, B.M. Defining Health in a Comprehensive Context: A New Definition of Integrative Health. *Am. J. Prev. Med.* **2017**, *53*, 134–137. [CrossRef]
9. The Academic Consortium for Integrative Medicine & Health. Available online: https://imconsortium.org/about/introduction/ (accessed on 1 October 2021).
10. Weeks, J. Five Eras and 125 Milestones in The Rise of Integrative Health and Medicine plus more. *Integr. Med.* **2017**, *16*, 26–28.
11. WHO. *WHO Global Report on Traditional and Complementary Medicine 2019*; World Health Organization: Geneva, Switzerland, 2019.
12. Bodeker, G.; Kronenberg, F. A Public Health Agenda for Traditional, Complementary, and Alternative Medicine. *Am. J. Public Health* **2002**, *92*, 1582–1591. [CrossRef]
13. World Health Organization (WHO). *WHO Traditional Medicine Strategy 2014–2023*; WHO: Geneva, Switzerland, 2013; Available online: https://www.who.int/publications/i/item/9789241506096 (accessed on 1 October 2021).
14. World Health Organization. Noncommunicable Diseases Country Profiles 2018. Available online: https://www.who.int/publications/i/item/ncd-country-profiles-2018 (accessed on 1 October 2021).
15. World Health Organization. Noncommunicable Diseases Fact Sheet. Available online: https://www.who.int/news-room/fact-sheets/detail/noncommunicable-diseases (accessed on 1 October 2021).
16. Cantlay, A.; Glyn, T.; Barton, N. Polypharmacy in the elderly. *InnovAiT Educ. Inspir. Gen. Pr.* **2016**, *9*, 69–77. [CrossRef]
17. Hajat, C.; Stein, E. The global burden of multiple chronic conditions: A narrative review. *Prev. Med. Rep.* **2018**, *12*, 284–293. [CrossRef]
18. Centers for Disease Control and Prevention. About Chronic Diseases. Available online: https://www.cdc.gov/chronicdisease/about/index.htm (accessed on 1 October 2021).
19. Buttorff, C.; Ruder, T.; Bauman, M. *Multiple Chronic Conditions in the United States*; Rand Corp: Santa Monica, CA, USA, 2017.
20. Martin, A.B.; Hartman, M.; Lassman, D.; Catlin, A. National Health Care Spending in 2019: Steady Growth for the Fourth Consecutive Year. *Health Aff.* **2020**, *40*, 1–11. [CrossRef]
21. Bloom, D.E.; Cafiero, E.T.; Jané-Llopis, E.; Abrahams-Gessel, S.; Bloom, L.R.; Fathima, S.; Feigl, A.B.; Gaziano, T.; Mowafi, M.; Pandya, A.; et al. *The Global Economic Burden of Noncommunicable Diseases*; World Economic Forum: Geneva, Switzerland, 2011.
22. Horrigan, B.; Lewis, S.; Abrams, D.I.; Pechura, C. Integrative Medicine in America—How Integrative Medicine is Being Practiced in Clinical Centers across the United States. *Glob. Adv. Health Med.* **2012**, *1*, 18–52. [CrossRef]
23. Kohl, W.K.; Dobos, G.; Cramer, H. Conventional and Complementary Healthcare Utilization Among US Adults With Cardiovascular Disease or Cardiovascular Risk Factors: A Nationally Representative Survey. *J. Am. Hear. Assoc.* **2020**, *9*, e014759. [CrossRef] [PubMed]
24. Greenlee, H.; DuPont-Reyes, M.J.; Rn, L.G.B.; Carlson, L.E.; Cohen, M.R.; Deng, G.; Johnson, J.A.; Mumber, M.; Seely, D.; Zick, S.M.; et al. Clinical practice guidelines on the evidence-based use of integrative therapies during and after breast cancer treatment. *CA Cancer J. Clin.* **2017**, *67*, 194–232. [CrossRef] [PubMed]
25. Qaseem, A.; Wilt, T.J.; McLean, R.M.; Forciea, M.A.; Clinical Guidelines Committee of the American College of Physicians; Denberg, T.D.; Barry, M.J.; Boyd, C.; Chow, R.D.; Fitterman, N.; et al. Noninvasive Treatments for Acute, Subacute, and Chronic Low Back Pain: A Clinical Practice Guideline From the American College of Physicians. *Ann. Intern. Med.* **2017**, *166*, 514–530. [CrossRef] [PubMed]
26. Melzer, J.; Deter, H.-C.; Uehleke, B. CAM in Psychiatry. *Evid.-Based Complement. Altern. Med.* **2013**, *2013*, 293248. [CrossRef]
27. Lakshmi, J.K.; Nambiar, D.; Narayan, V.; Sathyanarayana, T.N.; Porter, J.; Sheikh, K. Cultural consonance, constructions of science and co-existence: A review of the integration of traditional, complementary and alternative medicine in low- and middle-income countries. *Health Policy Plan.* **2014**, *30*, 1067–1077. [CrossRef]
28. Sierpina, V.S.; Dalen, J.E. The Future of Integrative Medicine. *Am. J. Med.* **2013**, *126*, 661–662. [CrossRef]
29. Xue, C.C. Traditional, complementary and alternative medicine: Policy and public health perspectives. *Bull. World Health Organ.* **2008**, *86*, 77–78. [CrossRef]
30. Barnes, J. Quality, efficacy and safety of complementary medicines: Fashions, facts and the future. Part I. Regulation and quality. *Br. J. Clin. Pharmacol.* **2003**, *55*, 226–233. [CrossRef]
31. Wenuganen, S.; Walton, K.; Katta, S.; Dalgard, C.; Sukumar, G.; Starr, J.; Travis, F.; Wallace, R.; Morehead, P.; Lonsdorf, N.; et al. Transcriptomics of Long-Term Meditation Practice: Evidence for Prevention or Reversal of Stress Effects Harmful to Health. *Medicina* **2021**, *57*, 218. [CrossRef]
32. Travis, F. On the Neurobiology of Meditation: Comparison of Three Organizing Strategies to Investigate Brain Patterns during Meditation Practice. *Medicina* **2020**, *56*, 712. [CrossRef]
33. Ali, S.; Ansari, M.; Alzohairy, M.; Almatroudi, A.; Alomary, M.; Alghamdi, S.; Rehman, S.; Khan, H. Natural Products and Nutrients against Different Viral Diseases: Prospects in Prevention and Treatment of SARS-CoV-2. *Medicina* **2021**, *57*, 169. [CrossRef] [PubMed]
34. Kshirsagar, S.; Rao, R. Antiviral and Immunomodulation Effects of Artemisia. *Medicina* **2021**, *57*, 217. [CrossRef] [PubMed]
35. Su, X.-Z.; Miller, L.H. The discovery of artemisinin and the Nobel Prize in Physiology or Medicine. *Sci. China Life Sci.* **2015**, *58*, 1175–1179. [CrossRef]
36. Sharma, H.; Wallace, R.K. Ayurveda and Epigenetics. *Medicina* **2020**, *56*, 687. [CrossRef] [PubMed]
37. Wallace, R. Ayurgenomics and Modern Medicine. *Medicina* **2020**, *56*, 661. [CrossRef] [PubMed]

38. Wallace, R. The Microbiome in Health and Disease from the Perspective of Modern Medicine and Ayurveda. *Medicina* **2020**, *56*, 462. [CrossRef]
39. Arteaga-Badillo, D.; Portillo-Reyes, J.; Vargas-Mendoza, N.; Morales-González, J.; Izquierdo-Vega, J.; Sánchez-Gutiérrez, M.; Álvarez-González, I.; Morales-González, Á.; Madrigal-Bujaidar, E.; Madrigal-Santillán, E. Asthma: New Integrative Treatment Strategies for the Next Decades. *Medicina* **2020**, *56*, 438. [CrossRef] [PubMed]
40. Gyawali, D.; Vohra, R.; Orme-Johnson, D.; Ramaratnam, S.; Schneider, R. A Systematic Review and Meta-Analysis of Ayurvedic Herbal Preparations for Hypercholesterolemia. *Medicina* **2021**, *57*, 546. [CrossRef] [PubMed]
41. Megas, I.-F.; Tolzmann, D.; Bastiaanse, J.; Fuchs, P.; Kim, B.-S.; Kröz, M.; Schad, F.; Matthes, H.; Grieb, G. Integrative Medicine and Plastic Surgery: A Synergy—Not an Antonym. *Medicina* **2021**, *57*, 326. [CrossRef]
42. Steinbaum, S. The Future of Women and Heart Disease in a Pandemic Era: Let's Learn from the Past. *Medicina* **2021**, *57*, 467. [CrossRef]
43. Jonas, W.; Rosenbaum, E. The Case for Whole-Person Integrative Care. *Medicina* **2021**, *57*, 677. [CrossRef] [PubMed]
44. Purushotham, A.; Hankey, A. Vegetarian Diets, Ayurveda, and the Case for an Integrative Nutrition Science. *Medicina* **2021**, *57*, 858. [CrossRef] [PubMed]
45. World Health Organization. WHO Coronavirus Disease (COVID-19) Dashboard. Available online: https://covid19.who.int/ (accessed on 1 October 2021).
46. Morens, D.M.; Fauci, A.S. Emerging Pandemic Diseases: How We Got to COVID-19. *Cell* **2020**, *182*, 1077–1092, Erratum in: **2020**, *183*, 837. [CrossRef] [PubMed]
47. Charaka Samhita. Available online: http://www.carakasamhitaonline.com/ (accessed on 1 October 2021).
48. Tillu, G.; Chaturvedi, S.; Chopra, A.; Patwardhan, B. Public Health Approach of Ayurveda and Yoga for COVID-19 Prophylaxis. *J. Altern. Complement. Med.* **2020**, *26*, 360–364. [CrossRef]
49. Sharma, H.; Clark, C. *Ayurvedic Healing: Contemporary Maharishi Ayurveda Medicine and Science*; Singing Dragon: London, UK, 2012.
50. Schneider, R.H.; Alexander, C.N.; Salerno, J.W.; Robinson, D.K.; Fields, J.Z.; Nidich, S.I. Disease Prevention and Health Promotion in the Aging with a Traditional System of Natural Medicine—Maharishi Vedic Medicine (MVM). *J. Aging Health* **2002**, *14*, 57–78. [CrossRef]
51. Federoff, H.J.; Gostin, L.O. Evolving from reductionism to holism: Is there a future for systems medicine? *JAMA* **2009**, *302*, 994–996. [CrossRef]
52. Luke, D.A.; Stamatakis, K.A. Systems Science Methods in Public Health: Dynamics, Networks, and Agents. *Annu. Rev. Public Health* **2012**, *33*, 357–376. [CrossRef]
53. Susruta. *Susruta Samhita, Sutra Sthana, 35/3*, 8th ed.; Vaidya Jadavaji Trikamji Acharya; Choukhamba Orientalia: Varanasi, India, 2005.
54. DeSalvo, K.; Hughes, B.; Bassett, M.; Benjamin, G.; Fraser, M.; Galea, S.; Gracia, J.N.; Howard, J. *Public Health COVID-19 Impact Assessment: Lessons Learned and Compelling Needs. NAM Perspectives. Discussion Paper*; National Academy of Medicine: Washington, DC, USA, 2021. [CrossRef]
55. World Health Organization & United Nations Children's Fund (UNICEF). *A Vision for Primary Health Care in the 21st Century: Towards Universal Health Coverage and the Sustainable Development Goals*; World Health Organization: Geneva, Switzerland, 2018.
56. Kasilo, O.M.J.; Wambebe, C.; Nikiema, J.-B.; Nabyonga-Orem, J. Towards universal health coverage: Advancing the development and use of traditional medicines in Africa. *BMJ Glob. Health* **2019**, *4*, e001517. [CrossRef]
57. Nsagha, D.S.; Ayima, C.W.; Nana-Njamen, T.; Assob, J.C. The Role of Traditional, Complementary/Alternative Medicine in Primary Healthcare, Adjunct to Universal Health Coverage in Cameroon: A Review of the Literature. *Am. J. Epidemiol.* **2020**, *8*, 37–47.
58. Onyambu, M.O.; Gikonyo, N.K.; Nyambaka, H.N.; Thoithi, G.N. A review of trends in herbal drugs standardization, regulation and integration to the national healthcare systems in Kenya and the globe. *Int. J. Pharmacogn. Chin. Med.* **2019**, *3*. [CrossRef]
59. James, P.B.; Wardle, J.; Steel, A.; Adams, J. Traditional, complementary and alternative medicine use in Sub-Saharan Africa: A systematic review. *BMJ Glob. Health* **2018**, *3*, e000895. [CrossRef] [PubMed]
60. Patwardhan, B. Health for India: Search for appropriate models. *J. Ayurveda Integr. Med.* **2012**, *3*, 173–174. [CrossRef] [PubMed]

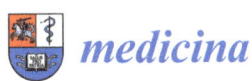 *medicina*

Perspective

The Case for Whole-Person Integrative Care

Wayne B. Jonas [1,*] **and Elena Rosenbaum** [2]

[1] Samueli Foundation, Alexandria, VA 22314, USA
[2] Department of Family and Community Medicine, Albany Medical College, Albany, NY 12208, USA; erosenbaum@communitycare.com
* Correspondence: Healing@samueli.org; Tel.: +1-7-03-647-7435

Abstract: *Rationale:* There is a need for medicine to deliver more whole-person care. This is a narrative review of several models of whole-person care and studies that illustrate the business case for whole-person models in primary care. *Objectives:* To provide an overview of what whole-person care models exist and explore evidence to support these models. *Study Selection:* Representative whole-person care models widely used in the United States are summarized and evaluated. Selected studies focused on outpatient primary care with examples from programs that integrate the delivery of conventional medical care, complementary and alternative medicine, and self-care within the context of social and cultural environments. *Methods:* Pubmed search conducted December 2020–February 2021. Two iterative searches using terms for "Whole Health Veterans Administration", "integrative medicine", "integrative health", "complementary and alternative medicine", and, as they related to the outcomes, of "health outcomes", "cost-effectiveness", "cost reduction", "patient satisfaction", and "physician satisfaction". Additional studies were identified from an initial search and the authors' experience of over 50 years. We looked for studies of whole-person care used in general primary care, those not using a single modality and only from United States practices. *Results:* A total of 125 (out of 1746) studies were found and met our inclusion criteria. We found that whole-person models of primary care exist, are quite heterogeneous in their approaches, and routinely report substantial benefits for improving the patient experience, clinical outcomes and in reducing costs. *Conclusions:* Evidence for the benefit of whole-person care models exist but definitions are quite heterogenous and unfocused. There is a need for more standardization of whole-person models and more research using whole systems approaches rather than reductionistic attempts using isolated components.

Keywords: integrative health; whole-person health; systems research; reductionism; complementary and alternative medicine; healing; healthcare transformation; overview

1. Introduction

For the last 100 years, healthcare has been dominated by the relentless application of a certain strategy in science known as reductionism. In this strategy the person is divided into ever smaller parts including organs, tissues, cells, organelles, proteins, and finally genetic material—RNA and DNA. This research strategy involves looking at how these parts influence each other and designing ways to control those parts. From this we have an explosion in knowledge of the parts of an individual and their mostly physical component interactions. This "knowledge of the parts" is then applied to a whole person by attempting to control these physical processes when they seem to be involved in disease. Treatment is framed almost entirely around controlling these component parts and attempting to balance the effectiveness of this control against the interference this control also places on normal, non-disease processes, producing unwanted effects.

Our theory is that in pursing the reductionistic strategy in science, we have neglected development of more "holistic" approaches of evaluation that provide more direct and relevant value for what matters in health care. Almost inevitably, the attempt to control one part of a complex system like a whole human being results in only partial effects (a small degree of efficacy) and adverse (unwanted) effects. Frequently, this produces more problems than it solves, and is fundamentally not designed to enhance the salutogenic and adaptogenic processes that rebalance a person's health as a whole [1,2]. In other words, the application of reductionism results in a focused attempt to control or remove the disease—to cure—rather than to restore the organism to optimal functioning—to heal.

Thus, there is a need to develop and use more "whole person" and "whole systems" strategies and evaluate their impact on health care outcomes, patient and provider experience and costs. This gap is now the focus of the strategic plan for the National Center for Complementary and Integrative Health (NCCIH), of the United States National Institutes of Health. [3] In his article we review some of these "whole person approaches" and evaluate their impact on the main outcomes desired in health care—clinical outcomes, experiences of care, and costs.

2. A Whole Person

A person is more than just their physical components or parts. They consist of the body and the external environment for sure but are also made up of at least three other dimensions including: (1) their behavior and lifestyle that interacts with the environment; (2) their social and emotional dimensions; and (3) their mental and spiritual dimensions, which bring meaning and purpose to life. These dimensions of what make up a human being have been defined by classic writers such as Abraham Maslow in the Hierarchy of Human Needs [4], Victor Frankel who demonstrated the importance of meaning for survival [5], and George Engel in his landmark work on the biopsychosocial model in biology and medicine [6].

How then can we develop health care that addresses the whole person in all his, her or their dimensions? Additionally, what evidence do we have that heath care models that incorporate whole person, rather than reductionistic models produce benefit on outcomes that matter, such as health outcomes, patient and provider experience and costs. In this narrative review, we describe several models of care that start from a holistic rather than a reductionistic perspective. We then review the selected literature for the impact these holistic approaches can have had on relevant outcomes. Our goal is to better, describe, define, and demonstrate the value of a new type of health care focused on the whole person.

3. Examples of Whole-Person Models

3.1. Optimal Healing Environments

Multiple models and operational frameworks have been created to conceptualize and deliver whole-person care. An example is the Optimal Healing Environment (OHE) framework developed by the Samueli Institute in 2003 [7]. Figure 1 illustrates this model. Several health care systems have used this framework for their operations and reported improved patient experience [8]. In addition, a comprehensive review of the business case benefits of this approach is published [9].

3.2. Total Force Fitness

Another example is the Total Force Fitness (TFF) model facilitated by the Samueli Institute and used by the US Military [10]. Figure 2 shows this model. TFF went beyond a medical environment to include physical, psychological, spiritual, social, and even economic aspects of human flourishing, integrated into a single framework and data collection system. This model sought to use a comprehensive whole-person framework for use in health care, as well as prevention and readiness within a military context. Multiple offshoots of this framework documented its value and are being applied in clinical settings such as the "Performance Triad" [11], in entire communities such as "Operation LiveWell", and the latest and most sophisticated version applied to the entire enterprise called the Holistic Health and Fitness (H2F) Program [12]. This program "recognizes that readiness depends on the proper combinations of physical fitness (such as strength, speed, and endurance) and foundational health (such as the cardiovascular, respiratory, immune, and hormonal systems), which are optimized through careful attention to nutritional readiness, mental readiness, spiritual readiness, and sleep readiness". HF2 aims to track the total health and function of a person in real-time to optimize function, not just treat disease.

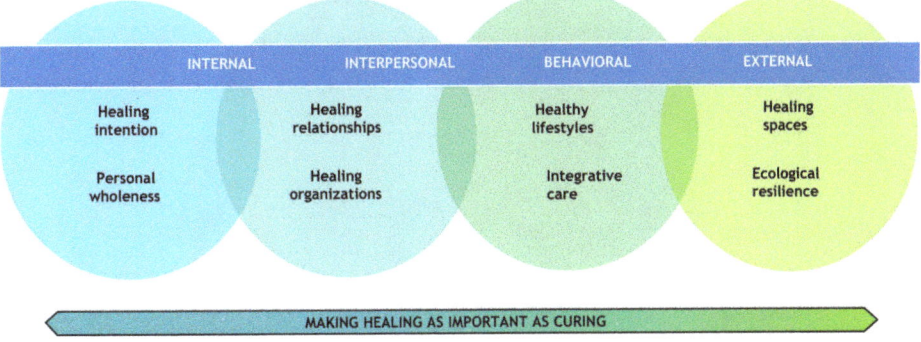

Figure 1. The Optimal Healing Environments Model.

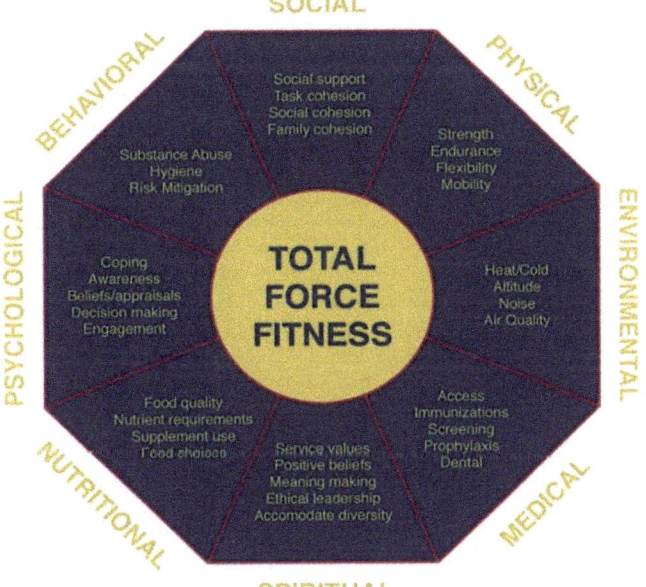

Figure 2. The Total Force Fitness Model.

3.3. Whole Health

Another, more recent model is currently being implemented in the Veteran's Health Administration (VHA) called Whole Health [13]. This approach starts with the mental and spiritual dimension, asking patients "what matters" to them in their life—their meaning and purpose—and then capturing 10 areas of behavior, lifestyle, and social support to create a "personal health plan" based on those assessments. Recent research on the outcomes from this model has found significant improvements in all major areas and will be reported on later in this review. Figure 3 illustrates this model.

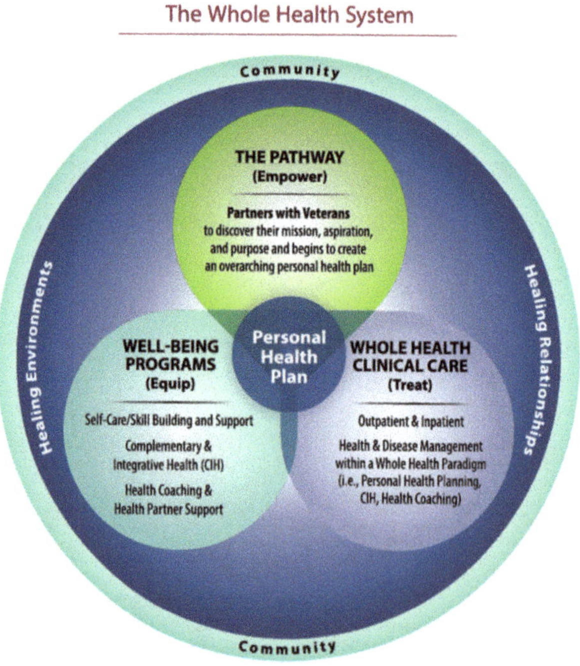

Figure 3. The VHA Whole Health Model.

3.4. Integrative Health

The latest evolution of what has been called complementary and alternative medicine is integrative health. Integrative health involves the optimal combination of all evidence-based approaches to help heal the person as a whole. Integrative care defines itself as the appropriate merger and integration of conventional care, drugless approaches, including complementary and alternative medicine (CAM), and behavior and lifestyle medicine. Integrative medicine and integrative health are being used by over 70 academic health centers in the U.S. and Canada, which have formed an organization called the Academic Consortium for Integrative Medicine and Health. The University of California, Irvine is the first major University to completely embrace this approach with others following [14,15]. Figure 4 illustrates this approach.

3.5. Advanced Primacy Care

Integrative health care is part of a larger type of whole-person primary care we have recently described as Advanced Primary Care [16]. Briefly this model begins with the basic transaction with the patient, the encounter, and the therapy, but then surrounds that transaction with three additional circles of care that enhance or enable whole-person care. In the first circle are the components of the Starfield model of primary care that includes first contact, comprehensive and continuous care. Then, a second circle using enhanced management systems for care is provided to better integrate care delivery. This circle includes chronic disease management, enhanced care coordination, pharmacy services, and the integration of mental health. The fourth and final circle brings in support for lifestyle change and CAM and a process for addressing the social and economic determinants of health. Integrative health has a role in supporting behavioral and lifestyle determinants. Figure 5 illustrates this model.

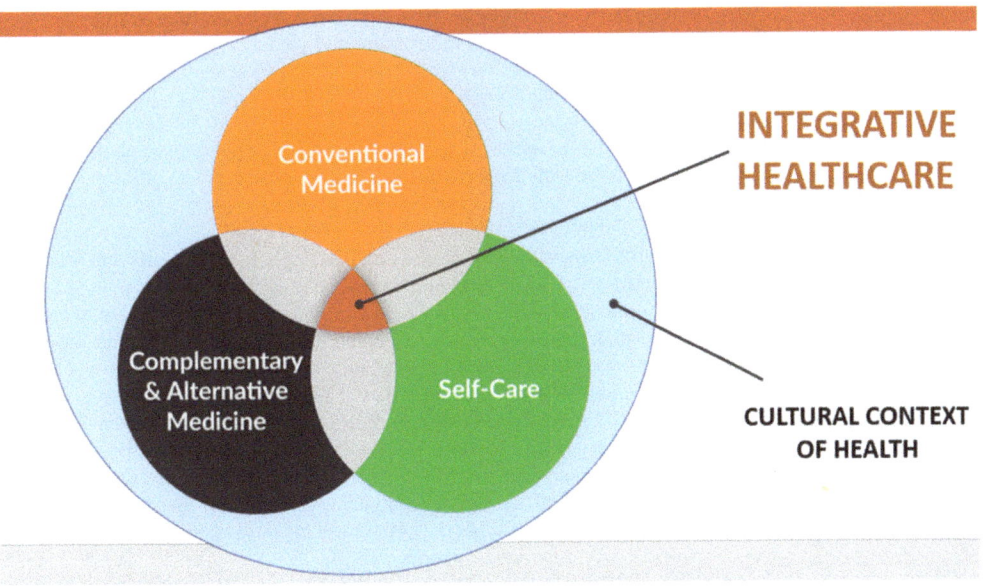

Figure 4. The Integrative Health Model.

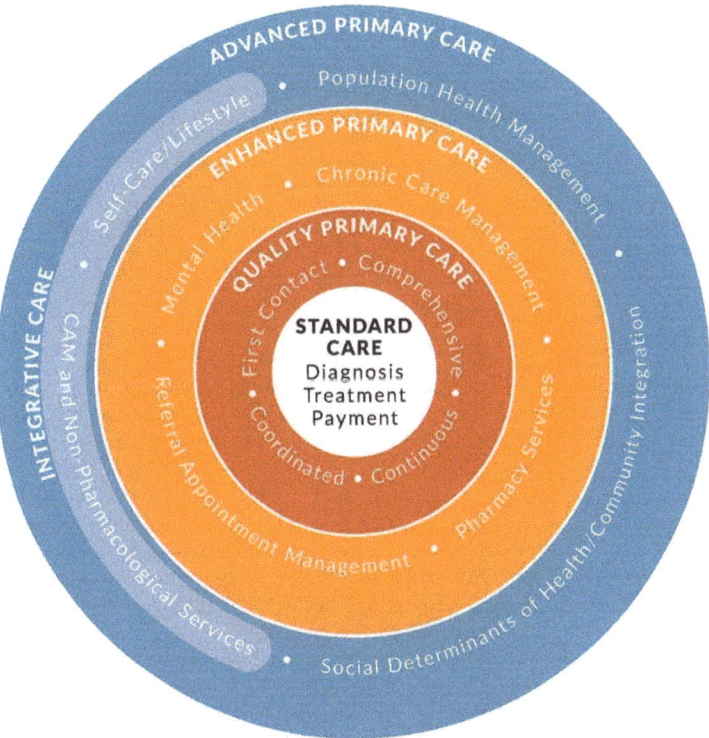

Figure 5. The Advanced Primary Care Model.

These models are only illustrative and not exhaustive of whole-person examples. To explore the impact that whole-person care models have on outcomes, we analyzed four aims of health care considered essential for quality. We used the outcomes described by the Institute for Healthcare Improvement called the Triple Aim [17,18] and added one additional aim (provider experience) to the analysis. The Triple Aim includes: (1) health improvement; (2) experiential outcomes in the form of patient satisfaction; and (3) cost reduction outcomes in the form of lowered costs per capita.

4. Materials and Methods

We selected studies focused on the models of whole-person care and included a few that emerged from the search based on broader health system data. We included relevant examples of programs with elements of coordinated delivery in at least three elements: conventional medical care, complementary and alternative medicine, and self-care within the social context of the patient. We looked for outcomes based on the Triple Aim criteria, plus the provider experience.

Two iterative Pubmed and Google searches were conducted between December 2020–May 2021 (last search done 15 May 2021) to seek studies looking at outcomes of whole-person outpatient primary care models. Search criteria used the search terms "Whole Health Veterans Administration", "integrative medicine", "integrative health", "complementary and alternative medicine", and, as they related to the outcomes, "health outcomes", "cost-effectiveness", "cost reduction", "patient satisfaction", "provider satisfaction", and "physician satisfaction". Inclusion criteria were models being in primary care, not done in a single sub-population or specially, not using a single modality or outcome measure, and only United States practices. After reviewing the citations from studies in the initial search, we conducted a second search, using the same criteria in Google.

To explore the business impact more clearly, we then conducted a deeper dive into the Veteran's Health System and Southcentral Foundation as existing models of whole-person care which have had extensive evaluation. We review and describe these findings in more detail.

5. Results

The first search resulted in 1764 references. Eighty-three met the criteria for screening. Nine articles from this initial search were included in this review. Forty-two additional studies were then screened. Twelve of these sources were included for a total of twenty-one studies that met all criteria from which this narrative review follows. See Table S1 for a list of the studies reviewed.

5.1. Evidence for Better Health Outcomes

The Veteran's Administration (VA) health system implemented Whole Health as part of the Comprehensive Addiction and Recovery Act to reduce rates of opioid addiction and improve chronic pain management using complementary and integrative health approaches. Piloted at 18 sites, Whole Health had benefits on all major aims, according to a two-year evaluation of 133,476 veterans who began receiving Whole Health services in fiscal years 2018 and 2019 [19]. Whole Health is a relationship-focused "approach to healthcare that empowers and equips people to take charge of their health and well-being and live their life to the fullest" [20] and incorporates self-care and complementary and integrative health approaches [20,21].

Whole Health System (WHS) was evaluated using the self-reported Veterans Health and Life Survey, a standard survey used to measure outcomes across the VA. This study found that veterans with chronic pain who received WHS, compared to those who received usual care, reported engaging in more healthy behaviors, being more involved with health care decisions, made small improvements in purpose in life, wellbeing and quality of life. They also made improvements in their ability to manage chronic pain as measured by the Perceived Stress Scale [20]. This evaluation also assessed the impact of Whole Health opioids use and on overall pharmacy costs. WHS users with chronic pain had larger decreases in opioid doses than veterans who received usual care. Decreases were largest in veterans who used more WHS [20].

A study was done of the University of Arizona Integrative Health Center integrative medicine adult primary care clinic. That clinic model combines conventional and complementary medical treatments, including nutrition, mind–body medicine, acupuncture, manual medicine, health coaching, educational classes, and groups. Results from a real-world observational evaluation of patient-reported outcomes (n = 177) showed improvements in mental, physical, and overall health, work productivity, and overall well-being [22]. Specifically, those who participated spent less time at work impaired, had better sleep, less fatigue and pain, more consumption of vegetables and physical activity, and improvements in self-reported quality of life (SF-12 in general health items, physical component, and mental component) and improvements in depression symptoms, anxiety symptoms, and mental wellbeing (measured by WHO-5, PHQ-2 and GAD-2 scores) [22].

Health coaching is a non-reductionistic delivery method for whole-person care models. Health coaches use their expertise in human behavior to help individuals set and achieve health goals and are an increasingly important component of whole-person integrative care teams. In a case series of 5 lifestyle programs at a large Western PA integrated delivery system, 14,591 UPMC health plan members self-selected to participate in a health coaching program. There was no comparison group. Self-reported results at 180 days demonstrated that health coaching helped 77% of participants reduce stress, 50.5% of participants increased physical activity, 65.2% of participants improved nutrition, 44.2% of participants lost weight and 7% of participants quit tobacco [23]. Other studies of health coaching demonstrate improvements in medication adherence. A non-blinded, randomized control trial of health coaching (n = 224) versus usual care (n = 217) demonstrated an increase in self-reported medication adherence, 10% improved concordance of reported medications compared with documented medications in the medical record, and a 17% decrease in medications listed in the medical record that were not reported by the patient [24]. An Integrative Health coaching program for individuals with Type 2 Diabetes focused on individuals' purpose in life and goals as a motivator for behavioral change. In a randomized control trial (n = 56), participants received 6 months of telephone coaching or usual care. Those receiving Integrative Health coaching had improved medication adherence, self- reported health, and improvements in hemoglobin A1c [25].

5.2. Evidence for Improved Patient Satisfaction

Regular users of integrative medicine like the "strong therapeutic relationship with a primary care provider who is a good listener and provides time, knowledge and understanding [26]". They believe that an approach that uses CAM and conventional medicine together is better than either alone [26]. Veterans at VA sites piloting the Whole Health System of care reported higher ratings of patient-centered care for discussing care goals and less difficulties in care with their provider [20]. The University of Arizona Integrative Health Center study results demonstrated that all patients (100%) reported that their practitioners treated them with respect. On a 10-point scale (1 = worst and 10 = best), 89% of patients rated overall satisfaction between 7 and 10 and 93% of patients rated trust in their practitioner between 7 and 10. Almost all patients (97%) would recommend the program to others [27].

A study was done evaluating the University of Michigan's Integrative Medicine Clinic. This clinic integrates conventional and complementary medicine using a whole-person model. A program evaluation of this clinic showed high patient satisfaction with the clinic. Patients were eligible for the study if they were seen at least 2 times in the clinic. Of the 274 patients initially surveyed, 85 completed the follow up questionnaire. More than half the patients rated their care as "excellent" or "best care ever" (37.6% and 24.7%, respectively). In resolving the primary issue, 55.3% of patients said the integrative medicine patient plan made "a significant difference" and 7.1% said that it "completely resolved my issue". In rating the impact of visits to the clinic on overall quality of life, 82.4% of patients reported at least some improvement [28].

Multiple studies have been done on the model developed and delivered by Southcentral Foundation (sometimes called the Nuka system). This system uses a relationship-based, whole-person model care for Native Alaskan people. The Foundation's approach includes calling and treating people as customer-owners rather than patients. This model has reported achieved excellent customer-owner satisfaction, with 96% satisfied with overall care and 95% who felt they had input into care decisions, and improved HEDIS measures [29]. These outcomes were a marked improvement over the more reductionistic, disease treatment approach taken for patients before the Nuka system was put in place.

5.3. Evidence for Lower Cost

Although more research is needed, there are instances of all or parts of whole-person integrative care that indicate promising cost implications. VA Whole Health Care health care costs were lower for 133,476 veterans who received WHS compared to those who received usual care. Results showed 12% to 24% lower costs in all categories except drugs, and the calculated total cost savings was $4845 (20%) less per person using WHS [19]. Although medication costs increased across the board, the increase in drug costs was 4.1% lower for those who participated in WHS [19] than those not enrolled in Whole Health. Drug costs increased less for comprehensive WHS users than for veterans who received usual care. Comprehensive WHS users had at least eight visits including both core WHS and complementary and integrative health services. In veterans with mental health conditions (PTSD, anxiety and/or depression), annual increases in drug costs were 3.5% for comprehensive WHS users compared with 12.5% for veterans who received usual care. In veterans with chronic conditions, annual increases in drug costs were 5.3% for comprehensive WHS users compared with 15.8% for veterans who received usual care [20].

Other evidence for cost savings of coordinated conventional and complementary and alternative care comes from Alternative Medicine, Inc. (AMI), an integrative medicine independent provider association under contract with a large HMO in metropolitan Chicago. Doctors of Chiropractic served as primary care physicians specializing in non-surgical/non-pharmacological approaches and consulting with medical physicians as necessary. Analysis of clinical and cost outcomes based on claims and patient surveys of over 21,743 member-months for 4 years were compared with conventional medicine IPA performance for the same HMO product in same region and period, showed lower costs for integrative medicine patients compared to those who received usual care. Per 1000 patients, integrative medicine patients had 43% fewer hospital admissions, 58.4% fewer hospital days, 43.2% fewer outpatient surgeries and procedures and 51.8% lower drug costs [30]. Claims analysis after 7 years demonstrated that compared to conventional medicine IPA performance, AMI's members had 60.2% fewer admissions, 59% fewer hospital days, 62% fewer outpatient surgeries and 85% lower pharmaceutical costs [31].

A study was done of the Maharishi Vedic (MV) approach, another multicomponent prevention program that integrates meditation, yoga, nutrition recommendations, supplements and breathing exercises. Researchers conducted a retrospective study using Blue Cross/Blue Shield Iowa data for patients who received care under the MV approach ($n = 693$), compared the statewide norm ($n = 600,000$) and a control group ($n = 4148$) getting non-holistic care. Four-year total medical expenditures for the MV approach group were 59% lower compared to statewide norm and 57% lower than the control group. Total medical expenses were 63% lower than the statewide norm at 11 years. Across ages and disease states health care utilization was lower for patients who received care under the MV approach [32].

We found several other program evaluations and randomized studies combining self-care with non-pharmacologic services and conventional care for individuals with chronic disease with most showing lower costs. We do not review all of those here but mention some of the major ones for illustration. The Multicenter Lifestyle Demonstration

Project reported that for persons with coronary artery disease, lifestyle changes plus yoga, meditation and progressive relaxation was medically effective and safe compared with revascularization surgery. Average cost savings of $29,529 was calculated for those who participated in the lifestyle change group [33]. The multicenter Diabetes Prevention Program for patients with prediabetes showed that lifestyle changes delayed development of diabetes and reduced incidence more than the drug metformin. Those in the lifestyle group had an 11-year delay and 20% lower total incidence of developing diabetes compared to a 3-year delay and 8% lower total incidence for those taking metformin compared to conventional care alone. The cost of lifestyle changes to society was about $8800 per quality-adjusted life-year (QALY) saved compared to about $29,900 for metformin [34].

Integration and coordination are essential to whole-person integrative care. Collaboration between health care and social services can improve health outcomes while decreasing costs. An example of a closed loop referral program is WellCare's that provides referrals to community-based public assistance programs, such as housing services and utility assistance, for 2718 participants insured through Medicare Advantage or Medicaid managed care in 14 states. Medical cost savings in the year after the needs were met, compared to those who had no needs met, were $1500 for participants with at least 1 social need met and about $2443 (10% lower) for participants with all social needs met [35].

Health coaching is an evidence-based process that assists patients in engaging and empowering them for their own health improvement through behavior change. It may reduce cost while improving health outcomes, independent of the specific treatment modality. Administrative claims data for high-cost commercial health plan members with multiple comorbidities and/or high adjusted clinical group risk scores were compared for members who received health coaching (n = 1161) and members who did not receive health coaching. Health coaching led to significant reductions in outpatient and total expenditures with estimated outpatient savings of $286 per person per month and estimated total cost savings of $412 per person per month [36].

5.4. Evidence for Improved Clinician Experience

Physicians who practice all or part of whole-person integrative care are less likely to burn out than other physicians. VA Whole Health Care evaluation demonstrated that clinical staff who are more involved with Whole Health were less likely to resign. All employees who were involved with Whole Health were more engaged and less likely to experience burnout. Employees reporting any involvement in Whole Health in 2019 identified their VA as a Best Place to Work and reported better leadership, intrinsic motivation, and being more engaged due to the behaviors of their supervisors [20].

In another example, physicians who perceived that their clinic was able to meet patients' social needs were less likely to be burned out according to an analysis of 1298 family physicians in ambulatory primary care settings [37]. Employee turnover at Southcentral Foundation, which provides relationship-based, whole-person care for Native Alaskan people, decreased by 15% from 2007 to 2015 [29].

Clinicians trained in complementary and alternative approaches appear to have improved satisfaction and wellbeing when integrated into usual care. Acupuncture training was significantly associated with decreased depersonalization of patients, a factor in burnout, according to a survey of 233 family physicians at the Uniformed Services Academy of Family Physicians 2017 conference [38]. Foundations in Integrative Health piloted a 32-h online competency-based interprofessional course in integrative health and evaluated results for 214 providers who completed the course. These providers had statistically significant improvements in their resiliency, changes in several wellness behaviors such as days engaged in an activity to manage stress, personal mind–body spiritual practices (breathing, spiritual rituals, and personal reflection), moderate, 30-min daily exercise, socializing with friends, and doing hobbies [39].

6. Discussion

In this review we have provided definitions and descriptions for several models and frameworks used to provide whole-person care rather than more reductionistic treatment models that address specific disease treatments only. In addition, we have explored the evidence of the impact of these models on four main types of outcomes—clinical, patient satisfaction, provider burn out and cost.

While most of these models demonstrated positive benefit in all these outcome areas, they are quite heterogenous and unfocused (See Table S1). There is no unified theory for whole-person care. Dimensions of what constitutes a whole person varied in different models, and they often had differing emphasis or strategic steps in their application, some using diet as major focus while others using mind–body approaches, for example. More work needs to be done to synthesize and simplify these models into more coherent systems. This might be done by studying the underlying mechanisms of healing, independent of looking at specific treatments for specific outcomes as is done in reductionism. Two lines of research may help improve this situation.

One research strategy for better understanding whole-person care is to look at so-called placebo response processes. Placebo effects cut across systems of care as they illuminate underlying mechanisms of healing that are agnostic to the specific treatments used. Mechanisms for placebo responses involve belief and expectation, classical conditioning, and social learning as they are embodied in the ritual of therapy [40]. The release of underlying healing processes by these mechanisms occurs across multiple conditions, irrespective of the modality or treatment being used. Thus, it is non disease specific and non-reductionistic. This research area may allow for are more complete understanding of whole-person healing and the integration of ancient traditional, complementary, conventional, allopathic, homeopathic or integrative systems, all of which utilize the placebo response. By studying the mechanisms of healing words and rituals, we may get to the core aspects of collective and individual healing across all health care systems [41].

A second area for research that could shed light on these fundamental processes of healing would be on non-instrumental approaches to healing. These go by a number of names such as intention, the biofield, subtle energies or consciousness and use ancient techniques such as laying on of hands, spiritual healing and more modern approaches such as Therapeutic or Healing Touch and Reiki [42,43]. This also includes more conventional approaches to healing such as psychotherapy, mind–body practices, and hypnosis in various forms. These are often collectively referred to as "vitalist" approaches. Researching these non-instrumental approaches by examining "healing presence" and communication processes in the patient-provider encounter could shed light on fundamental processes of whole-person healing and how they work independent of the specific interventions that use a drug, pill, needle or knife linked to a specific outcome. [44] More research on the impact of these health models is needed.

7. Conclusions

Current approaches to health care rest on reductionistic research strategies that seek treatments found by isolating and studying parts of a human being and then applying them for their "specific effects". This is the basis of so-called evidence-based medicine. However, people are not just a collection of their parts. They are complex, dynamic, interactive systems that need to be studied and treated using whole person, ecological models. This review explored several examples of such holistic models and found improved outcomes from their use on patient satisfaction, health outcomes, and on reduced costs and reduced provider burnout. While there is increasing evidence for the benefit of these models, there is a need for more and better research using whole system strategies. We need to explore and standardize our understanding of healing and use both research and delivery strategies more aligned with the nature of actual human beings.

Supplementary Materials: The following are available online at https://www.mdpi.com/article/10.3390/medicina57070677/s1, Table S1: Studies included in narrative review.

Author Contributions: Conceptualization, W.B.J.; methodology, W.B.J. and E.R.; validation, W.B.J. and E.R.; formal analysis, W.B.J. and E.R.; investigation, W.B.J. and E.R.; data curation, W.B.J. and E.R.; writing—original draft preparation, W.B.J. and E.R.; writing—review and editing, W.B.J. and E.R. Both authors have read and agreed to the published version of the manuscript.

Funding: This research received no external funding.

Conflicts of Interest: The authors do not have any relevant financial relationships with any commercial interests.

References

1. Giordano, J.; Jonas, W. Asclepius and hygieia in dialectic: Philosophical, ethical and educational foundations of an integrative medicine. *Integr. Med. Insights* **2007**, *2*, 53–60. [CrossRef]
2. Jonas, W.; Chez, R.; Smith, K.; Sakallaris, B. Salutogenesis: The defining concept for a new healthcare system. *Glob. Adv. Health Med.* **2014**, *3*, 82–91. [CrossRef] [PubMed]
3. Available online: https://www.nccih.nih.gov/about/offices/od/director/past-messages/considering-whole-person-health-as-we-develop-nccihs-next-strategic-plan (accessed on 24 June 2021).
4. Maslow, A. *Motivation and Personality*; Harper: New York, NY, USA, 1954; ISBN 978-0-06-041987-5.
5. Frankl, V. *Man's Search for Ultimate Meaning*; Ingram Publisher Services: La Vergne, TN, USA, 2000; ISBN 978-0-7382-0354-6.
6. Borrell-Carrio, F. The biopsychosocial model 25 years later: Principles, practice, and scientific inquiry. *Ann. Fam. Med.* **2004**, *2*, 576–582. [CrossRef]
7. Chez, R.; Pelletier, K.; Jonas, W. Toward optimal healing environments in health care: Second American Samueli Symposium. *J. Altern. Complement. Med.* **2004**, *10* (Suppl. 1). [CrossRef]
8. Christianson, J.; Finch, M.; Findlay, B.; Goertz, C.; Jonas, W. *Reinventing the Patient Experience: Strategies for Hospital Leaders*; Health Administration Press: Chicago, IL, USA, 2007.
9. Sakallaris, B.R.; Macallister, L.; Smith, K.; Mulvihill, D.L. The business case for optimal healing environments. *Glob. Adv. Health Med.* **2016**, *5*, 94–102. [CrossRef] [PubMed]
10. Jonas, W.; Deuster, P.; O'Connor, F.; Macedonia, C. *Total Force Fitness for the 21st Century: A New Paradigm*; Oxford University Press: New York, NY, USA, 2010.
11. Available online: https://p3.amedd.army.mil/ (accessed on 11 June 2021).
12. Available online: https://armypubs.army.mil/epubs/DR_pubs/DR_a/ARN30714-FM_7-22-000-WEB-1.pdf (accessed on 30 March 2021).
13. Available online: https://www.va.gov/wholehealth/ (accessed on 11 June 2021).
14. Available online: https://ssihi.uci.edu/about-us/ (accessed on 30 March 2021).
15. Available online: https://www.prnewswire.com/news-releases/new-medical-school-to-be-established-in-northwest-arkansas-as-part-of-alice-waltons-vision-for-whole-health-301240755.html (accessed on 11 June 2021).
16. Jonas, W. A New Model of Care to Return Holism to Family Medicine. *J. Fam. Pract.* **2020**, *69*. [CrossRef]
17. Available online: http://www.ihi.org:80/Engage/Initiatives/TripleAim/Pages/MeasuresResults.aspx (accessed on 11 June 2021).
18. Berwick, D.M.; Nolan, T.W.; Whittington, J. The Triple Aim: Care, Health, And Cost. *Health Aff.* **2008**, *27*, 759–769. [CrossRef] [PubMed]
19. Cover Commission. Creating Options for Veterans' Expedited Recovery: Final Report 2020. Available online: https://www.va.gov/COVER/docs/COVER_Commission-Final-Report-2020-01-24.PDF (accessed on 11 June 2021).
20. Bokhour, B.; Hyde, J.; Zeliadt, S.; Mohr, H. Whole Health System of Care Evaluation—A Progress Report on Outcomes of the WHS Pilot at 18 Flagship Sites. *Cent. Eval. Patient Cent. Care VA EPCC-VA* **2020**, *3*. Available online: https://vdocument.in/reader/full/whole-health-system-of-care-evaluation-feb-18-2020-a-whole-health-system (accessed on 11 June 2021).
21. Gaudet, T.; Kligler, B. Whole Health in the Whole System of the Veterans Administration: How Will We Know We Have Reached This Future State? *J. Altern. Complement. Med.* **2019**, *25*, S7–S11. [CrossRef] [PubMed]
22. Crocker, R.L.; Hurwitz, J.T.; Grizzle, A.J.; Abraham, I.; Rehfeld, R.; Horwitz, R.; Weil, A.T.; Maizes, V. Real-World Evidence from the Integrative Medicine Primary Care Trial (IMPACT): Assessing Patient-Reported Outcomes at Baseline and 12-Month Follow-Up. *Evid. Based Complement. Alternat. Med.* **2019**, *2019*, 1–9. [CrossRef]
23. Budzowski, A.R.; Parkinson, M.D.; Silfee, V.J. An Evaluation of Lifestyle Health Coaching Programs Using Trained Health Coaches and Evidence-Based Curricula at 6 Months Over 6 Years. *Am. J. Health Promot.* **2019**, *33*, 912–915. [CrossRef] [PubMed]
24. Thom, D.H.; Willard-Grace, R.; Hessler, D.; DeVore, D.; Prado, C.; Bodenheimer, T.; Chen, E. The Impact of Health Coaching on Medication Adherence in Patients with Poorly Controlled Diabetes, Hypertension, and/or Hyperlipidemia: A Randomized Controlled Trial. *J. Am. Board Fam. Med.* **2015**, *28*, 38–45. [CrossRef]
25. Wolever, R.Q.; Dreusicke, M.; Fikkan, J.; Hawkins, T.V.; Yeung, S.; Wakefield, J.; Duda, L.; Flowers, P.; Cook, C.; Skinner, E. Integrative Health Coaching for Patients with Type 2 Diabetes. *Diabetes Educ.* **2010**, *36*, 629–639. [CrossRef]

26. McCaffrey, A.M.; Pugh, G.F.; O'Connor, B.B. Understanding Patient Preference for Integrative Medical Care: Results from Patient Focus Groups. *J. Gen. Intern. Med.* **2007**, *22*, 1500–1505. [CrossRef] [PubMed]
27. Crocker, R.L.; Grizzle, A.J.; Hurwitz, J.T.; Rehfeld, R.A.; Abraham, I.; Horwitz, R.; Weil, A.; Maizes, V. Integrative Medicine Primary Care: Assessing the Practice Model through Patients' Experiences. *BMC Complement. Altern. Med.* **2017**, *17*, 490. [CrossRef] [PubMed]
28. Myklebust, M.; Pradhan, E.K.; Gorenflo, D. An Integrative Medicine Patient Care Model and Evaluation of Its Outcomes: The University of Michigan Experience. *J. Altern. Complement. Med.* **2008**, *14*, 821–826. [CrossRef]
29. Eby, D. Internationally Heralded Approaches to Population Health Driven by Alaska Native/American Indian/Native American Communities. Presented at the Institute of Healthcare Improvement 28th National Forum on Quality Improvement and Healthcare, Orlando, FL, USA, 4–7 December 2016.
30. Sarnat, R.L.; Winterstein, J. Clinical and Cost Outcomes of an Integrative Medicine IPA. *J. Manipulative Physiol. Ther.* **2004**, *27*, 336–347. [CrossRef] [PubMed]
31. Sarnat, R.L.; Winterstein, J.; Cambron, J.A. Clinical utilization and cost outcomes from an integrative medicine independent physician association: An additional 3-year update. *J. Manipulative Physiol. Ther.* **2007**, *30*, 263–269. [CrossRef] [PubMed]
32. Orme-Johnson, D.W.; Herron, R.E. An innovative approach to reducing medical care utilization and expenditures. *Am. J. Manag. Care* **1997**, *3*, 135–144.
33. Ornish, D. Avoiding Revascularization with Lifestyle Changes: The Multicenter Lifestyle Demonstration Project. *Am. J. Cardiol.* **1998**, *82*, 72–76. [CrossRef]
34. Herman, W.H.; Hoerger, T.J.; Brandle, M.; Hicks, K.; Sorensen, S.; Zhang, P.; Hamman, R.F.; Ackermann, R.T.; Engelgau, M.M.; Ratner, R.E.; et al. The Cost-Effectiveness of Lifestyle Modification or Metformin in Preventing Type 2 Diabetes in Adults with Impaired Glucose Tolerance. *Ann. Intern. Med.* **2005**, *142*, 323–332. [CrossRef] [PubMed]
35. Pruitt, Z.; Emechebe, N.; Quast, T.; Taylor, P.; Bryant, K. Expenditure Reductions Associated with a Social Service Referral Program. *Popul. Health Manag.* **2018**, *21*, 469–476. [CrossRef]
36. Jonk, Y.; Lawson, K.; O'Connor, H.; Riise, K.S.; Eisenberg, D.; Dowd, B.; Kreitzer, M.J. How Effective Is Health Coaching in Reducing Health Services Expenditures? *Med. Care* **2015**, *53*, 133–140. [CrossRef]
37. De Marchis, E.; Knox, M.; Hessler, D.; Willard-Grace, R.; Olayiwola, J.N.; Peterson, L.E.; Grumbach, K.; Gottlieb, L.M. Physician Burnout and Higher Clinic Capacity to Address Patients' Social Needs. *J. Am. Board Fam. Med.* **2019**, *32*, 69–78. [CrossRef] [PubMed]
38. Crawford, P.F.; Rupert, J.; Jackson, J.T.; Walkowski, S.; Ledford, C.J.W. Relationship of Training in Acupuncture to Physician Burnout. *J. Am. Board Fam. Med.* **2019**, *32*, 259–263. [CrossRef] [PubMed]
39. Brooks, A.J.; Maizes, V.; Billimek, J.; Blair, J.; Chen, M.-K.; Goldblatt, E.; Kilgore, D.; Klatt, M.; Kligler, B.; Koithan, M.S.; et al. Professional Development in Integrative Health through an Interprofessional Online Course in Clinical Settings. *Explore* **2020**. [CrossRef]
40. Colloca, L.; Barsky, A.J. Placebo and Nocebo Effects. *N. Engl. J. Med.* **2020**, *382*, 554–561. [CrossRef]
41. Jonas, W.B. Reframing Placebo in Research and Practice. *Phil. Trans. R. Soc. B* **2011**, *366*, 1896–1904. [CrossRef]
42. Jonas, W.B.; Crawford, C.C. *Healing, Intention, and Energy Medicine: Science, Research Methods, and Clinical Implications*; Churchill Livingstone: New York, NY, USA, 2003; ISBN 9780443072376.
43. Jain, S.; Ives, J.; Jonas, W.; Hammerschlag, R.; Muehsam, D.; Vieten, C.; Vicario, D.; Chopra, D.; King, R.P.; Guarneri, E. Biofield Science and Healing: An Emerging Frontier in Medicine. *Glob. Adv. Health Med.* **2015**, *4*. [CrossRef]
44. Jain, S. *Healing Ourselves: Biofield Science and the Future of Health*; Sounds True: Louisville, CO, USA, 2021; ISBN 978-1-68364-433-0.

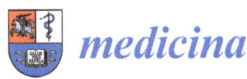

Review

The Microbiome in Health and Disease from the Perspective of Modern Medicine and Ayurveda

Robert Keith Wallace

Department of Physiology and Health, Maharishi International University, Fairfield, IA 52556, USA; kwallace@miu.edu

Received: 12 August 2020; Accepted: 9 September 2020; Published: 11 September 2020

Abstract: The role of the microbiome in health and disease helps to provide a scientific understanding of key concepts in Ayurveda. We now recognize that virtually every aspect of our physiology and health is influenced by the collection of microorganisms that live in various parts of our body, especially the gut microbiome. There are many external factors which influence the composition of the gut microbiome but one of the most important is diet and digestion. Ayurveda and other systems of traditional health have for thousands of years focused on diet and digestion. Recent research has helped us understand the connection between the microbiome and the many different prevention and therapeutic treatment approaches of Ayurveda.

Keywords: microbiome; Ayurveda; gut bacteria; diet; lifestyle; disease; prevention; integrative medicine

1. Introduction

DNA sequencing technology and bioinformatics have made it possible to evaluate the composition of the diverse community of bacteria, archaea, fungi, viruses, and other organisms that form the microbiome. A growing body of research has now correlated the microbiome with a wide variety of diseases [1–4]. The microbiome is present in many parts of the body but the largest collection of over 30 trillion bacteria is in the gut [5].

The gut microbiome participates in vital processes including digestion, energy homeostasis and metabolism, the synthesis of vitamins and other nutrients, and the development and regulation of immune function. It also contributes to the production of numerous compounds that enter the blood and affect various tissues and organs of the body [3,4].

An important consideration is the recognition of the enormous variation in the gut microbiota composition in each individual, as well as in each area of the digestive tract. Throughout the intestines there are specific niches that house individual microbial communities, which can be immunologically more active than others. A balanced and diverse microbiome is critical for maintaining health and immunological balance [6,7].

When the microbiome is in balance it contributes to many health benefits, but when out of balance, it can cause problems in the gut and other areas of the body. Dysbiosis arises when the delicate and elaborate ecology of microbial communities are disrupted by internal or external factors. A disrupted microbiome is characterized by the overgrowth of one or more of the different microbial colonies. A complex interaction between the microbiome and immune systems may result in an inflammatory state [8,9]. An imbalanced microbiome has been associated with a number of gastrointestinal diseases including irritable bowel syndrome (IBS) and inflammatory bowel disorder (IBD) [10–12]. Conditions such as asthma, atopy, childhood obesity, and autism spectrum have been correlated with excess antibiotic use and a resulting alteration in the microbiome in childhood [13–16]. Numerous other conditions such as obesity, autoimmune disorders, cardiovascular disease, cancer, and neurological disorders have also been linked with changes in the microbiome [1–4,17–19].

Diet can rapidly alter the composition of the microbiome [20–23]. A western diet high in meat products, providing nutrients such as choline and carnitine, can cause certain gut bacteria to produce trimethylamine (TMA). TMA is absorbed into the bloodstream and then oxidized in the liver to form trimethylamine-N-oxide (TMAO). High levels of TMAO have been suggested to contribute to cardiovascular disease by interfering with cholesterol metabolism and transportation, foam cell formation, and platelet aggregation [24–34].

Gut bacteria may also affect cardiovascular disease by a decrease in fiber intake. Dietary fiber is a rich source of food for gut bacteria and its reduction can lead to a decreased bacterial production of the short chain fatty acid butyrate. This change can lead to dysbiosis and local inflammation in the gut lining, resulting in impaired gut barrier function and the possible leakage of bacterial toxins, such as lipopolysaccharides, into the bloodstream [30–34].

There are other microorganism communities throughout the body which can contribute to health and disease. At one time, the lung was considered a sterile organ, but we now recognized that it has its own microbiome which extends into the lower lung. There is cross talk between the lung and gut microbiomes, which could be relevant to patients with COVID 19 that display gastrointestinal symptoms [35–38].

The gut microbiome also affects the brain and mental health. The basis for this interaction is the gut–brain axis, which consists of the brain, immune system, endocrine system, enteric nervous system (ENS), enteroendocrine system (EEC), and the gut bacteria. There is a bidirectional flow of information between the gut and brain. The most direct is through the vagus nerve, which is an important and long nerve in the body that regulates many internal functions. A less direct means of communication is through different chemical messengers, such as neurotransmitters, hormones, and peptides. The gut produces numerous peptides and neurotransmitters. Many of these are also found in the brain. The secretion of these gut-derived chemicals can be influenced by the composition of the gut microbiome. In addition, the gut microbiome can also produce its own unique array of chemical messengers, that go into the bloodstream and affect different parts of the body. There is also research showing that gut microbes can activate immune cells in the gut wall, which causes the release of proinflammatory cytokines and ultimately may affect the permeability of the blood–brain barrier [39–41]. Animal studies have shown that a disrupted microbiome can cause anxiety-like and depression-like behaviors [42,43]. A new field of psychobiotics has even emerged, which utilizes probiotics to affect moods and behavior in humans [44].

While the precise manner in which the microbiome participates in these many disease states is still not completely clear, there are currently a number of therapeutic approaches that are now being tested in clinical trials including diet, prebiotics, probiotics, antibiotics, and fecal microbiome transplantation (FMT) [45–47]. Recent studies, for example, have utilized personalized nutritional advice based on microbiome data and other factors [48–50]

2. Ayurveda

Hippocrates, the father of modern western medicine, is famous for his expression "All disease begins in the gut." Ayurveda places great importance on proper diet and digestion, as well as on all aspects of lifestyle. Some researchers consider Ayurveda to be an ancient science of epigenetics [51]. The Ayurvedic practitioners might not have understood the precise nutrigenomic mechanics of how food can affects gene expression [52], but they did recognize that each individual has his or her own unique psychophysiological constitution, which is affected by diet, digestion, lifestyle, stress management, and environmental factors [53].

Ayurveda describes the functioning of our mind and body in terms of three main doshas—the governing principles of the physiology—Vata, Pitta, and Kapha [54]. In a previous paper, we have reviewed the research on the physiological, biochemical, and genetic correlates of each of the doshas. As we explain, the category of Vata dosha includes processes responsible for movement at all levels of the physiology, excretion of wastes, and also cognition. The primary location of Vata, according to

Ayurveda, is in the colon, where most of the gut microbiome is located. Pitta dosha is responsible for such functions as digestion, metabolism, thermoregulation, and energy homeostasis and resides in the mid gut area. Kapha dosha governs the growth and maintenance of structure and its primary location is in the chest area. Genetic research shows a significant difference between each dosha type and gene expression. Genes related to cell cycles were upregulated in the Vata types whereas genes in the immune response pathways were upregulated in the Pitta type, and genes in the immune signaling pathways were upregulated in Kapha types. Each dosha type is suggested to display its own style of brain functioning [55,56]. In Ayurveda, one of the first stages of an assessment of a person's health is to determine the distribution of the three doshas at birth, which is called Prakriti. In addition, an assessment is made of the state of balance of the doshas, which is called Vikriti. In fact, one can have a dominant Vata Prakrti at birth, but at the time of the diagnosis, the primary imbalance may be in Pitta due to some environmental factor.

In Figure 1, we illustrate that the microbiome is integral to both modern medicine and Ayurveda. We elaborate on this concept throughout the article.

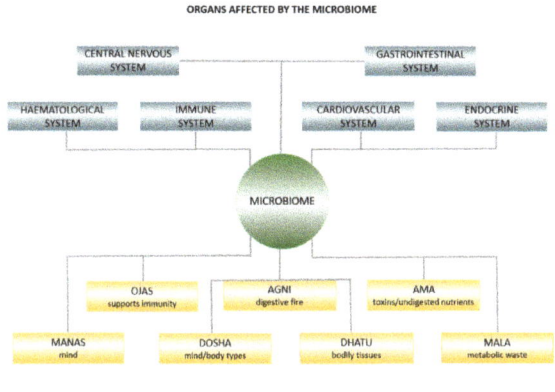

Figure 1. Ayurvedic anatomy affected by the microbiome.

3. Prakriti and Gut Bacteria

One study has examined the relationship between Prakriti and the composition of the microbiome. The researchers found that three main Prakriti types, Vata, Pitta, or Kapha, had a unique microbiome composition [57]. The population studied were from the same region and had similar dietary habits. The main bacteria of all the subjects were from the phyla Bacteroidetes and Firmicutes. There were distinct differences between the Vata, Pitta, or Kapha groups in less common bacteria. The extreme Pitta individuals, for example, had more butyrate producing microbes which might help protect them from inflammatory diseases. The extreme Kapha women had larger amounts of a type of bacteria called *Prevotella copri*, which has been associated with patients who have rheumatoid arthritis and insulin resistance. A more recent paper analyzes how the concept of Prakriti can be used as a stratifier of the gut microbiome [58].

4. Ayurveda Herbs and Spices and the Microbiome

Ayurveda considers food as medicine. It uses spices and herbs to help create and maintain balance in the physiology, and to treat specific disorders. Recent research shows that both ginger and a herbal preparation called Triphala can have beneficial effects on the microbiome. Triphala consists of three fruits: Emblica officinalis (Amalaki), Terminalia bellerica (Bibhitaki), and Terminalia chebula (Haritaki). It is a fundamental component of Ayurvedic gastrointestinal and rejuvenation treatment programs, particularly to help improve elimination. Studies have found that Triphala has different potential clinical applications which include appetite stimulation and a reduction in hyperacidity and constipation. It also has a number of inherent biological properties such as anti-inflammatory, immunomodulatory, antibacterial, antimutagenic, adaptogenic, hypoglycemic, antineoplastic, chemoprotective and radioprotective, and antioxidant activities. In the study, it was shown that the polyphenols in Triphala modulate the human gut microbiome and thereby promote the growth of beneficial Bifidobacteria and Lactobacillus while inhibiting the growth of undesirable gut microbes. The authors also suggest that the bioactivity of Triphala is elicited by gut microbiota that generate a variety of anti-inflammatory compounds [59].

Turmeric is another Ayurvedic preparation which has been found to affect digestion and the microbiome. Turmeric and its active ingredient curcumin have been the subject of thousands of peer-reviewed and published biomedical studies, with hundreds of potential preventive and therapeutic applications on such diseases as ulcerative colitis, stomach ulcers, osteoarthritis, heart disease, cancer, and neurodegenerative disorders [60,61]. Interestingly, the active ingredient of turmeric, curcumin, has been shown to be biological active but because of its poor bioavailability and inability to reach target tissues, it has not been found to be effective in clinical trials [62,63]. It may also be ineffective because we no longer have the synergic effects of the other ingredients. It is suggested that curcumin may restore dysbiosis of the gut microbiome and as a result have a neuroprotective effect, however, future research is needed to know how curcumin actually affects the microbiome in different individuals [64,65].

There are many other important Ayurveda herbs and preparations that need to be further studied. One of the most important categories are Rasayanas which are designed to lengthen the lifespan [66]. Once again, future research will be needed to examine the specific effects of Rasayana on the microbiome.

5. Ama and Leaky Gut Syndrome

Ayurveda explains that most diseases are caused by an accumulation of ama or undigested food. Ama literally means "uncooked food," but it can be understood from a scientific perspective as endogenous toxins resulting from imbalanced or incomplete digestion. Ama can be formed as a result of reduced Agni, or digestive power. Agni has a number of different meanings and not only relates to digestive enzymes but also to the metabolic process in the different tissues or dhatus of the body [67]. Ama is initially formed in the digestive tract, but at a later stage of disease it can leak into the bodily tissues and turn into Amavisha, a reactive form of ama, that leads to tissue disruption and chronic inflammation and disease.

It has been suggested that compromised mucosal integrity, such as a disruption in the tight junctions, leads to dysbiosis, resulting in the formation of Ama [68]. Ama is also produced at other levels of the physiology, including the cellular level. Excessive formation of free radicals contributes to the formation of Ama. A variety of free radicals and reactive oxygen species (ROS) are produced during cellular metabolism. Excessive amounts of these reactive molecules can cause damage, starting the disease process. The ability to control their concentrations may be helpful for the prevention and treatment of many disorders.

Antioxidants "scavenge" free radicals and ROS and render them harmless. Antioxidants can be lipid- or water-soluble; some are produced in the body and others are obtained from food or dietary supplements. Natural antioxidants range from vitamins to enzymes to herbal mixtures. Powerful antioxidants are present in the bioflavonoids found in concentrated form in Rasayanas. The use of these Rasayanas, might be helpful in neutralizing the excessive free radical activity that contributes to Ama formation. However, it is not clear if accumulated Ama in the body can be removed by the use of Rasayanas and antioxidants alone. Other Ayurvedic methodologies may be required to eradicate accumulated Ama. Rasayanas are best administered after a detoxification treatment such as panchakarma and are utilized to neutralize ongoing damage to the physiology and regenerate the system [68].

It is interesting to interpret the meaning of Ama in terms of recent findings. Remarkable progress has been made in understanding the mechanisms of leaky gut syndrome in celiac patients. In celiac disease, the tight junctions that hold the cells of the gut wall together become loose, and as a result, undigested food and harmful substances "leak" through the gut wall and into the bloodstream, causing inflammation. The exact mechanism of this process involves a product of gluten called gliadin, which interacts with receptors on the surface of the cells in the small intestine, causing the production of zonulin. Zonulin then causes the proteins, which bind tight junctions, to relax and allow unwanted substances to enter the bloodstream. In celiac patients, this process is exaggerated and can ultimately result in a harmful autoimmune reaction [69,70]. A disruption in the gut microbiome has been associated with problems in the gut barrier. It is suggested that gut dysbiosis may cause the release of zonulin but the exact mechanisms are complex and still under investigation [71,72].

6. Biorhythms and Gut Bacteria

Ayurveda clearly identifies daily, seasonal, and lifetime rhythms. Each day, for example, consists of a sequence of periods, which are characterized by Vata, Pitta, or Kapha. The day starts with a Kapha period from 6 am to 10 am, then a Pitta period from 10 am to 2 pm, and then a Vata period from 2 pm to 6 pm. Next is another Kapha period from 6 pm to 10 pm, a Pitta from 10 pm to 2 am and finally a Vata from 2 am to 6 am. Each season is represented by either one dosha or a combination of doshas: late autumn and winter are cold and dry and correspond to the Vata dosha. Summer is hot and naturally corresponds to Pitta dosha. Spring is cold and wet and corresponds to Kapha dosha. The daily routine is called dinacharya and the seasonal routine is called ritucharya.

Modern medicine also recognizes the importance of daily rhythms to your health and the 2017 Nobel Prize in Physiology and Medicine was awarded for research on the genetic basis of biological rhythms. From bacteria to humans, almost all forms of life have an internal "biological clock," which maintains an approximately 24 h rhythm. When external signals of light and dark are introduced unnaturally, the master clock becomes confused and this creates health problems. Shift workers, for instance, have been shown to have a higher incidence of cancer, cardiovascular disease, digestive disorders, and obesity, as well as psychiatric and neurodegenerative diseases [73].

One of the most important timing issues for the body, which has been seen in research on animals and humans, is when you eat. If you eat within 2 h before you normally go to sleep, it can desynchronize the circadian rhythms of certain cells in the intestine and liver from those in the rest of your body [74].

Gut bacteria also have biological rhythms. One study created jet lag in mice by forcing these normally nocturnal animals to stay awake during the day. When the researchers transferred the gut bacteria from jet-lagged mice into germ-free mice, the recipient mice developed both obesity and glucose intolerance [75]. A number of studies have shown that time-restricted feeding and eating frequency affects the composition of the microbiome [76]. Recent research on the gut bacteria reveals not only the presence of a daily rhythm, but also seasonal biorhythms [77,78]. The relationship between the circadian rhythms and gut microbiota appears to be bidirectional and may have important influences on health [79–82].

Ayurvedic recommendations of specific diets at specific times may relate to the seasonal rhythms of the microbiome. Over the winter, for example, Kapha and Ama are said to build up in the body. Early spring is described as the ideal time to rebalance Kapha and reduce Ama to prevent toxins and excess mucus from creating congestion and allergies. Foods that are primarily Kapha in nature—heavy, greasy, and mucus forming—tend to increase both Kapha and Ama. Ayurveda recommends reducing or eliminating Kapha foods during this time, which might help to heal the gut and reboot the microbiome [83].

7. Probiotic Enemas and Bastis

Probiotic enemas have been suggested to help cure certain neurological disorders [84]. Probiotics that are taken orally must pass through your stomach and the small intestine, which is not ideal because stomach acid and digestive enzymes destroy many of the valuable probiotic bacteria long before they reach the colon. A probiotic enema, however, provides an almost instantaneous route to the colon, where most of the gut bacteria live.

The Ayurvedic term for enema is basti, and bastis are a valuable part of the deep purification and detox treatment program known as panchakarma, which, as we mentioned, cleanses the body of impurities and promotes health and longevity. There are many types of bastis: some are for purification, others for elimination, others strengthen the tissues and provide valuable nutrients. Bastis use ingredients such as sesame oil, medicated ghee, buttermilk, lassi, many different combinations of herbs, and in special cases, bone broth. A search of Pub Med shows a number of published studies on different types of bastis that have been used for various clinical applications [85–92].

These studies, however, do not mention the use of bastis as a means to modify or reboot the gut bacteria. By studying how bastis affect gut bacteria composition we might gain a better scientific understanding of the mechanisms of their beneficial actions on specific health conditions. We already know that sesame oil has a positive effect on colon cells, and on certain beneficial bacteria [93,94].

In a more recent study, the metabolomic profile was taken after a 6-day panchakarma treatment. The experimental group consisted of healthy male and female subjects whose treatment program included herbs, vegetarian diet, meditation, yoga, and massage. The results showed that 12 plasma phosphatidylcholines decreased after treatment in the experimental group as compared to the control group of 54 subjects. There were changes in metabolites across many pathways such as phospholipid biosynthesis, choline metabolism, and lipoprotein metabolism, with statistically significant changes in the plasma levels of phosphatidylcholines, sphingomyelins and others in just 6 days. It is unclear whether the lipid metabolites were modulated by the gut microbiome or by the external agents such as herbs, vegetarian diet, meditation, yoga, and massage [95].

The study of panchakarma and other Ayurvedic purification treatments is an important area of future research. It would also be useful to compare the modern use of fecal transplant treatment with all the different types of basti treatments.

8. The Gut–Brain Axis and Ojas

The gut–brain axis, as we described earlier, consists of a number of major systems in the body, as well as the gut bacteria. The brain communicates to the gut through either nerves or through hormones and chemical messengers. The gut–brain axis includes the enteric nervous system (ENS), enteroendocrine system (EEC) and the gut bacteria, which all produce different chemicals. The ENS produces more than 30 neurotransmitters. Almost 90% of all the serotonin in the body is produced by cells in the gut, as well as 50% of the dopamine [39–41,96].

According to Ayurveda, the digestion and gut play leading roles in immunity. Ayurveda speaks about a substance or a process called Ojas, the finest product of healthy digestion, which strengthens the immune system and has many beneficial effects on the mind and body.

Can Ojas be identified by modern science? In Ayurveda there is a description of seven basic tissues or dhatus and three waste products or malas. The tissues roughly correspond to the tissues as discussed in modern physiology and the waste products include feces, urine, and sweat. The tissues are important because digestion includes the transformation of food into each of these tissues and ultimately to Ojas. It is unclear what this means in terms of modern science. It might correspond to a metabolic process that involves specific precursors which come from a well-functioning digestive system and a balance microbiome.

There are several possible candidates for Ojas. One is serotonin, a key regulator of mood, sleep, appetite, and other brain functions. As we mentioned, the gut produces most of the serotonin in the body, which circulates throughout your bloodstream and influences not only your immune system, but your heart rate, blood clotting, intestinal motility, pulmonary arteries, heart, brain, and mammary glands, as well as the cell growth of liver and bone cells [97]. One of the key precursors of serotonin is tryptophan, an essential amino acid, which is obtained through the normal digestion of certain foods.

Ojas is described as being beneficial to all parts of the body so we might ask if excess serotonin has any deleterious effects. An overabundance of serotonin due to drugs can lead to a number of damaging symptoms, including anxiety, sweating, sleep disturbance, appetite changes, headaches, confusion and lethargy, dilated pupils, rapid heart rate, etc. [98]. Additionally, individuals with social phobia have been shown to have excess serotonin [99].

Another interesting candidate is a chemical called butyric acid, which, as we mentioned, is a by-product of the gut bacteria and has numerous beneficial effects, including improvement of immunity [100].

Ojas is described in the Ayurvedic texts as having many properties, such as its ability to coordinate the junction between the mind and body. Some of these effects may not be covered by either serotonin or butyric acid. The exact nature of Ojas remains an ongoing research project.

9. Stress, Ayurveda, and Psychobiotics

Stress can have many deleterious effects. When the brain triggers the adrenal glands to release cortisol, it goes into the bloodstream and affects both the gut and the gut bacteria. Cortisol can increase the intestinal permeability, which results in a leaky gut. It can also shut down the activity of the gut immune system [71,101].

Ayurveda uses a wide variety of approaches to improve the mind or manas and to alleviate the effects of stress. One of these is meditation, which is an integral part of both Ayurveda and its sister discipline, yoga. The Transcendental Meditation (TM) program introduced by Maharishi Mahesh Yogi over fifty years ago has been shown to have many distinct physiological changes, including a reduction in cortisol, as well as beneficial effects on mental and physical health [102–107]. To date, we know of no studies which have examined the effect of meditation on the gut microbiome.

Ayurveda has long explained that disturbances in our mental state, which are usually associated with a Vata imbalance, can be traced to problems in the nervous system and the gut. It recommends specific herbs such as Ashwagandha and Brahmi, which may interact with the microbiome. It also has a long tradition of using natural probiotics such as lassi. Modern research on the microbiome validates this concept, showing that depression and anxiety may be linked to a disrupted microbiome and may be improved through the use of probiotics.

One brain imaging study showed that women react differently to stimuli depending on the type of bacteria they have in their gut. The same researchers had previously shown that diet could affect the brain. They gave subjects either a psychobiotic (a probiotic mixture that is used for mental health) or a placebo. They then showed the subjects images of frightened faces while measuring brain activity. The subjects taking the placebo showed a normal stress response with specific areas of the brain responsible for emotions being activated. Subjects receiving the psychobiotic showed a reduced stress response in these same areas of the brain [108,109].

10. The Future of Ayurveda and Modern Medicine

We are living in a transitional moment in medicine. New studies are emerging that will help us make better choices. The field of integrative medicine represents an important achievement since it combines the best of modern medicine with the best of traditional system of natural health, such as Ayurveda. Integrative medicine benefits greatly from research on the microbiome because it helps us better understand the ancient practices of Ayurveda in the light of modern science [110].

Funding: This research did not receive any specific grant from funding agencies in the public, commercial, or not-for-profit sectors. A grant from the Wege Foundation helped pay for publication costs.

Acknowledgments: Thanks to Roxanne Medeiros for creating the graphic.

Conflicts of Interest: The author declares no conflict of interest.

References

1. Zheng, D.; Liwinski, T.; Elinav, E. Interaction between microbiota and immunity in health and disease. *Cell Res.* **2020**, *30*, 492–506. [CrossRef]
2. Malla, M.A.; Dubey, A.; Kumar, A.; Yadav, S.; Hashem, A.; Abd Allah, E.F. Exploring the Human Microbiome: The Potential Future Role of Next-Generation Sequencing in Disease Diagnosis and Treatment. *Front. Immunol.* **2019**, *9*, 2868. [CrossRef] [PubMed]
3. Mohajeri, M.H.; Brummer, R.J.M.; Rastall, R.A.; Weersma, R.K.; Harmsen, H.J.M.; Faas, M.; Eggersdorfer, M. The Role of the Microbiome for Human Health: From Basic Science to Clinical Applications. *Eur. J. Nutr.* **2018**, *57*, 1–14. [CrossRef]
4. Armour, C.R.; Nayfach, S.; Pollard, K.S.; Sharpton, T.J. A Metagenomic Meta-Analysis Reveals Functional Signatures of Health and Disease in the Human Gut Microbiome. *mSystems* **2019**, *4*. [CrossRef] [PubMed]
5. Sender, R.; Fuchs, S.; Milo, R. Revised Estimates for the Number of Human and Bacteria Cells in the Body. *PLoS Biol.* **2016**, *14*, e1002533. [CrossRef] [PubMed]
6. Tong, M.; Li, X.; Parfrey, L.W.; Roth, B.; Ippoliti, A.; Wei, B.; Borneman, J.; Mcgovern, D.P.B.; Frank, D.N.; Li, E.; et al. A Modular Organization of the Human Intestinal Mucosal Microbiota and Its Association with Inflammatory Bowel Disease. *PLoS ONE* **2013**, *8*, e80702. [CrossRef]
7. Huttenhower, C.; Gevers, D.; Knight, R.; Abubucker, S.; Badger, J.H.; Chinwalla, A.T.; Creasy, H.H.; Earl, A.M.; FitzGerald, M.G.; Fulton, R.S.; et al. Structure, Function and Diversity of the Healthy Human Microbiome. *Nature* **2012**, *486*, 207–214. [CrossRef]
8. Sommer, F.; Backhed, F. The gut microbiota engages different signaling pathways to induce Duox2 expression in the ileum and colon epithelium. *Mucosal Immunol.* **2015**, *8*, 372–379. [CrossRef]
9. Geuking, M.B.; Köller, Y.; Rupp, S.; McCoy, K.D. The interplay between the gut microbiota and the immune system. *Gut Microbes* **2014**, *5*, 411–418. [CrossRef]
10. De Palma, G.; Collins, S.M.; Bercik, P. The microbiota-gut-brain axis in functional gastrointestinal disorders. *Gut Microbes* **2014**, *5*, 419–429. [CrossRef]
11. Kennedy, P.J.; Cryan, J.F.; Dinan, T.G.; Clarke, G. Irritable bowel syndrome: A microbiome-gut-brain axis disorder? *World J. Gastroenterol.* **2014**, *20*, 14105–14125. [CrossRef] [PubMed]
12. Khan, I.; Ullah, N.; Zha, L.; Bai, Y.; Khan, A.; Zhao, T.; Che, T.; Zhang, C. Alteration of Gut Microbiota in Inflammatory Bowel Disease (IBD): Cause or Consequence? IBD Treatment Targeting the Gut Microbiome. *Pathogens* **2019**, *8*, 126. [CrossRef] [PubMed]
13. Francino, M.P. Antibiotics and the Human Gut Microbiome: Dysbioses and Accumulation of Resistances. *Front. Microbiol.* **2016**, *6*, 1543. [CrossRef] [PubMed]
14. Mueller, N.T.; Whyatt, R.; Hoepner, L.; Oberfield, S.; Dominguez-Bello, M.G.; Widen, E.M.; Hassoun, A.; Perera, F.; Rundle, A. Prenatal exposure to antibiotics, cesarean section and risk of childhood obesity. *Int. J. Obes.* **2015**, *39*, 665–670. [CrossRef]
15. Arrieta, M.C.; Stiemsma, L.T.; Amenyogbe, N.; Brown, E.M.; Finlay, B. The intestinal microbiome in early life: Health and disease. *Front. Immunol.* **2014**, *5*, 427. [CrossRef]
16. Kozyrskyj, A.L.; Bahreinian, S.; Azad, M.B. Early life exposures: Impact on asthma and allergic disease. *Curr. Opin. Allergy Clin. Immunol.* **2011**, *11*, 400–406. [CrossRef]
17. Burcelin, R. Gut microbiota and immune crosstalk in metabolic disease. *Mol. Metab.* **2016**, *5*, 771–781. [CrossRef]
18. Patterson, E.; Ryan, P.M.; Cryan, J.F.; Dinan, T.G.; Ross, R.P.; Fitzgerald, G.F.; Stanton, C. Gut microbiota, obesity and diabetes. *Postgrad. Med. J.* **2016**, *92*, 286–300. [CrossRef]
19. Sha, S.; Ni, L.; Stefil, M.; Dixon, M.; Mouraviev, V. The human gastrointestinal microbiota and prostate cancer development and treatment. *Investig. Clin. Urol.* **2020**, *61*, S43–S50. [CrossRef]
20. Conlon, M.A.; Bird, A.R. The Impact of Diet and Lifestyle on Gut Microbiota and Human Health. *Nutrients* **2015**, *7*, 17–44. [CrossRef]
21. Sakkas, H.; Bozidis, P.; Touzios, C.; Kolios, D.; Athanasiou, G.; Athanasopoulou, E.; Gerou, I.; Gartzonika, C. Nutritional Status and the Influence of the Vegan Diet on the Gut Microbiota and Human Health. *Medicina* **2020**, *56*, 88. [CrossRef]
22. Redondo-Useros, N.; Nova, E.; González-Zancada, N.; Díaz, L.E.; Gómez-Martínez, S.; Marcos, A. Microbiota and Lifestyle: A Special Focus on Diet. *Nutrients* **2020**, *12*, 1776. [CrossRef] [PubMed]

23. Matsushita, M.; Fujita, K.; Nonomura, N. Influence of Diet and Nutrition on Prostate Cancer. *Int. J. Mol. Sci.* **2020**, *21*, 1447. [CrossRef] [PubMed]
24. Roncal, C.; Martínez-Aguilar, E.; Orbe, J.; Ravassa, S.; Fernandez-Montero, A.; Saenz-Pipaon, G.; Ugarte, A.; Mendoza, A.E.-H.D.; Rodriguez, J.A.; Fernández-Alonso, S.; et al. Trimethylamine-N-Oxide (TMAO) Predicts Cardiovascular Mortality in Peripheral Artery Disease. *Sci. Rep.* **2019**, *9*. [CrossRef] [PubMed]
25. Kanitsoraphan, C.; Rattanawong, P.; Charoensri, S.; Senthong, V. Trimethylamine N-Oxide and Risk of Cardiovascular Disease and Mortality. *Curr. Nutr. Rep.* **2018**, *7*, 207–213. [CrossRef]
26. Wang, Z.; Klipfell, E.; Bennett, B.J.; Koeth, R.; Levison, B.S.; Dugar, B.; Feldstein, A.E.; Britt, E.B.; Fu, X.; Chung, Y.-M.; et al. Gut Flora Metabolism of Phosphatidylcholine Promotes Cardiovascular Disease. *Nature* **2011**, *472*, 57–63. [CrossRef]
27. Tang, W.W.; Wang, Z.; Levison, B.S.; Koeth, R.A.; Britt, E.B.; Fu, X.; Wu, Y.; Hazen, S.L. Intestinal Microbial Metabolism of Phosphatidylcholine and Cardiovascular Risk. *N. Engl. J.* **2013**, *368*, 1575–1584. [CrossRef]
28. Senthong, V.; Wang, Z.; Li, X.S.; Fan, Y.; Wu, Y.; Tang, W.H.W.; Hazen, S.L. Intestinal Microbiota-Generated Metabolite Trimethylamine-N-Oxide and 5-Year Mortality Risk in Stable Coronary Artery Disease: The Contributory Role of Intestinal Microbiota in a COURAGE-Like Patient Cohort. *J. Am. Heart Assoc.* **2016**, *5*. [CrossRef]
29. Zeisel, S.H.; Warrier, M. TrimethylamineN-Oxide, the Microbiome, and Heart and Kidney Disease. *Annu. Rev. Nutr.* **2017**, *37*, 157–181. [CrossRef]
30. Yoshida, N.; Yamashita, T.; Hirata, K.-I. Gut Microbiome and Cardiovascular Diseases. *Diseases* **2018**, *6*, 56. [CrossRef]
31. Trøseid, M.; Andersen, G.Ø.; Broch, K.; Hov, J.R. The Gut Microbiome in Coronary Artery Disease and Heart Failure: Current Knowledge and Future Directions. *EBioMedicine* **2020**, *52*, 102649. [CrossRef] [PubMed]
32. Kazemian, N.; Mahmoudi, M.; Halperin, F.; Wu, J.C.; Pakpour, S. Gut Microbiota and Cardiovascular Disease: Opportunities and Challenges. *Microbiome* **2020**, *8*. [CrossRef] [PubMed]
33. Tang, W.W.; Bäckhed, F.; Landmesser, U.; Hazen, S.L. Intestinal Microbiota in Cardiovascular Health and Disease. *J. Am. Coll. Cardiol.* **2019**, *73*, 2089–2105. [CrossRef] [PubMed]
34. Sata, Y.; Marques, F.Z.; Kaye, D.M. The Emerging Role of Gut Dysbiosis in Cardio-Metabolic Risk Factors for Heart Failure. *Curr. Hypertens. Rep.* **2020**, *22*. [CrossRef]
35. Zhang, D.; Li, S.; Wang, N.; Tan, H.-Y.; Zhang, Z.; Feng, Y. The Cross-Talk between Gut Microbiota and Lungs in Common Lung Diseases. *Front. Microbiol.* **2020**, *11*, 301. [CrossRef]
36. Loverdos, K.; Bellos, G.; Kokolatou, L.; Vasileiadis, I.; Giamarellos, E.; Pecchiari, M.; Koulouris, N.; Koutsoukou, A.; Rovina, N. Lung Microbiome in Asthma: Current Perspectives. *J. Clin. Med.* **2019**, *8*, 1967. [CrossRef]
37. Gao, Q.Y.; Chen, Y.X.; Fang, J.Y. 2019 Novel Coronavirus Infection and Gastrointestinal Tract. *J. Dig. Dis.* **2020**, *21*, 125–126. [CrossRef]
38. Zuo, T.; Zhang, F.; Lui, G.C.; Yeoh, Y.K.; Li, A.Y.; Zhan, H.; Wan, Y.; Chung, A.; Cheung, C.P.; Chen, N.; et al. Alterations in Gut Microbiota of Patients With COVID-19 During Time of Hospitalization. *Gastroenterology* **2020**. [CrossRef]
39. Lyon, L. All disease begins in the gut': Was Hippocrates right? *Brain* **2018**, *141*, e20. [CrossRef]
40. Carabotti, M.; Scirocco, A.; Maselli, M.A.; Severi, C. The gut-brain axis: Interactions between enteric microbiota, central and enteric nervous systems. *Ann. Gastroenterol.* **2015**, *28*, 203–209.
41. Mu, C.; Yang, Y.; Zhu, W. Gut Microbiota: The Brain Peacekeeper. *Front. Microbiol.* **2016**, *7*. [CrossRef] [PubMed]
42. Lach, G.; Schellekens, H.; Dinan, T.G.; Cryan, J.F. Anxiety, Depression, and the Microbiome: A Role for Gut Peptides. *Neurotherapeutics* **2017**, *15*, 36–59. [CrossRef] [PubMed]
43. Dinan, T.G.; Cryan, J.F. Melancholic Microbes: A Link between Gut Microbiota and Depression? *Neurogastroenterol. Motil.* **2013**, *25*, 713–719. [CrossRef]
44. Bermúdez-Humarán, L.G.; Salinas, E.; Ortiz, G.G.; Ramirez-Jirano, L.J.; Morales, J.A.; Bitzer-Quintero, O.K. From Probiotics to Psychobiotics: Live Beneficial Bacteria Which Act on the Brain-Gut Axis. *Nutrients* **2019**, *11*, 890. [CrossRef] [PubMed]
45. Cani, P.D. Human Gut Microbiome: Hopes, Threats and Promises. *Gut* **2018**, *67*, 1716–1725. [CrossRef] [PubMed]

46. Barko, P.; Mcmichael, M.; Swanson, K.; Williams, D. The Gastrointestinal Microbiome: A Review. *J. Vet. Intern. Med.* **2017**, *32*, 9–25. [CrossRef]
47. Hills, R.D.; Pontefract, B.A.; Mishcon, H.R.; Black, C.A.; Sutton, S.C.; Theberge, C.R. Gut Microbiome: Profound Implications for Diet and Disease. *Nutrients* **2019**, *11*, 1613. [CrossRef]
48. Zeevi, D.; Korem, T.; Zmora, N.; Israeli, D.; Rothschild, D.; Weinberger, A.; Ben-Yacov, O.; Lador, D.; Avnit-Sagi, T.; Lotan-Pompan, M.; et al. Personalized Nutrition by Prediction of Glycemic Responses. *Cell* **2015**, *163*, 1079–1094. [CrossRef]
49. Mendes-Soares, H.; Raveh-Sadka, T.; Azulay, S.; Edens, K.; Ben-Shlomo, Y.; Cohen, Y.; Ofek, T.; Bachrach, D.; Stevens, J.; Colibaseanu, D.; et al. Assessment of a Personalized Approach to Predicting Postprandial Glycemic Responses to Food Among Individuals Without Diabetes. *JAMA Netw. Open* **2019**, *2*. [CrossRef]
50. Chen, P.B.; Black, A.S.; Sobel, A.L.; Zhao, Y.; Mukherjee, P.; Molparia, B.; Moore, N.E.; Muench, G.R.A.; Wu, J.; Chen, W.; et al. Directed Remodeling of the Mouse Gut Microbiome Inhibits the Development of Atherosclerosis. *Nat. Biotechnol.* **2020**. [CrossRef]
51. Sharma, H. Ayurveda: Science of life, genetics, and epigenetics. *AYU* **2016**, *37*, 87–91. [CrossRef] [PubMed]
52. Bordoni, L.; Gabbianelli, R. Primers on nutrigenetics and nutri(epi)genomics: Origins and development of precision nutrition. *Biochimie* **2019**, *160*, 156–171. [CrossRef] [PubMed]
53. Sharma, H.; Meade, J.G. *Dynamic DNA*; SelectBooks: New York, NY, USA, 2018.
54. Dash, B.; Sharma, R.K. *Charaka Samhita*; Caukhambha Orientalia: Varanasi, India, 1995.
55. Prasher, B.; Negi, S.; Aggarwal, S.; Mandal, A.K.; Sethi, T.P.; Deshmukh, S.R.; Purohit, S.G.; Sengupta, S.; Khanna, S.; Mohammad, F.; et al. Whole Genome Expression and Biochemical Correlates of Extreme Constitutional Types Defined in Ayurveda. *J. Transl. Med.* **2008**, *6*, 48. [CrossRef] [PubMed]
56. Travis, F.T.; Wallace, R.K. Dosha brain-types: A neural model of individual differences. *J. Ayurveda Integr. Med.* **2015**, *6*, 280–285. [CrossRef] [PubMed]
57. Chauhan, N.S.; Pandey, R.; Mondal, A.K.; Gupta, S.; Verma, M.K.; Jain, S.; Ahmed, V.; Patil, R.; Agarwal, D.; Girase, B.; et al. Western Indian Rural Gut Microbial Diversity in Extreme Prakriti Endo-Phenotypes Reveals Signature Microbes. *Front. Microbiol.* **2018**, *9*, 118. [CrossRef]
58. Jnana, A.; Murali, T.S.; Guruprasad, K.P.; Satyamoorthy, K. Prakriti phenotypes as a stratifier of gut microbiome: A new frontier in personalized medicine? [published online ahead of print, 2020 Jul 24]. *J. Ayurveda Integr. Med.* **2020**, S0975-947630041-3. [CrossRef]
59. Peterson, C.T.; Denniston, K.; Chopra, D. Therapeutic Uses of Triphala in Ayurvedic Medicine. *J. Altern. Complement. Med.* **2017**, *23*, 607–614. [CrossRef]
60. Aggarwal, B.B.; Yuan, W.; Li, S.; Gupta, S.C. Curcumin-Free Turmeric Exhibits Anti-Inflammatory and Anticancer Activities: Identification of Novel Components of Turmeric. *Mol. Nutr. Food Res.* **2013**, *57*, 1529–1542. [CrossRef]
61. Mcfadden, R.-M.T.; Larmonier, C.B.; Shehab, K.W.; Midura-Kiela, M.; Ramalingam, R.; Harrison, C.A.; Besselsen, D.G.; Chase, J.H.; Caporaso, J.G.; Jobin, C.; et al. The Role of Curcumin in Modulating Colonic Microbiota During Colitis and Colon Cancer Prevention. *Inflamm. Bowel Dis.* **2015**, *21*, 2483–2494. [CrossRef]
62. Nelson, K.M.; Dahlin, J.L.; Bisson, J.; Graham, J.; Pauli, G.F.; Walters, M.A. The Essential Medicinal Chemistry of Curcumin. *J. Med. Chem.* **2017**, *60*, 1620–1637. [CrossRef]
63. Lopresti, A.L. The Problem of Curcumin and Its Bioavailability: Could Its Gastrointestinal Influence Contribute to Its Overall Health-Enhancing Effects? *Adv. Nutr.* **2018**, *9*, 41–50. [CrossRef] [PubMed]
64. Shen, L.; Liu, L.; Ji, H.-F. Regulative Effects of Curcumin Spice Administration on Gut Microbiota and Its Pharmacological Implications. *Food Nutr. Res.* **2017**, *61*, 1361780. [CrossRef] [PubMed]
65. Di Meo, F.; Margarucci, S.; Galderisi, U.; Crispi, S.; Peluso, G. Curcumin, Gut Microbiota, and Neuroprotection. *Nutrients* **2019**, *11*, 2426. [CrossRef] [PubMed]
66. Guruprasad, K.P.; Dash, S.; Shivakumar, M.B.; Shetty, P.R.; Raghu, K.S.; Shamprasad, B.R.; Udupi, V.; Acharya, R.V.; Vidya, P.B.; Nayak, J.; et al. Influence of Amalaki Rasayana on Telomerase Activity and Telomere Length in Human Blood Mononuclear Cells. *J. Ayurveda Integr. Med. Med.* **2017**, *8*, 105–112. [CrossRef] [PubMed]
67. Agrawal, A.K.; Yadav, C.R.; Meena, M.S. Physiological aspects of Agni. *AYU* **2010**, *31*, 395–398. [CrossRef] [PubMed]
68. Sharma, H. Leaky gut syndrome, dysbiosis, ama, free radicals, and natural antioxidants. *AYU* **2009**, *30*, 88–105.

69. Fasano, A. Zonulin, Regulation of Tight Junctions, and Autoimmune Diseases. *Ann. N. Y. Acad. Sci.* **2012**, *1258*, 25–33. [CrossRef]
70. Sturgeon, C.; Fasano, A. Zonulin, a Regulator of Epithelial and Endothelial Barrier Functions, and Its Involvement in Chronic Inflammatory Diseases. *Tissue Barriers* **2016**, *4*. [CrossRef]
71. Kelly, J.R.; Kennedy, P.J.; Cryan, J.F.; Dinan, T.G.; Clarke, G.; Hyland, N.P. Breaking down the barriers: The gut microbiome, intestinal permeability and stress-related psychiatric disorders. *Front. Cell. Neurosci.* **2015**, *9*, 392. [CrossRef]
72. Fasano, A. All disease begins in the (leaky) gut: Role of zonulin-mediated gut permeability in the pathogenesis of some chronic inflammatory diseases. *F1000Research* **2020**, *9*. [CrossRef]
73. Kecklund, G.; Axelsson, J. Health Consequences of Shift Work and Insufficient Sleep. *BMJ* **2016**, i5210. [CrossRef] [PubMed]
74. Zarrinpar, A.; Chaix, A.; Panda, S. Daily Eating Patterns and Their Impact on Health and Disease. *Trends Endocrinol. Metab.* **2016**, *27*, 69–83. [CrossRef] [PubMed]
75. Thaiss, C.A.; Zeevi, D.; Levy, M.; Zilberman-Schapira, G.; Suez, J.; Tengeler, A.C.; Abramson, L.; Katz, M.N.; Korem, T.; Zmora, N.; et al. Transkingdom Control of Microbiota Diurnal Oscillations Promotes Metabolic Homeostasis. *Cell* **2014**, *159*, 514–529. [CrossRef] [PubMed]
76. Kaczmarek, J.L.; Thompson, S.V.; Holscher, H.D. Complex interactions of circadian rhythms, eating behaviors, and the gastrointestinal microbiota and their potential impact on health. *Nutr. Rev.* **2017**, *75*, 673–682. [CrossRef]
77. Smits, S.A.; Leach, J.; Sonnenburg, E.D.; Gonzalez, C.G.; Lichtman, J.S.; Reid, G.; Knight, R.; Manjurano, A.; Changalucha, J.; Elias, J.E.; et al. Seasonal Cycling in the Gut Microbiome of the Hadza Hunter-Gatherers of Tanzania. *Science* **2017**, *357*, 802–806. [CrossRef]
78. Davenport, E.R.; Mizrahi-Man, O.; Michelini, K.; Barreiro, L.B.; Ober, C.; Gilad, Y. Seasonal Variation in Human Gut Microbiome Composition. *PLoS ONE* **2014**, *9*. [CrossRef] [PubMed]
79. Deaver, J.A.; Eum, S.Y.; Toborek, M. Circadian Disruption Changes Gut Microbiome Taxa and Functional Gene Composition. *Front. Microbiol.* **2018**, *9*, 737. [CrossRef]
80. Voigt, R.; Forsyth, C.; Green, S.; Engen, P.; Keshavarzian, A. Circadian Rhythm and the Gut Microbiome. *Int. Rev. Neurobiol.* **2016**, 193–205. [CrossRef]
81. Paulose, J.K.; Wright, J.M.; Patel, A.G.; Cassone, V.M. Human Gut Bacteria Are Sensitive to Melatonin and Express Endogenous Circadian Rhythmicity. *PLoS ONE* **2016**, *11*, e146643. [CrossRef]
82. Reynolds, A.C.; Paterson, J.L.; Ferguson, S.A.; Stanley, D.; Wright, K.P.; Dawson, D. The Shift Work and Health Research Agenda: Considering Changes in Gut Microbiota as a Pathway Linking Shift Work, Sleep Loss and Circadian Misalignment, and Metabolic Disease. *Sleep Med. Rev.* **2017**, *34*, 3–9. [CrossRef]
83. Wallace, R.K.; Wallace, S.; Stenberg, S.; Davis, J.; Farley, A. *The Rest and Repair Diet*; Dharma Publications: Fairfield, IA, USA, 2019.
84. Perlmutter, D.; Loberg, K. *The Brain Maker: The Power of Gut Microbes to Heal and Protect Your Brain for Life*; Little Brown and Company: Boston, MA, USA, 2015.
85. Kadus, P.A.; Vedpathak, S.M. Comparative Study of Anuvasana Basti with Constant and Escalating Dose as an Alternative to Snehapana in Purvakarma of Vamana and Virechana. *J. Ayurveda Integr. Med.* **2017**, *8*, 194–199. [CrossRef]
86. Anu, M.; Kunjibettu, S.; Archana, S.; Dei, L. Management of Premature Contractions with Shatavaryadi Ksheerapaka Basti—A Case Report. *AYU* **2017**, *38*, 148. [CrossRef]
87. Pooja, B.; Bhatted, S. A Standard Controlled Clinical Study on Virechana Karma and Lekhana Basti in the Management of Dyslipidemia (Medoroga). *AYU* **2016**, *37*, 32. [CrossRef] [PubMed]
88. Kadus, P.; Vedpathak, S. Anuvasan Basti in Escalating Dose Is an Alternative for Snehapana before Vamana and Virechana: Trends from a Pilot Study. *J. Ayurveda Integr. Med.* **2014**, *5*, 246. [CrossRef]
89. Shukla, G.; Bhatted, S.; Dave, A.; Shukla, V. Efficacy of Virechana and Basti Karma with Shamana Therapy in the Management of Essential Hypertension: A Comparative Study. *AYU* **2013**, *34*, 70. [CrossRef] [PubMed]
90. Auti, S.; Thakar, A.; Shukla, V.; Ravishankar, B. Assessment of Lekhana Basti in the Management of Hyperlipidemia. *AYU* **2013**, *34*, 339. [CrossRef] [PubMed]
91. Swapnil, S.; Anup, B.; Ashok, B.; Ravishankar, B.; Shukla, V. Evaluation of Anti-Hyperlipidemic Activity of Lekhana Basti in Albino Rats. *AYU* **2013**, *34*, 220. [CrossRef]

92. Baria, R.; Pandya, D.; Joshi, N. Clinical Efficacy of Panchamuladi Kaala Basti (Enema) in the Management of Amavata (Rheumatoid Arthritis). *AYU* **2011**, *32*, 90. [CrossRef]
93. Periasamy, S.; Hsu, D.-Z.; Chandrasekaran, V.R.M.; Liu, M.-Y. Sesame Oil Accelerates Healing of 2,4,6-Trinitrobenzenesulfonic Acid–Induced Acute Colitis by Attenuating Inflammation and Fibrosis. *J. Parenter. Enteral. Nutr.* **2012**, *37*, 674–682. [CrossRef]
94. Hou, R.; Lin, M.; Wang, M.; Tzen, J. Increase of Viability of Entrapped Cells of Lactobacillus Delbrueckii Ssp. Bulgaricus in Artificial Sesame Oil Emulsions. *J. Dairy Sci.* **2003**, *86*, 424–428. [CrossRef]
95. Peterson, C.T.; Lucas, J.; John-Williams, L.S.; Thompson, J.W.; Moseley, M.A.; Patel, S.; Peterson, S.N.; Porter, V.; Schadt, E.E.; Mills, P.J.; et al. Identification of Altered Metabolomic Profiles Following a Panchakarma-Based Ayurvedic Intervention in Healthy Subjects: The Self-Directed Biological Transformation Initiative (SBTI). *Sci. Rep.* **2016**, *6*, 6. [CrossRef]
96. Cani, P.D.; Knauf, C. How Gut Microbes Talk to Organs: The Role of Endocrine and Nervous Routes. *Mol. Metab.* **2016**, *5*, 743–752. [CrossRef] [PubMed]
97. Herr, N.; Bode, C.; Duerschmied, D. The Effects of Serotonin in Immune Cells. *Front. Cardiovasc. Med.* **2017**, *4*. [CrossRef] [PubMed]
98. Boyer, E.W.; Shannon, M. The serotonin syndrome. *N. Engl. J. Med.* **2005**, *352*, 1112–1120. [CrossRef] [PubMed]
99. Frick, A.; Åhs, F.; Engman, J.; Jonasson, M.; Alaie, I.; Björkstrand, J.; Frans, Ö.; Faria, V.; Linnman, C.; Appel, L.; et al. Serotonin Synthesis and Reuptake in Social Anxiety Disorder. *JAMA Psychiatry* **2015**, *72*, 794. [CrossRef] [PubMed]
100. Corrêa-Oliveira, R.; Fachi, J.L.; Vieira, A.; Sato, F.T.; Vinolo, M.A.R. Regulation of Immune Cell Function by Short-Chain Fatty Acids. *Clin. Transl. Immunol.* **2016**, *5*. [CrossRef] [PubMed]
101. Foster, J.A.; Rinaman, L.; Cryan, J.F. Stress & the Gut-Brain Axis: Regulation by the Microbiome. *Neurobiol. Stress* **2017**, *7*, 124–136. [CrossRef]
102. Wallace, R.K. Physiological Effects of Transcendental Meditation. *Science* **1970**, *167*, 1751–1754. [CrossRef]
103. Wallace, R.; Benson, H.; Wilson, A. A Wakeful Hypometabolic Physiologic State. *Am. J. Physiol.* **1971**, *221*, 795–799. [CrossRef]
104. Travis, F.; Shear, J. Focused Attention, Open Monitoring and Automatic Self-Transcending: Categories to Organize Meditations from Vedic, Buddhist and Chinese Traditions. *Conscious. Cogn.* **2010**, *19*, 1110–1118. [CrossRef]
105. Nidich, S.; Mills, P.J.; Rainforth, M.; Heppner, P.; Schneider, R.H.; Rosenthal, N.E.; Salerno, J.; Gaylord-King, C.; Rutledge, T. Non-Trauma-Focused Meditation versus Exposure Therapy in Veterans with Post-Traumatic Stress Disorder: A Randomised Controlled Trial. *Lancet Psychiatry* **2018**, *5*, 975–986. [CrossRef]
106. Barnes, V.; Orme-Johnson, D. Clinical and Pre-Clinical Applications of the Transcendental Meditation Program® in the Prevention and Treatment of Essential Hypertension and Cardiovascular Disease in Youth and Adults. *Curr. Hypertens Rev.* **2006**, *2*, 207–218. [CrossRef] [PubMed]
107. Schneider, R.H.; Grim, C.E.; Rainforth, M.V.; Kotchen, T.; Nidich, S.I.; Gaylord-King, C.; Salerno, J.W.; Kotchen, J.M.; Alexander, C.N. Stress Reduction in the Secondary Prevention of Cardiovascular Disease. *Circ. Cardiovasc. Qual. Outcomes* **2012**, *5*, 750–758. [CrossRef] [PubMed]
108. Tillisch, K.; Mayer, E.A.; Gupta, A.; Gill, Z.; Brazeilles, R.; Nevé, B.L.; Vlieg, J.E.V.H.; Guyonnet, D.; Derrien, M.; Labus, J.S. Brain Structure and Response to Emotional Stimuli as Related to Gut Microbial Profiles in Healthy Women. *Psychosom. Med.* **2017**, *79*, 905–913. [CrossRef] [PubMed]
109. Tillisch, K.; Labus, J.; Kilpatrick, L.; Jiang, Z.; Stains, J.; Ebrat, B.; Guyonnet, D.; Legrain–Raspaud, S.; Trotin, B.; Naliboff, B.; et al. Consumption of Fermented Milk Product With Probiotic Modulates Brain Activity. *Gastroenterology* **2013**, *144*. [CrossRef]
110. Wallace, R.K.; Wallace, S. *Gut Crisis*; Dharma Publications: Fairfield, IA, USA, 2017.

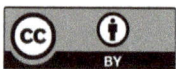

© 2020 by the author. Licensee MDPI, Basel, Switzerland. This article is an open access article distributed under the terms and conditions of the Creative Commons Attribution (CC BY) license (http://creativecommons.org/licenses/by/4.0/).

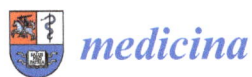

Review

Ayurveda and Epigenetics

Hari Sharma [1,*] and Robert Keith Wallace [2,*]

1. Ohio State Integrative Medicine, Department of Family and Community Medicine, College of Medicine, The Ohio State University, Columbus, OH 43221, USA
2. Department of Physiology and Health, Maharishi International University, Fairfield, IA 52556, USA
* Correspondence: sharma.2@osu.edu (H.S.); kwallace@miu.edu (R.K.W.)

Received: 5 November 2020; Accepted: 8 December 2020; Published: 11 December 2020

Abstract: Ayurveda is a comprehensive, natural health care system that originated in the ancient Vedic times of India. Epigenetics refers to the external modification of DNA that turns genes on and off, affecting gene expression. This occurs without changes in the basic structure of the DNA. This gene expression can have transgenerational effects. The major factors that cause epigenetic changes are lifestyle and behavior, diet and digestion, stress, and environmental factors. Ayurveda addresses these factors, thereby affecting the Deha (body) Prakriti (psychophysiological constitution), which corresponds to the phenotype, and indirectly the Janma (birth) Prakriti, which corresponds to the genotype. Thus, it is proposed that epigenetics is an important mechanism of Ayurveda. This correlation and understanding will lead to better communication and understanding with the current medical system, and lead to better integration of both sciences in the management of optimal health. In addition, research on Ayurvedic modalities affecting gene expression will further increase correlation and understanding between the current medical system and Ayurveda.

Keywords: Ayurveda; epigenetics; genotype; phenotype; Prakriti; doshas

1. Introduction

Ayurveda is a comprehensive, natural system of health care that originated in the ancient Vedic times of India. Ayurveda is a Sanskrit term that translates as the "Science of Life." Sanskrit was the main language used in communication and teaching in the ancient Vedic times. In the context of current knowledge, many of the original concepts of Veda (translates as "knowledge") and Ayurveda are not clearly understood, and this results in varied interpretations in current communication. Additionally, many of the terms originally used cannot be properly translated in current terminology, and some terms have no corresponding counterparts in English, which results in confusion and misunderstanding. This article proposes a correlation of the ancient Ayurvedic concepts and terminology with the current understanding of cellular physiology. Topics covered include genotype and phenotype and their correlation with Janma (birth) Prakriti and Deha (body) Prakriti (psychophysiological Ayurvedic constitution), and epigenetics and its correlation as an important mechanism of Ayurveda.

The difference between living and non-living entities is the presence of deoxyribonucleic acid (DNA) in living species. In the living species, the difference between them is in the order of the bases (adenine–thymine, guanine–cytosine) in the DNA [1]. All nucleated cells contain DNA. The combination of DNA creates genes. It is estimated that humans have approximately 20,000 genes. Less than 2% of these are coding genes that express themselves and are known as the genotype. The genotype refers to the part of the genetic makeup that determines specific characteristics of an individual. It is stable and non-changing unless there is toxic damage. The genotype is responsible for the development of the phenotype of the individual [1]. The phenotype refers to the physical properties of an individual—appearance, development, and behavior. Whatever one does in one's life—knowingly or unknowingly—affects the phenotype and changes the expression of the genotype accordingly.

The four major factors affecting the phenotype are lifestyle and behavior, diet and digestion, stress, and environmental factors [1].

2. Genotype and Phenotype in Ayurveda

In Ayurvedic terms, the Janma Prakriti or birth Prakriti does not change and is the foundation of the psychophysiological constitution or Deha Prakriti (body Prakriti), which changes and is dynamic. The genotype corresponds to Ayurvedic birth Prakriti and the phenotype corresponds to Ayurvedic Deha Prakriti. Disturbance in the Deha Prakriti is known as Vikriti in Ayurveda, which correlates with disorders and diseases in the current medical system. Manohar has described the presence of vivid accounts in the ancient Ayurvedic texts about the inheritance of diseases and the genetic basis for the transmission of such diseases from parents to progeny [2]. The Ayurvedic understanding that Deha Prakriti has a genetic basis has been corroborated by current scientific research. For example, the phosphoglucomutase 1 (*PGM1*) gene has been correlated with Pitta Prakriti (one of the Prakriti types) [3]. Research on human leucocyte antigen (*HLA*) gene polymorphism showed a reasonable correlation between HLA type and Prakriti type [4].

According to Ayurveda, there are three governing principles of the physiology, known as doshas. The three doshas are Vata, Pitta, and Kapha. Vata governs motion, flow, and communication, including the flow of the blood, the beating of the heart, the transmission of nerve impulses, etc. Pitta regulates digestion, metabolism, and transformation. Kapha governs the structure of the body. These three doshas make up the psychophysiological constitution. In the process of DNA expression, the two strands of DNA separate and the knowledge present in the strand is replicated and comes out as messenger ribonucleic acid (mRNA). The knowledge carried in mRNA is then utilized by transfer RNA (tRNA), which lines up the designated amino acids to form the specified protein (Figure 1). It is proposed that mRNA, tRNA, and protein have features and properties that represent Vata, Pitta, and Kapha at the cellular level. Messenger RNA corresponds with Vata (transmission of information), tRNA corresponds with Pitta (transformation), and protein corresponds with Kapha (structure) [1] (Figure 1).

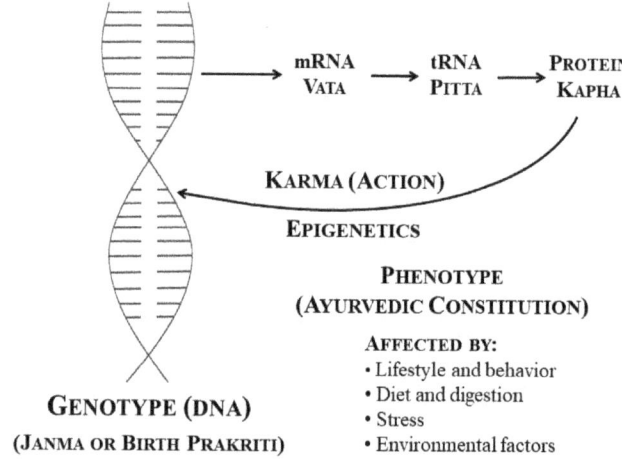

Figure 1. DNA and cellular function and correlation with Ayurveda. mRNA, messenger ribonucleic acid; tRNA, transfer ribonucleic acid; DNA, deoxyribonucleic acid. Modified and reprinted from [1], with permission from SelectBooks, 2018.

3. Epigenetics and Ayurveda

Epigenetics refers to the external modification of DNA that turns genes on and off, affecting gene expression. This occurs without changes in the DNA sequence. This process produces a change in the phenotype without a change in the genotype [1]. In brief, DNA methylation, histone modification, chromatin remodeling, and micro RNA (miRNA) are involved in modifying DNA expression. DNA methylation is a process in which methyl groups are added to the DNA molecule. This process changes the activity of the DNA [5]. Histones are proteins that DNA wraps around in the nucleus, forming chromatin. This process condenses DNA into a more compact form and protects the DNA structure and sequence. Chromatin can condense or it can relax, thereby changing the expression of DNA. Histones play a major role in the condensation and relaxation of chromatin and thereby affect DNA expression [6]. Chromatin remodeling refers to the rearrangement of chromatin from a condensed state to a transcriptionally accessible state, allowing transcription factors or other DNA-binding proteins to access DNA and control gene expression [7]. MicroRNA refers to small non-coding RNA molecules that "silence" or stop the functioning of mRNA [8].

It is estimated that 90% of life is controlled by epigenetics—the changes in gene expression brought about by what one does in one's life. Whatever is done to the phenotype or Ayurvedic psychophysiological constitution (Deha Prakriti) is relayed back to the DNA, which changes its expression accordingly. Thus, the process of epigenetics represents action (Karma—the Sanskrit word for "action") on the level of the cells (Figure 1). In the field of physics, this is represented by Newton's Third Law of Motion: For every action there is an equal and opposite reaction. Another way of putting it is the Biblical saying "As you sow, so shall you reap." Every cell is going through this process. Factors that cause epigenetic changes affect DNA expression and this can also be transmitted to the progeny [9].

As mentioned previously, there are four major factors that affect one's life. These factors are addressed in Ayurveda for maintaining health and preventing disease. They are lifestyle and behavior, diet and digestion, stress, and environmental factors. If an individual's actions are in the positive direction, Deha Prakriti remains balanced and health is maintained. If actions are not in the positive direction, Deha Prakriti becomes imbalanced, creating Vikriti, and disease manifests. This whole process occurs through the mechanism of epigenetics. These epigenetic changes can be reversed [10]. Ayurveda addresses the factors that cause epigenetic changes, and it thereby affects both the phenotype and expression of the genotype in a positive manner. Thus, it is proposed that epigenetics is an important mechanism of Ayurveda [1,11].

A further correlation between epigenetics and Ayurveda relates to the personalized nature of the process of epigenetics and the health care system of Ayurveda. Each individual holds their health in their own hands. Through the process of epigenetics, their actions affect their health in a direct and very personal way, which can help prevent disease or lead to disease. Ayurveda is a prevention-oriented system of health care that provides detailed recommendations that are personalized for each individual based on their unique Prakriti and Vikriti.

4. Research on the Four Major Factors that Cause Epigenetic Changes

A growing body of evidence demonstrates the importance of the four major factors that cause epigenetic changes in the expression of DNA [10,12]. It has been identified that diet, obesity, physical activity, tobacco smoking, alcohol consumption, environmental pollutants, psychological stress, and working the night shift might modify epigenetic patterns [13]. For example, polyphenols, which are natural compounds widely found in plant foods, have been shown to modify the activity of DNA methyltransferases, histone acetylases, and histone deacetylases, inducing reversibility of epigenetic dysregulation. Epigenetic biomarkers of obesity, including genes involved in adipogenesis, methylation patterns of obesity-related genes, and inflammation genes could help predict susceptibility and prevent obesity. Physical activity has been associated with higher methylation in peripheral blood lymphocytes of long interspersed nucleotide element-1 (LINE-1) elements, which are a class of repeated sequences that are highly repeated in the human genome. Low methylation in these elements is associated with inflammatory responses and chromosomal instability [13].

Regarding tobacco smoking, cigarette smoke condensate decreases nuclear levels of certain histone modifications in respiratory epithelial cells, with these alterations being similar to changes in histone modifications found in lung cancer tissues. With regard to alcohol consumption, a population-based case–control study showed the association between LINE-1 hypomethylation in blood leukocyte DNA and gastric cancer was stronger among individuals who were current alcohol drinkers. An occupational study examined the effects of exposure to air pollution, specifically particulate matter and metal components, on miRNA expression in workers at an electric-furnace steel plant. It was found that two miRNAs related to oxidative stress and inflammation were overexpressed and positively correlated with the levels of lead exposure and oxidative DNA damage [13].

Regarding psychological stress, research has shown hypermethylation of the glucocorticoid receptor gene in suicide victims with a history of childhood abuse, but not in controls or suicide victims who did not experience childhood abuse. Several epidemiological studies have shown that working the night shift can have negative effects on the health and well-being of workers. A study on a population of night-shift workers showed alterations in blood DNA methylation, including changes in gene-specific methylation of inflammatory genes [13]. The following is further research on the four major factors that cause epigenetic changes.

4.1. Lifestyle and Behavior

Epigenetic dysregulations may play an important role in the onset, progression, and pathogenesis of various human disorders and diseases, including cancer and cardiovascular, neurodegenerative, and autoimmune diseases [14]. A study on men with prostate cancer showed that a lifestyle intervention program that included meditation, breathing exercises, aerobic exercise, and a vegetarian diet changed the expression of 500 genes, including the downregulation of disease-promoting genes involved in tumor formation [15]. A study on patients with coronary artery disease showed that a lifestyle modification program that included stress management, aerobic exercise, and a vegetarian diet resulted in successful and sustained modulation of gene expression that ameliorated cardiovascular risk [16]. A study on the impact of a health promotion intervention that included increased physical activity and increased intake of fruits/vegetables impacted patterns of DNA methylation in gene regions related to immune cell metabolism, tumor suppression, and overall aging [17]. Two additional studies have shown a linkage between exercise and DNA methylation, with concordant health-enhancing changes in the phenotype [18,19].

4.2. Diet and Digestion

Dietary nutrients and bioactive food components are epigenetic regulators that modify gene expression. Diet can modify epigenetic mechanisms by regulating DNA methylation, histone modifications, chromatin remodeling, and changes in miRNA expression [10,20]. For example, foods that contain B vitamins can influence DNA methylation [21]. Curcumin, one of the components of *Curcuma longa* L. (turmeric), is a histone deacetylase inhibitor, as demonstrated in B cell non-Hodgkin lymphoma cells. The expression levels of several histone deacetylase enzymes were downregulated following curcumin treatment. The dysfunction of histone deacetylases is associated with the manifestation of several different types of cancer [22]. In breast cancer cells, curcumin significantly downregulated both estrogen receptor alpha (ERα) and p53 protein levels, with a concomitant decrease in breast cancer cell viability. Both ERα and p53 are known to contribute to the formation and progression of hormone-dependent breast cancer [23].

In addition to curcumin, other bioactive food components have been shown to modulate epigenetic events, with epigenetic targets that are associated with breast cancer prevention and therapy. These bioactive ingredients include dietary polyphenols, epigallocatechin gallate from green tea, genistein from soybean, isothiocyanates from plant foods, resveratrol from grapes, and sulforaphane from cruciferous vegetables [24]. These bioactive food components have shown similar results in other types of cancer [25]. In light of these findings, an "epigenetics diet" has been proposed, which would utilize these bioactive dietary compounds to neutralize epigenetic aberrations as a form of cancer treatment, and be utilized as cancer prevention [26].

In Ayurveda, optimal digestion is considered to be of prime importance in maintaining health. A nutritious diet will not have the maximum impact in promoting health unless the digestive capacity is optimal. Balanced Agni (digestive fire) is critical for proper digestion to occur. If the Agni is not functioning properly, the food will not be properly digested and this can lead to the production of Ama, a toxic byproduct of incomplete digestion that is linked to disorders and diseases. Research has found that the response to food intake and individual nutrients includes epigenetic events [27]. Bile acids, which are necessary for lipid digestion and absorption, are also signaling molecules. Bile acid synthesis is transcriptionally regulated in relation to the fasted-to-fed cycle. The underlying mechanisms include chromatin remodeling at promoters of key genes involved in their metabolism [27].

Herbs have been shown to exhibit epigenetic mechanisms [28]. A study on herbs showed that 36% interacted with histone-modifying enzymes and 56% of these promoted chromatin condensation [29]. Withaferin A, a component of *Withania somnifera (L.) Dunal* (Ashwagandha), has been shown to downregulate DNA methyltransferases and histone deacetylase in breast cancer cells and induce apoptosis of these cells [30,31].

4.3. Stress

Exposure to stressors can change epigenetic marks, or tags, and influence the way genes are expressed [32]. Stress-associated epigenetic changes have been correlated with depression [33]. Feelings of anger, stress, frustration, and fear cause the DNA to become shorter and tighter, and switch off many codes. In contrast, feelings of gratitude, love, and appreciation cause the DNA to relax, and the strands unwind and begin to express [34]. A pilot study on telomerase gene expression in hypertensive patients showed that stress reduction through meditation and lifestyle modifications increased telomerase gene expression [35]. In light of these research studies, stress management can be viewed as a crucial requirement for health and well-being. In this regard, Ayurveda has long included a thorough understanding of meditation as a technique for stress management and the development of consciousness.

4.4. Environmental Factors

Environmental factors can alter gene expression through epigenetic mechanisms [10]. Research has shown that environmental toxicants such as diesel exhaust particles, cigarette smoke, and inorganic arsenate can silence certain tumor suppressor genes, resulting in carcinogenesis [36]. Chronic sun exposure causes epigenetic changes in the skin. Hypomethylation was seen in sun-exposed epidermis samples from older individuals [37].

Epigenetic changes can affect future generations. Nutrition abnormalities, environmental toxicants, and environmental stress can promote epigenetic alterations that are transmitted to subsequent generations, resulting in disease [9]. It has been shown that exposure to air pollution during gestation affects the gestating mother, her embryo, and its developing germ line, thereby influencing the third generation's phenotype [38]. Many effects of traumatic stress can be transmitted to future generations, even when individuals from these generations are not exposed to a traumatic stressor [39].

As mentioned previously, Ayurveda addresses the four major factors that cause epigenetic changes, for the maintenance of health and prevention of disease. As a comprehensive system of health care, there are multiple aspects of Ayurveda that relate to these four factors. For example, Dinacharya (daily routine) recommends the optimal times for getting up in the morning, eating, exercising, meditating, etc., to stay in tune with the natural rhythms of nature that support optimal health. Ratricharya (night routine) recommends the optimal time to go to bed to ensure a good night's sleep, which is considered one of the main pillars of health in Ayurveda. It is this aspect of Ayurveda that recommends against working the night shift, due to the adverse physiological changes that can result. Ritucharya (seasonal routine) includes recommendations for each season, e.g., eating cooling foods during the summer and minimizing hot, spicy foods.

Other areas of Ayurveda that provide health-promoting recommendations include Ahara-Vihara (diet and guidelines for eating), Sadvritta (social and personal behavior), Manasa Tivra (mental stress) and Manas Vritti (mental fluctuations), and Paryavarana (environment, including home and workplace). With regard to Manas (mind), mental fluctuations are created by the incoming information received through the five senses (sight, hearing, taste, touch, and smell). An overload of this sensory input can cause stress, strain, and imbalance in the mind. Through the mind–body connection, this imbalance can lead to physical disorders.

Ayurveda has various recommendations for stress management and resilience. Increasing Bala and Ojas is important in this regard. Bala refers to strength, including physical strength, mental strength, and strong immunity. Ojas is the end-product of perfect digestion and metabolism at the cellular or tissue level. Ojas maintains and enhances immunity. It also nourishes and sustains the dhatus (tissues) of the body [40]. One of the recommendations for reducing mental stress and increasing Bala and Ojas to increase resilience is Vedic meditation, which utilizes a technique that goes beyond the mind and deep into the inner being, which is a place of peace and bliss. Research has demonstrated the health benefits of this type of meditation [41].

5. Conclusions

In conclusion, it is proposed that the genotype and phenotype correspond to Ayurvedic Janma (birth) Prakriti and Deha (body) Prakriti (psychophysiological constitution), respectively. Imbalance or disorder of the Deha Prakriti is known as Vikriti and corresponds to disorders and diseases in the current medical system. It is proposed that mRNA, tRNA, and protein have features and properties that represent the three governing principles of the physiology or Ayurvedic doshas—Vata, Pitta, and Kapha—at the cellular level. There are four major factors that affect the phenotype or Deha Prakriti in a positive or negative way, depending on what one does in one's life. These four factors are lifestyle and behavior, diet and digestion, stress, and environmental factors. These factors produce changes in the phenotype or Deha Prakriti that affect the expression of the genotype, the Janma (birth) Prakriti, without changing its basic structure. Ayurveda addresses these four major factors of life and thereby affects both the phenotype and genotype in a positive way through the process of epigenetics. Thus, it is proposed that epigenetics is an important mechanism of Ayurveda. This correlation and understanding of the process of healing and health maintenance will improve the understanding and communication between Ayurveda and the current medical system, and lead to better integration of both sciences in the management of optimal health. In addition, research on Ayurvedic modalities affecting gene expression will further increase the correlation and understanding between the current medical system and Ayurveda.

Funding: A grant from the Wege Foundation provided for publication costs.

Conflicts of Interest: The authors declare no conflict of interest.

References

1. Sharma, H.; Meade, J.G. *Dynamic DNA*; SelectBooks: New York, NY, USA, 2018.
2. Manohar, P.R. Medical Genetics in Classical Ayurvedic Texts: A Critical Review. *Indian J. Hist. Sci.* **2016**, *51*, 417–422. [CrossRef]
3. Govindaraj, P.; Nizamuddin, S.; Sharath, A.; Jyothi, V.; Rotti, H.; Raval, R.; Nayak, J.; Bhat, B.K.; Prasanna, B.V.; Shintre, P.; et al. Genome-wide Analysis Correlates Ayurveda Prakriti. *Sci. Rep.* **2015**, *5*, 15786. [CrossRef] [PubMed]
4. Patwardhan, B.; Joshi, K.; Chopra, A. Classification of Human Population Based on HLA Gene Polymorphism and the Concept of Prakriti in Ayurveda. *J. Altern. Complement. Med.* **2005**, *11*, 349–353.

5. Moore, L.D.; Le, T.; Fan, G. DNA Methylation and its Basic Function. *Neuropsychopharmacology* **2013**, *38*, 23–38. [CrossRef]
6. Fan, J.; Krautkramer, K.A.; Feldman, J.L.; Denu, J.M. Metabolic Regulation of Histone Post-translational Modifications. *ACS Chem. Biol.* **2015**, *10*, 95–108. [CrossRef]
7. Kumar, R.; Li, D.-Q.; Müller, S.; Knapp, S. Epigenomic Regulation of Oncogenesis by Chromatin Remodeling. *Oncogene* **2016**, *35*, 4423–4436. [CrossRef]
8. Lu, T.X.; Rothenberg, M.E. MicroRNA. *J. Allergy Clin. Immunol.* **2018**, *141*, 1202–1207. [CrossRef]
9. Skinner, M.K. Environmental Stress and Epigenetic Transgenerational Inheritance. *BMC Med.* **2014**, *12*, 153. [CrossRef]
10. Abdul, Q.A.; Yu, B.P.; Chung, H.Y.; Jung, H.A.; Choi, J.S. Epigenetic Modifications of Gene Expression by Lifestyle and Environment. *Arch. Pharm. Res.* **2017**, *40*, 1219–1237. [CrossRef]
11. Sharma, H. Ayurveda: Science of Life, Genetics, and Epigenetics. *AYU* **2016**, *37*, 87–91. [CrossRef]
12. Moore, D.S. Behavioral Epigenetics. *Wires Syst. Biol. Med.* **2017**, *9*, 1333. [CrossRef] [PubMed]
13. Alegria-Torres, J.A.; Baccarelli, A.; Bollati, V. Epigenetics and Lifestyle. *Epigenomics* **2011**, *3*, 267–277. [CrossRef] [PubMed]
14. Haluskova, J. Epigenetic Studies in Human Diseases. *Folia Biol. (Praha)* **2010**, *56*, 83–96. [PubMed]
15. Ornish, D.; Magbanua, M.J.M.; Weidner, G.; Weinberg, V.; Kemp, C.; Green, C.; Mattie, M.D.; Marlin, R.; Simko, J.; Shinohara, K.; et al. Changes in Prostate Gene Expression in Men Undergoing an Intensive Nutrition and Lifestyle Intervention. *Proc. Natl. Acad. Sci. USA* **2008**, *105*, 8369–8374. [CrossRef]
16. Blackburn, H.L.; McErlean, S.; Jellema, G.L.; van Laar, R.; Vernalis, M.N.; Ellsworth, D.L. Gene Expression Profiling During Intensive Cardiovascular Lifestyle Modification: Relationships with Vascular Function and Weight Loss. *Genom. Data* **2015**, *4*, 50–53. [CrossRef]
17. Hibler, E.; Huang, L.; Andrade, J.; Spring, B. Impact of a Diet and Activity Health Promotion Intervention on Regional Patterns of DNA Methylation. *Clin. Epigenetics* **2019**, *11*, 133. [CrossRef]
18. Lindholm, M.E.; Marabita, F.; Gomez-Cabrero, D.; Rundqvist, H.; Ekström, T.J.; Tegnér, J.; Sundberg, C.J. An Integrative Analysis Reveals Coordinated Reprogramming of the Epigenome and the Transcriptome in Human Skeletal Muscle after Training. *Epigenetics* **2014**, *9*, 12. [CrossRef]
19. Rönn, T.; Volkov, P.; Davegårdh, C.; Dayeh, T.; Hall, E.; Olsson, A.H.; Nilsson, E.; Tornberg, A.; Nitert, M.D.; Eriksson, K.-F.; et al. A Six Months Exercise Intervention Influences the Genome-wide DNA Methylation Pattern in Human Adipose Tissue. *PLoS Genet.* **2013**, *9*. [CrossRef]
20. Choi, S.-W.; Friso, S. Epigenetics: A New Bridge Between Nutrition and Health. *Adv. Nutr.* **2010**, *1*, 8. [CrossRef]
21. Mahmoud, A.M.; Ali, M.M. Methyl Donor Micronutrients that Modify DNA Methylation and Cancer Outcome. *Nutrients* **2019**, *11*, 608. [CrossRef]
22. Liu, H.-L.; Chen, Y.; Cui, G.-H.; Zhou, J.-F. Curcumin, a Potent Anti-tumor Reagent, is a Novel Histone Deacetylase Inhibitor Regulating B-NHL Cell Line Raji Proliferation. *Acta Pharmacol. Sin.* **2005**, *26*, 603–609. [CrossRef] [PubMed]
23. Hallman, K.; Aleck, K.; Dwyer, B.; Lloyd, V.; Quigley, M.; Sitto, N.; Siebert, A.E.; Dinda, S. The Effects of Turmeric (Curcumin) on Tumor Suppressor Protein (p53) and Estrogen Receptor (ERα) in Breast Cancer Cells. *Breast Cancer (Dove. Med. Press)* **2017**, *9*, 153–161. [CrossRef] [PubMed]
24. Khan, S.I.; Aumsuwan, P.; Khan, I.A.; Walker, L.A.; Dasmahapatra, A.K. Epigenetic Events Associated with Breast Cancer and their Prevention by Dietary Components Targeting the Epigenome. *Chem. Res. Toxicol.* **2012**, *25*, 61–73. [CrossRef] [PubMed]
25. Shukla, S.; Meeran, S.M.; Katiyar, S.K. Epigenetic Regulation by Selected Dietary Phytochemicals in Cancer Chemoprevention. *Cancer Lett.* **2014**, *355*, 9–17. [CrossRef]
26. Lewis, K.A.; Tollefsbol, T.O. The Influence of an Epigenetics Diet on the Cancer Epigenome. *Epigenomics* **2017**, *9*, 1153–1155. [CrossRef]
27. De Fabiani, E.; Mitro, N.; Gilardi, F.; Galmozzi, A.; Caruso, D.; Crestani, M. When Food Meets Man: The Contribution of Epigenetics to Health. *Nutrients* **2010**, *2*, 551–571. [CrossRef]
28. El-Beshbishy, H.A.; Hassan, M.H.; Aly, H.A.A.; Doghish, A.S.; Alghaithy, A.A.A. Crocin "Saffron" Protects Against Beryllium Chloride Toxicity in Rats through Diminution of Oxidative Stress and Enhancing Gene Expression of Antioxidant Enzymes. *Ecotoxicol. Environ. Saf.* **2012**, *83*, 47–54. [CrossRef]

29. Anwar, M.A.; Al Disi, S.S.; Eid, A.H. Anti-hypertensive Herbs and their Mechanisms of Action: Part II. *Front. Pharmacol.* **2016**, *7*, 50. [CrossRef]
30. Royston, K.J.; Udayakumar, N.; Lewis, K.; Tollefsbol, T.O. A Novel Combination of Withaferin A and Sulforaphane Inhibits Epigenetic Machinery, Cellular Viability and Induces Apoptosis of Breast Cancer Cells. *Int. J. Mol. Sci.* **2017**, *18*, 1092. [CrossRef]
31. Royston, K.J.; Paul, B.; Nozell, S.; Rajbhandari, R.; Tollefsbol, T.O. Withaferin A and Sulforaphane Regulate Breast Cancer Cell Cycle Progression through Epigenetic Mechanisms. *Exp. Cell Res.* **2018**, *368*, 67–74. [CrossRef]
32. Zannas, A.S.; West, A.E. Epigenetics and the Regulation of Stress Vulnerability and Resilience. *Neuroscience* **2014**, *264*, 157–170. [CrossRef] [PubMed]
33. Park, C.; Rosenblat, J.D.; Brietzke, E.; Pan, Z.; Lee, Y.; Cao, B.; Zuckerman, H.; Kalantarova, A.; McIntyre, R.S. Stress, Epigenetics and Depression: A Systematic Review. *Neurosci. Biobehav. Rev.* **2019**, *102*, 139–152. [CrossRef] [PubMed]
34. Lancer, D. The Healing Power of Eros. *Int. J. Emerg. Ment. Health* **2015**, *17*, 213–218.
35. Duraimani, S.; Schneider, R.H.; Randall, O.S.; Nidich, S.I.; Xu, S.; Ketete, M.; Rainforth, M.A.; Gaylord-King, C.; Salerno, J.W.; Fagan, J. Effects of Lifestyle Modification on Telomerase Gene Expression in Hypertensive Patients: A Pilot Trial of Stress Reduction and Health Education Programs in African Americans. *PLoS ONE* **2015**, *10*. [CrossRef] [PubMed]
36. Panahi, Y.; Beiraghdar, F.; Amirhamzeh, A.; Poursaleh, Z.; Saadat, A.; Sahebkar, A. Environmental Toxicant Exposure and Cancer: The Role of Epigenetic Changes and Protection by Phytochemicals. *Curr. Pharm. Des.* **2016**, *22*, 130–140. [CrossRef]
37. Vandiver, A.R.; Irizarry, R.A.; Hansen, K.D.; Garza, L.A.; Runarsson, A.; Li, X.; Chien, A.L.; Wang, T.S.; Leung, S.G.; Kang, S.; et al. Age and Sun Exposure-related Widespread Genomic Blocks of Hypomethylation in Nonmalignant Skin. *Genome Biol.* **2015**, *16*, 80. [CrossRef]
38. Shukla, A.; Bunkar, N.; Kumar, R.; Bhargava, A.; Tiwari, R.; Chaudhury, K.; Goryacheva, I.Y.; Mishra, P.K. Air Pollution Associated Epigenetic Modifications: Transgenerational Inheritance and Underlying Molecular Mechanisms. *Sci. Total Environ.* **2019**, *656*, 760–777. [CrossRef]
39. Jawaid, A.; Roszkowski, M.; Mansuy, I.M. Transgenerational Epigenetics of Traumatic Stress. *Prog. Mol. Biol. Transl. Sci.* **2018**, *158*, 273–298.
40. Sharma, H.; Clark, C. *Ayurvedic Healing: Contemporary Maharishi Ayurveda Medicine and Science*; Singing Dragon: London, UK, 2012.
41. Sharma, H. Meditation: Process and Effects. *AYU* **2015**, *36*, 233–237. [CrossRef]

Publisher's Note: MDPI stays neutral with regard to jurisdictional claims in published maps and institutional affiliations.

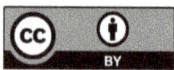

© 2020 by the authors. Licensee MDPI, Basel, Switzerland. This article is an open access article distributed under the terms and conditions of the Creative Commons Attribution (CC BY) license (http://creativecommons.org/licenses/by/4.0/).

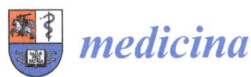

Article

Transcriptomics of Long-Term Meditation Practice: Evidence for Prevention or Reversal of Stress Effects Harmful to Health

Supaya Wenuganen [1], Kenneth G. Walton [1,2], Shilpa Katta [3,4], Clifton L. Dalgard [4], Gauthaman Sukumar [4], Joshua Starr [4], Frederick T. Travis [5], Robert Keith Wallace [1], Paul Morehead [1], Nancy K. Lonsdorf [1], Meera Srivastava [4,*] and John Fagan [1,6,*]

1. Department of Physiology and Health, Maharishi International University, Fairfield, IA 52556, USA; wenuganen@miu.edu (S.W.); kwalton@miu.edu (K.G.W.); kwallace@miu.edu (R.K.W.); pmorehead@miu.edu (P.M.); healthoffice@drlonsdorf.com (N.K.L.)
2. Institute for Prevention Research, Fairfield, IA 52556, USA
3. Cancer Genomics Research Laboratory (CGR), Division of Cancer Epidemiology and Genetics, NCI Leidos Biomedical Research, Inc., Gaithersburg, MD 20877, USA; shilpareddy.20k@gmail.com
4. Department of Anatomy, Physiology, and Genetics, Uniformed Services University of the Health Sciences, Bethesda, MD 20814, USA; clifton.dalgard@usuhs.edu (C.L.D.); gauthaman.sukumar.ctr@usuhs.edu (G.S.); joshua.starr.ctr@usuhs.edu (J.S.)
5. Center for Brain, Cognition, and Consciousness, Maharishi International University, Fairfield, IA 52557, USA; ftravis@miu.edu
6. Health Research Institute, Fairfield, IA 52556, USA
* Correspondence: meera.srivastava@usuhs.edu (M.S.); john.fagan@HRILabs.org (J.F.)

Abstract: *Background and Objectives*: Stress can overload adaptive mechanisms, leading to epigenetic effects harmful to health. Research on the reversal of these effects is in its infancy. Early results suggest some meditation techniques have health benefits that grow with repeated practice. This study focused on possible transcriptomic effects of 38 years of twice-daily Transcendental Meditation® (TM®) practice. *Materials and Methods*: First, using Illumina® BeadChip microarray technology, differences in global gene expression in peripheral blood mononuclear cells (PBMCs) were sought between healthy practitioners and tightly matched controls ($n = 12$, age 65). Second, these microarray results were verified on a subset of genes using quantitative polymerase chain reaction (qPCR) and were validated using qPCR in larger TM and control groups ($n = 45$, age 63). Bioinformatics investigation employed Ingenuity® Pathway Analysis (IPA®), DAVID, Genomatix, and R packages. *Results*: The 200 genes and loci found to meet strict criteria for differential expression in the microarray experiment showed contrasting patterns of expression that distinguished the two groups. Differential expression relating to immune function and energy efficiency were most apparent. In the TM group, relative to the control, all 49 genes associated with inflammation were downregulated, while genes associated with antiviral and antibody components of the defense response were upregulated. The largest expression differences were shown by six genes related to erythrocyte function that appeared to reflect a condition of lower energy efficiency in the control group. Results supporting these gene expression differences were obtained with qPCR-measured expression both in the well-matched microarray groups and in the larger, less well-matched groups. *Conclusions*: These findings are consistent with predictions based on results from earlier randomized trials of meditation and may provide evidence for stress-related molecular mechanisms underlying reductions in anxiety, post-traumatic stress disorder (PTSD), cardiovascular disease (CVD), and other chronic disorders and diseases.

Keywords: chronic stress; transcendental meditation; gene expression; energy metabolism; biological aging; epigenetic effects; allostatic load

Citation: Wenuganen, S.; Walton, K.G.; Katta, S.; Dalgard, C.L.; Sukumar, G.; Starr, J.; Travis, F.T.; Wallace, R.K.; Morehead, P.; Lonsdorf, N.K.; et al. Transcriptomics of Long-Term Meditation Practice: Evidence for Prevention or Reversal of Stress Effects Harmful to Health. *Medicina* 2021, 57, 218. https://doi.org/10.3390/medicina57030218

Academic Editors: Robert H. Schneider, Mahadevan Seetharaman and Vaidutis Kučinskas

Received: 1 December 2020
Accepted: 22 February 2021
Published: 1 March 2021

Publisher's Note: MDPI stays neutral with regard to jurisdictional claims in published maps and institutional affiliations.

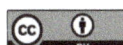

Copyright: © 2021 by the authors. Licensee MDPI, Basel, Switzerland. This article is an open access article distributed under the terms and conditions of the Creative Commons Attribution (CC BY) license (https://creativecommons.org/licenses/by/4.0/).

1. Introduction

McEwen and Akil [1] recently outlined major steps of progress from 50 years of research on the neurobiology of stress. The concept of stress responses as adaptive mechanisms capable of being overworked or overloaded, thereby producing an "allostatic load" that increases propensity for disease, is one of many contributions from the McEwen laboratory [1,2]. Repeated exposure to even mild stressors can constrain adaptive mechanisms, contributing to cardiometabolic, cognitive, and behavioral disorders [1–3]. Such approaches to modeling physiological dysregulation predict not only illness but also longevity [4,5]. Moreover, psychosocial stress is associated with elevated oxidative stress [6,7], a further contributor to disease and aging. The high prevalence of stress-related diseases naturally motivates the search for effective interventions.

Accumulated research on the standardized Transcendental Meditation® (TM®) technique suggests it can reduce unwanted effects of stress. This technique was revived from the ancient Vedic tradition and made available to the world at large by Maharishi Mahesh Yogi starting in the 1950s [8,9]. The first research on physiological effects appeared in 1970 [10]. As reported and reviewed by others, investigations of the TM program as a therapeutic intervention have reported benefits for PTSD [11–13], anxiety disorders [14], and risk factors for cardiovascular disease (CVD) [15–18]. Moreover, studies on healthcare utilization suggest reductions in a wide spectrum of diseases [19,20]. Evidence supports the conclusion that the automatic self-transcending nature of this technique bears primary responsibility for these effects [21,22].

Research on long-term molecular and cellular effects of stress that relate to disease and aging has focused on the immune system and mitochondrial energy production. Early investigations found differences affecting glucocorticoid and inflammatory signaling [23]. Further research led to the discovery of a "Conserved Transcriptional Response to Adversity (CTRA)" accompanying severe or chronic stress [24,25]. The CTRA involves upregulation of pro-inflammatory genes and downregulation of antiviral and antibody components of the defense response [26].

Energy metabolism also is a key component of stress responses and adaptation [27], and mitochondrial energy production is affected by stress [28,29]. Both chronic stress and aging are associated with reductions in mitochondrial function and energy efficiency [30,31].

Some mind–body interventions have been reported to decrease or reverse such effects of stress [32–34], including effects on the "epigenetic clock", a reproducible biomarker of biological aging [35]. However, meditation studies and other mind–body intervention research, especially studies examining transcriptomic effects, have tended to be of short duration [36,37]. This leaves a gap in our knowledge of effects deriving from decades-long practice of these programs. Based on prior research indicating that effects of the TM program are cumulative, we hypothesized that long-term practice would produce transcriptomic differences connected to the program's stress-reducing and health-promoting benefits. Results of this study appear to support that hypothesis. Due to budgetary constraints and to this being the first of its kind, the study is exploratory, not definitive, in nature. Nevertheless, it employs the three steps characterizing gene expression comparisons, namely a discovery step (microarray comparison [38]), a verification and validation step applying a quantitatively more accurate approach (qPCR) to a sample of genes, and a functional analysis showing consistency with prior research on stress effects and meditation. The results appear to provide promising avenues for further investigation.

2. Materials and Methods

2.1. Research Design and Participants

This study used DNA microarray transcriptomics and qPCR technologies in peripheral blood mononuclear cells (PBMCs) to compare non-practitioner control groups and TM practitioner groups. First, two demographically well-matched small groups were selected from a larger pool of volunteers for the microarray analysis (Table 1). Later, qPCR analysis of 15 genes selected from those differentially expressed in the microarray was used to test the reproducibility of the microarray results in the larger pool of 45 volunteers. All study participants were recruited through advertising on the campus of Maharishi International University and in public places in or near Fairfield, Iowa. The design and methods were approved by the University's Institutional Review Board. Following both written and oral descriptions of the study, participants gave signed consent prior to participation.

Table 1. Demographic Matching of Control and Transcendental Meditation® (TM) Groups for Microarray Analysis.

Demographic Variables	Control Group	TM Group
n	6	6
Age (years ± SD)	65.0 ± 4.9	64.5 ± 5.4
Sex (number of males)	4	5
Non-vegetarians (number of)	5	5
Non-smokers (number of)	6	6
Non-drinkers (number of)	6	6
Moderate exercisers (number of)	6	6
Subjective SES * (mean)	3.0	3.1

* Subjective socioeconomic status (SES), using a 5-point scale from 1 for "lower class" to 5 for "upper class".

To reduce genetic variation, study participants were limited to self-identified white males and females. Prospective participants were excluded if they reported a doctor-identified history of diabetes, nerve damage, heart attack, coronary heart disease, stroke, kidney failure, cancer, any other life-threatening illness, a major psychiatric disorder, or substance abuse. In addition, candidates for the control group were excluded if they had ever been instructed in the TM program. Practitioners of the TM program were excluded if they had not regularly practiced the program twice a day or usually twice a day.

The meditation program consisted of the standard TM technique [9] practiced in the microarray TM group for 458 ± 49 months, with later addition of the TM-Sidhi® program, also practiced twice daily in this group, for 406 ± 50 months. The TM-Sidhi program, like the TM program, is drawn from the ancient Vedic tradition and is said to promote more rapid incorporation of the benefits of TM practice into daily life [9]. As with the small groups for microarray analysis, the larger groups used for qPCR analysis were not significantly different in age (Table 2). The TM group was notably higher in the number of vegetarians and tended to be higher in other indicators of healthy lifestyle. Subjective socioeconomic status (SES) data were not available. TM in this qPCR study was practiced for 475 ± 40 months, and the TM-Sidhi program for 396 ± 44 months.

Table 2. Demographic Matching of Control and TM Groups for qPCR Validation Analysis.

Demographic Variables	Control Group	TM Group
n	22	23
Age (years ± SD)	62.2 ± 4.64	63.6 ± 3.92
Sex (number of males)	10	14
Non-vegetarians (number of)	20	8
Non-smokers (number of)	17	23
Non-drinkers (number of)	17	21
Moderate exercisers (number of)	18	23
Subjective SES *	N/A	N/A

* Subjective SES data were not available for these participants.

2.2. PBMC Preparation

Blood was drawn in random order from 4–6 participants a day between 10 AM and 4 PM by a certified phlebotomist using a 19-gauge butterfly needle. A total of 16 mL was drawn in two collection tubes (BD Vacutainer® CPT™ Mononuclear Cell Preparation Tube). The buffy coat containing the PBMCs was harvested according to the manufacturer's instructions, and the cell pellet was stored at −80 °C.

2.3. RNA Extraction, Concentration Measurement, and Integrity Check

RNA was extracted from the buffy coat employing the RNAzol B Kit (Ambion®). RNA concentration was estimated using a UV absorption ratio method [39]. Ratios above 1.7 were considered sufficiently pure for the sample to be used for microarray and qPCR analyses. RNA integrity was analyzed by automated electrophoresis on microfluidic labchips using the Experion™ System (Bio-Rad). RNA Quality Indicator (RQI) values considered acceptable were in the range $7 < RQI \leq 10$. Samples meeting the criterion for integrity were selected for array-based expression profiling.

2.4. Whole-Genome mRNA Expression Using Bead-Based Array

Total RNA samples from matched TM and control groups were shipped on dry ice to the Genomics Core at the University of Chicago, Chicago, IL, for genome-wide mRNA expression profiling using Illumina® Gene Expression BeadChip technology. A minimum amount of 50 ng of total RNA for each sample was labeled using the Illumina TotalPrep™ RNA Labeling Kit (Ambion). Labeled samples were incubated on Illumina HumanHT-12v4 Expression BeadChips containing probes for 47,231 features and imaged using the Illumina iScan system. Raw data from the iScan were converted using the GenomeStudio software package and Gene Expression Module (Illumina), resulting in identification of 16,247 genes and loci.

Microarray data were subjected to statistical analysis using R BioConductor (lumi and BeadArray) packages that include methods correcting for Type 1 and Type 2 errors [40]. Differential expression for each individual gene was considered acceptable if it met comparatively strict criteria, i.e., ratio of TM and control group gene-expression values (normalized by the quantile method) ≥ 2.0 and p-value for differential expression ≤ 0.05. A heat map with hierarchical clustering was created from data on the differentially expressed genes using the average linkage method and the Pearson distance metric to show how data aggregated. This analysis was performed in R version 2.11.1 with the gplots package using hclust and heapmap.2 functions [41]. Networks with molecular paths plausibly affected by practice of the TM program were identified using Ingenuity® Pathway Analysis (IPA®) software [42].

To assign functional annotations for differentially expressed genes, gene ontological enrichment analysis was performed through the DAVID database, a free online web-based tool. Differentially expressed genes submitted to DAVID were sorted into lists of ranked genes under enriched gene ontological process terms. The p-values displayed are a DAVID adjustment of the Fisher exact test p-value from testing for a significantly higher number of genes in the submitted list belonging to the group of genes, compared with all genes in the human genome [43].

A similar approach was used in the disease association analysis, in this case using Genomatix. Genomatix is data-mining software for extracting and analyzing gene relationships from literature databases such as NCBI PubMed and annotation data such as Gene Ontology. The software calculates overrepresentation of specific biological terms within the input and ranks genes related to specific diseases in the output. The program calculates p-values in a similar manner to that described for the DAVID online tool.

2.5. qPCR Analysis

Target genes chosen for validation of the microarray results included genes representing the main findings of the microarray component, including key relationships to health and aging. The primers were designed using Primer BLAST and were purchased from IDT® Technologies (http://www.idtdna.com/site, accessed 5 January 2014). The target genes, the reference gene, and their primer sequences are shown in Table S1: Primer Sequences for qPCR Reactions.

First, for each participant, complementary DNA (cDNA) was constructed from the extracted RNA employing the iScript™ cDNA Synthesis Kit (Bio-Rad). Each cDNA reaction mixture of 20 μL contained 1 μg of the RNA template and 10 μL of master mix (containing 1.0 μL iScript reverse transcriptase solution, 4.0 μL of 5× iScript mix, and 5 μL nuclease-free water). The PCR reaction was run in the GeneAmp® PCR 9700 systen (Applied Biosystems) in the following steps: 5 min at 25 °C; 30 min at 42 °C; 3.5 min at 85 °C, and hold at 4 °C.

Second, the qPCR experiment was conducted using the SsoFast™ EvaGreen® Supermix (Bio-Rad). Each reaction contained 5 μL 1× SsoFast EvaGreen supermix, a final concentration of 320 nM each of forward primer and reverse primer, 5 ng cDNA template, and 2.9 μL nuclease-free water in a 10-μL final volume. Finally, samples were assayed in quadruplicate in a 320-well reaction plate using a C1000 thermal cycler (Bio-Rad) combined with a CFX 384 Real-Time System (Bio-Rad) in the following cycling steps: 1. Enzyme activation: 95 °C, 30 s, 1 cycle; 2. Denaturation: 95 °C, 3 s, 40 cycles; 3. Annealing/Extension: 58 °C, 5 s, 40 cycles; 4. Melt curve: 65–95 °C (in 0.5 °C increments, 5 s/step), 1 cycle.

The relative expression level of each gene ("fold difference") was calculated using the $(2.0^{(\Delta\Delta Ct)})$ method [44]. Statistical analysis was performed using ANOVA in SPSS. An alpha level of $p \leq 0.05$ was adopted for statistical significance.

3. Results

3.1. Differential Expression, Heat Map, and Clustering Analysis from the Microarray Study

Gene expression profiles for the 200 genes and loci that met the cut-off criteria are shown in Figure 1. The majority of these (136) were downregulated in the TM group. Numerical gene expression data, including expression ratios and *p*-values for all 200 genes and loci, are available in Table S2: Differentially Expressed Genes and Loci. The hierarchical clustering analysis based on Pearson correlation distances showed distinct expression patterns for each group. One gene, *SLC6A4*, coding for the serotonin reuptake transporter, whose *p*-value exceeded the chosen ≤ 0.05 cut-off by a small margin (actual $p = 0.057$), was included because of its known importance in stress-related mechanisms and health. The expression ratios of all genes and loci met the criterion of ≥ 2.0.

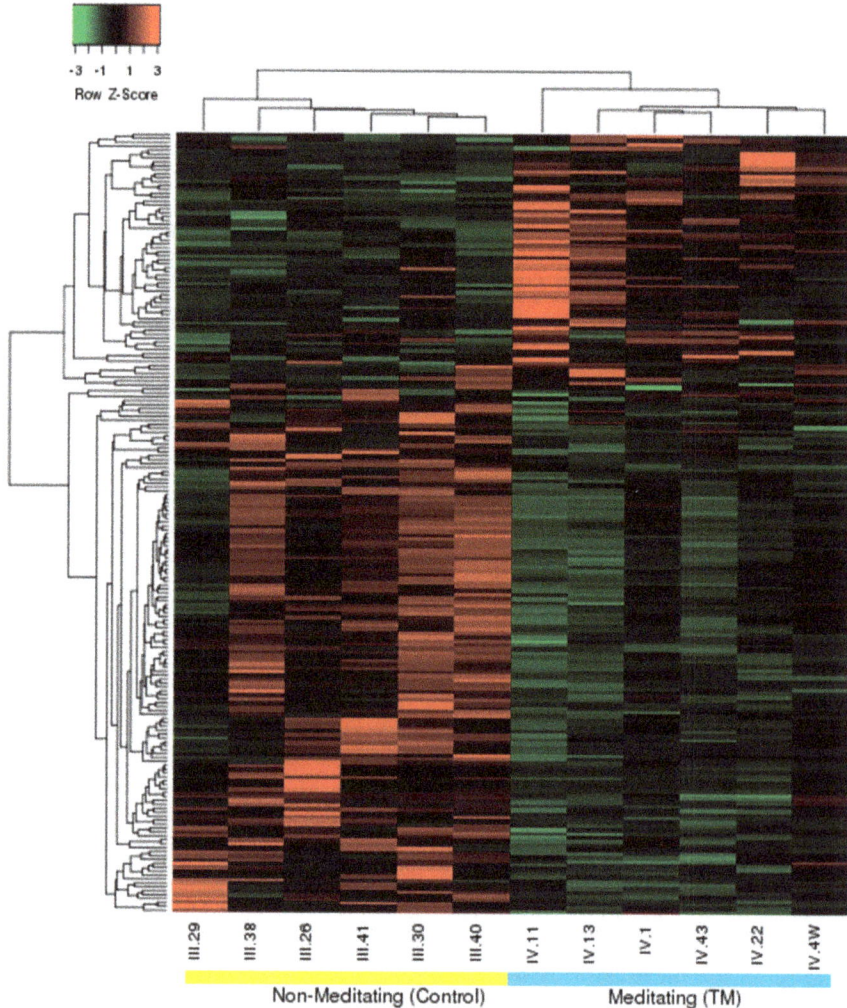

Figure 1. Heat map and hierarchical clustering of differentially expressed genes. The figure shows the relative expression of genes across participants, with hierarchical clustering of genes (rows) and participants (columns). Each colored bar indicates the degree to which the Z-score-normalized expression for that gene is either greater than (red) or less than (green) the median value for the gene.

3.2. qPCR Validation of Microarray Data

Verification and validation of the microarray data were conducted on 15 key genes selected from the 200. Verification of microarray data on these selected genes compared microarray output to results obtained with qPCR (Table 3). Preliminary validation (Table 4) involved larger groups that were less well-matched demographically (see Table 2) than those in the microarray comparison (see Table 1).

Table 3. Comparison of Microarray Output with qPCR Output in the Small Groups.

	Microarray Output (N = 12)		qPCR Output (N = 10 *)	
		Genes Downregulated in the TM Group Relative to the Control Group		
Gene	p-Value	Expression Ratio **	p-Value	"Fold Difference" ***
AHSP	0.002	5.45	<0.001	14.58
ALOX12	0.006	2.45	0.071	2.76
CD22	0.037	2.48	0.248	2.01
ITGB3	0.013	2.11	0.015	3.15
ITGB5	0.006	2.00	0.019	2.47
LMNA	0.004	2.16	0.063	2.35
MYL9	0.017	2.88	0.161	2.01
SOCS3	0.030	2.33	0.003	6.50
TAL1	0.002	2.36	0.073	2.19
		Genes Upregulated in the TM Group Relative to the Control Group		
CDKN1C	0.017	2.79	0.003	2.28
CXCL10	0.014	2.89	0.084	2.33
HES4	0.047	2.00	0.748	1.12
IGFBP7	0.026	2.08	0.449	1.43
IL1B	0.012	3.54	0.126	1.77
TLR4	0.002	2.23	0.741	1.11

* TM participant 4 W lacked sufficient RNA for qPCR, so a demographically matched control (40) was dropped from the qPCR analysis, leaving $N = 10$. ** ratio of normalized mean expression values, reciprocal in the case of downregulation in TM. *** "Fold Difference" = $2^{(\Delta\Delta Ct)}$; Ct = threshold cycle.

Table 4. qPCR Determination of Relative Gene Expression (Ct) and "Fold Difference" * in Larger Groups.

		Genes Downregulated in the TM Group Relative to the Control Group						
Gene	Group	Mean Ct	Std. Dev.	N	df	F	p-Value	"Fold Difference" *
AHSP	Control	32.5668	2.1561	22	1	12.674	0.001	3.86
	TM	34.5163	1.4674	23				
ALOX12	Control	30.6055	0.7140	22	1	3.194	0.081	1.44
	TM	31.1267	1.1756	23				
CD22	Control	30.7102	0.8499	22	1	1.482	0.230	1.29
	TM	31.0753	1.1344	23				
ITGB3	Control	26.4452	0.7939	22	1	4.031	0.051	1.52
	TM	27.0511	1.1830	23				
ITGB5	Control	30.9789	0.6233	22	1	5.938	0.019	1.41
	TM	31.4723	0.7281	23				
LMNA	Control	29.8050	0.7014	22	1	3.546	0.066	1.37
	TM	30.2638	0.9137	23				
MYL9	Control	27.1693	0.6926	22	1	1.792	0.188	1.31
	TM	27.5611	1.1940	23				
SOCS3	Control	31.4033	0.9121	22	1	10.626	0.002	2.17
	TM	32.5206	1.3372	23				
TAL1	Control	30.7461	0.6561	22	1	3.441	0.070	1.35
	TM	31.1823	0.8969	23				

Table 4. Cont.

Gene	Group	Mean Ct	Std. Dev.	N	df	F	p-Value	"Fold Difference" *
		Genes Upregulated in the TM Group Relative to the Control Group						
CDKN1C	Control	30.2448	0.7156	22	1	2.085	0.156	1.24
	TM	29.9343	0.7260	23				
CXCL10	Control	32.7365	0.9466	22	1	12.950	0.001	2.03
	TM	31.7125	0.9613	23				
HES4	Control	34.1132	0.6820	22	1	1.044	0.313	1.16
	TM	34.3267	0.7179	23				
IGFBP7	Control	29.8499	0.8188	22	1	1.805	0.186	1.27
	TM	29.5057	0.8956	23				
IL1B	Control	31.4125	1.0132	22	1	1.655	0.205	1.28
	TM	31.0576	0.8328	23				
TLR4	Control	29.0808	0.7732	22	1	0.782	0.381	1.15
	TM	28.8832	0.7260	23				

* "Fold Difference" = $2^{(\Delta\Delta Ct)}$; Ct = threshold cycle.

3.3. Top Networks

Principal networks that reflect possible causal and functional significance were found by applying IPA to the 200 genes. The network with the highest p-score, along with its top functions and diseases, is shown in Figure 2. The network with the second highest p-score is shown in Figure 3 (Additional networks with lower p-scores are shown in Figures S1–S3: Networks 3–5). Each network includes molecules central to the network (core molecules) and other molecules that affect or are affected by the core molecules. Network 1 (Figure 2), with a p-score of 37 (i.e., $p = 1 \times 10^{-37}$), is strongly related to stress, inflammation, and the defense response. The largest number of connections are to the NF-κB complex and the interferon alpha complex.

Three differentially expressed genes in Network 1—*IL1B* and *TLR4* (upregulated in the TM group) and *SOCS3* (downregulated in the TM group)—are connected not only to the NF-κB complex but also to interferons alpha and gamma, immunoglobulin, and other core molecules. The major themes of this network are cell-to-cell signaling and interaction, hematologic system development and function, and inflammatory response. Key canonical pathways (CPs) are highlighted in the figure.

Core molecules of Network 2 (p-score 28; Figure 3) include the P38 mitogen-activated protein kinases (P38 MAPKs), which are responsive to many stressors and are involved in apoptosis, autophagy, and cell differentiation; AKT, also known as protein kinase B (PKB), important in signaling pathways regulating cell growth, proliferation, differentiation, and survival; IgG, a key protein activating the complement system for eliminating pathogens; and CAV1, a plasma membrane protein important in coupling integrins to the Ras-ERK pathway and promoting cell cycle progression. CAV1 also connects with a central class of histones (Histone H3) involved in the regulation of glucocorticoid signaling and other genes. The major themes of Network 2 are cellular morphology, cell-to-cell signaling and interaction, and hematopoiesis.

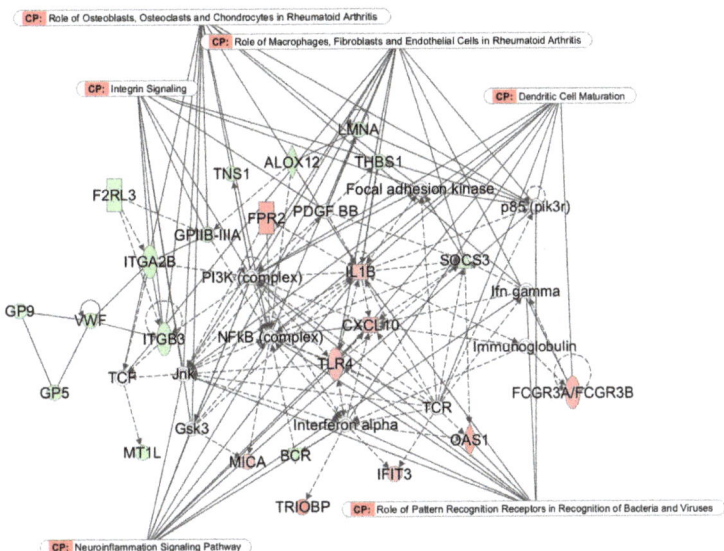

Figure 2. Network 1 (p-score 37): Cell-to-cell signaling and interaction, hematologic system development and function, and inflammatory response. Nodes without color denote non-significant genes, solid lines denote direct connections, and dotted lines denote indirect connections. Genes color-coded in red are upregulated and those in green are downregulated in the TM group. CP indicates canonical pathways.

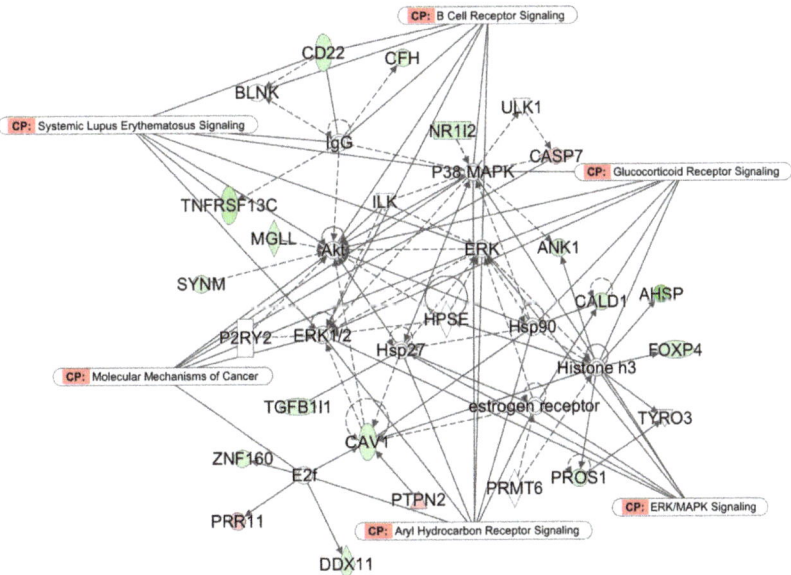

Figure 3. Network 2 (p-score 28): Cellular morphology, cell-to-cell signaling and interaction, and hematopoiesis. Nodes without color denote non-significant genes, solid lines denote direct connections, and dotted lines denote indirect connections. Genes color-coded in red are upregulated and those in green are downregulated in the TM group. CP indicates canonical pathways.

3.4. Gene Ontological Process Terms

Analysis of gene ontological process terms enriched in the 200 differentially expressed genes revealed 12 terms that were statistically significant and potentially meaningful in relation to known effects of the TM program (Table 5).

Table 5. Gene Ontological Process Terms.

Term	p-Value	Genes Downregulated in the TM Group
Blood Coagulation	8.40×10^{-8}	F2RL3, CAV1, ITGB3, MMRN1, GP9, VWF, GP5, GP6, THBS1, TREML1, PROS1, ALOX12, ITGA2B, HBD
Cell Activation	1.30×10^{-4}	F2RL3, CAV1, BCR, SNCA, TNFRSF13C, PAWR, ITGB3, GP9, VWF, GP5, GP6, THBS1, TREML1, WNT7A, ALOX12, ITGA2B
Response to Stress	1.70×10^{-4}	SLC8A3, F2RL3, CAV1, CDC14B, SNCA, SLC6A4, FSTL1, PAWR, ITGB3, MMRN1, TRIM10, GP9, GP5, ALAS2, GP6, DDX11, PLOD2, CFH, MGLL, THBS1, HBD, BCR, PTPRF, SOCS3, LMNA, HBA2, HBA1, PTPRN, VWF, SH2D3C, TGFB1I1, TREML1, PROS1, ITGA2B, ALOX12
Exocytosis	4.00×10^{-4}	VWF, ANK1, BCR, SNCA, SYTL4, ITGB3, THBS1, MMRN1, PROS1, ITGA2B
Cell Adhesion	8.70×10^{-4}	CAV1, PTPRF, CALD1, TNFRSF13C, ITGB5, ITGB3, PAWR, MMRN1, GP9, KIFC3, VWF, GP5, CD22, CNTNAP2, SGCE, TGFB1I1, LAMC1, THBS1, JAM3, ALOX12, ITGA2B
Hematopoiesis	1.30×10^{-3}	TAL1, ALAS2, AHSP, BCL11A, ZNF160
Term	p-Value	Genes Upregulated in the TM Group
Defense Response	2.40×10^{-4}	OAS1, CCL4L1, CXCL10, MICA, CASP5, FPR2, IFIT3, IL1B, LILRB2, METRNL, PTPN2, TLR4, VNN1
Response to External Stimuli	3.30×10^{-4}	CCL4L1, CXCL10, MICA, ATF3, BATF3, CASP5, FPR2, IFIT3, IL1B, LILRB2, METRNL, KCNJ2, PTPN2, TLR4
Inflammatory Response	9.30×10^{-4}	CCL4L1, CXCL10, FPR2, IL1B, METRNL, PTPN2, TLR4, VNN1
Immune System Processes	1.20×10^{-3}	OAS1, CCL4L1, CXCL10, FCGR3B, MICA, FPR2, IFIT3, IL1B, LILRB2, PTPN2, TLR4, VNN1
Homeostatic Processes	1.90×10^{-3}	CXCL10, CKB, FPR2, IL1B, METRNL, KCNJ2, PTPN2, SLC31A2, SLC4A8, TLR4, UTS2
Cell Chemotaxis	2.50×10^{-2}	GPR44, CCRL2, FPR2, CXCL10

3.5. Gene Classification Based on Associated Disease

Groupings of differentially expressed genes based on associated diseases are shown in Table 6. Sixty-two genes were related to hematologic diseases, 26 to coronary artery disease, 34 to diabetes complications, 49 to inflammation, and 64 to CVD. All these disease-related genes were downregulated in the TM group relative to the control group.

Table 6. Differentially Expressed Genes Classified According to Associated Diseases (All Downregulated in the TM Group Relative to Control Group).

Disease	p-Value	Genes
Hematologic Diseases	1.5×10^{-10}	TRIM10, VPREB3, CFH, MGP, F2RL3, AHSP, TAL1, ITGB3, HBD, GATM, HRASLS, TMCC2, OSBP2, TNFRSF13C, PTCRA, DMTN, GP9, TNS1, CAV1, JAM3, CMTM5, BCL11A, SOCS3, SNCA, HBA2, SH2D3C, PTPRN, NR1I2, TGFB1I1, HDC, HBM, DDX11, PAWR, ITGB5, LMNA, ITGA2B, CABP5, THBS1, FOXP4, HBA1, ANK1, GP5, MAP1A, SLC35D3, CALD1, CD22, SLC4A1, BCR, LAMC1, ALOX12, HOMER2, TREML1, ALAS2, CA1, ABCB4, XK, EBF1, PTPRF, MMRN1, PLOD2, VWF, GP6
Coronary Artery Disease	9.7×10^{-8}	CFH, MGP, F2RL3, ITGB3, MGLL, TNFRSF13C, CAV1, JAM3, SOCS3, PNOC, FSTL1, NDUFAF3, NR1I2, LMNA, ITGA2B, THBS1, HBA1, GP5, CALD1, PEAR1, EBF1, PTPRF, SLC6A4, VWF, GP6, FHL1
Diabetes Complications	2.2×10^{-7}	CFH, MGP, F2RL3, ITGB3, GATM, SGCE, DMTN, CAV1, SOCS3, PNOC, FSTL1, HBA2, NDUFAF3, PTPRN, TGFB1I1, HDC, CNTNAP2, LMNA, ITGA2B, THBS1, SELENBP1, HBA1, ANK1, GP5, CALD1, CD22, SLC4A1, LAMC1, ALOX12, CA1, PTPRF, SLC6A4, VWF, GP6
Inflammation	7.1×10^{-6}	CFH, MGP, CTDSPL, F2RL3, TAL1, ITGB3, MGLL, GATM, HRASLS, SLC8A3, TNFRSF13C, DMTN, WNT7A, GP9, CAV1, JAM3, SOCS3, SNCA, PNOC, FSTL1, HBA2, SH2D3C, PTPRN, NR1I2, HDC, PAWR, ITGB5, LMNA, ITGA2B, THBS1, SELENBP1, HBA1, ANK1, GP5, MAP1A, CALD1, CD22, SLC4A1, BCR, ALOX12, TREML1, ALAS2, CA1, ABCB4, EBF1, PTPRF, SLC6A4, MMRN1, VWF
Cardiovascular Disease	4.4×10^{-4}	VPREB3, CFH, MGP, CTDSPL, F2RL3, AHSP, TAL1, ITGB3, HBD, MGLL, GATM, HRASLS, SGCE, SLC8A3, TNFRSF13C, DMTN, WNT7A, GP9, CAV1, JAM3, CMTM5, SOCS3, SNCA, PNOC, FSTL1, HBA2, NDUFAF3, PTPRN, NR1I2, TGFB1I1, HDC, DDX11, PAWR, CNTNAP2, ITGB5, LMNA, ITGA2B, THBS1, SELENBP1, FOXP4, HBA1, ANK1, GP5, MAP1A, CALD1, CD22, SLC4A1, BCR, LAMC1, ALOX12, PEAR1, ALAS2, CA1, ABCB4, XK, EBF1, PTPRF, SLC6A4, MMRN1, PLOD2, ZNF160, VWF, GP6, FHL1

3.6. Top Genes Upregulated in the Control Group, and Erythropoiesis-Related Genes

Table 7 shows the top six genes upregulated in the control group, along with four genes known to be related to erythropoiesis. As described in the Discussion, these top six genes are mainly involved in erythrocyte function.

Table 7. Top Six Upregulated Genes in the Control Group and Upregulation of Genes Controlling Erythropoiesis.

Gene	Control Mean	Control SD	TM Mean	TM SD	Expression Ratio	p-Value
HBM	93.53	57.09	9.53	15.76	9.8	0.004
SLC4A1	72.47	49.02	8.13	10.54	8.9	0.002
ALAS2	631.43	579.80	78.12	67.67	8.1	0.002
CA1	85.37	77.98	12.40	9.03	6.9	0.002
AHSP	203.13	186.36	37.27	20.60	5.5	0.002
HBD	586.23	457.93	139.48	59.29	4.2	0.002
GATA1	19.22	8.31	11.17	4.27	1.7	0.049
GATA2	33.72	6.23	21.82	9.74	1.6	0.030
TAL1	64.28	9.70	27.18	6.22	2.4	0.002
EPOR	83.67	11.01	70.27	14.03	1.2	0.108

4. Discussion

These results show first that the gene expression patterns obtained from the microarray analysis of small, demographically well-matched groups differ from each other in a manner consistent with expectations from prior research. Second, the qPCR results examining the relative expression of a sample of 15 key genes in these small groups as well as in larger, less well-matched groups appeared to uphold the trend of the microarray results. This was despite the poor demographic matching in the larger groups. Third, these expression differences appear to have functional confirmation from known stress effects on health and aging.

Several precautions concerning interpretation deserve mention. Because the group size for the validation step was relatively small, conclusions regarding possible TM effects cannot be generalized to larger populations without further confirming studies. A second precaution is that the control groups did not perform an activity that might qualify as a placebo for the twice-daily practice of TM programs for 38 years. Thirdly, it is possible that the two groups compared by microarray may have differed consistently in some unknown or poorly controlled variable.

The first important strength of the study is the finding of 200 genes in the discovery (microarray) component despite the use of comparatively strict inclusion criteria (expression ratio ≥ 2.0 and p-value ≤ 0.05). This ratio cut-off is quite high. Only 275 genes and loci (out of a total 16,247 in our study) reached the ratio criterion, while 2041 met the p-value criterion.

The second important strength is the existence of characteristic gene expression patterns for the two groups. The patterns are clear enough to be detected visually (Figure 1). More importantly, these patterns were derived objectively using hierarchical clustering analysis of the 200 genes, with data input consisting only of gene name, expression level, and participant signifier. The patterns derived are distinct and likely reflect functional differences rather than random differences in gene expression. These distinct patterns, combined with the random order of blood sampling and processing across both participants and days, argue against a transient stress or stimulus as the possible cause of between-group differences.

The third and greatest strength lies in the fulfillment of predictions based on prior investigations. Many transcriptomic effects of chronic or extreme stress are known [23–25,45], and prior evidence exists for at least partial reversal of some of these effects by mind–body interventions [36], including by other techniques of meditation [32,33]. Furthermore, independent evidence exists showing that the TM program can reverse long-lasting effects of stress such as symptoms of PTSD [11–13], risk factors for CVD [15–18], chronically high levels of stress-related hormones [17,46,47], and low efficiency of energy metabolism [48]. Taken together, these prior studies predict that transcriptomic patterns associated with stress, such as the CTRA and low energy efficiency (see Introduction), should be prevented or reversed after long-term practice of this program.

In the TM group, evidence of prevention or reversal of the CTRA can be seen first in the IPA network analysis of microarray data. Among the 14 genes in Network 1 (see Figure 2) that were downregulated in the TM group relative to the control group, 11 were associated with inflammation in the disease association analysis. On the other hand, among the 10 genes in Network 1 that were upregulated in the TM group, 7 were associated with the defense response in the analysis by gene ontological process term enrichment.

Further indications that the TM group expresses a low-inflammation trait comes from the individual genes. The pro-inflammatory genes in Network 1 were either direct (e.g., *SOCS3*) or indirect (e.g., *ITGB3*) target genes of NF-κB. Expression of suppressor of cytokine signaling 3 (*SOCS3*) is known to correlate directly with pro-inflammatory cytokine levels [49], as are expression levels of integrin genes (*ITGB3*, *ITGB5*, and *ITGA2B*) [50]. A relative downregulation of these and 45 other genes related to inflammatory disease was found in the TM group, consistent with prevention or reversal of the primary, pro-inflammatory component of the CTRA.

Based on the upregulation of genes related to disease resistance, e.g., those in the defense response and immune system processes categories from the analysis of gene ontological process term enrichment, seven of which also appear in Network 1, the TM group appeared to have enhanced antiviral, antibacterial, and anti-cancer activities, once again opposite to the CTRA pattern. The roles of specific differentially expressed genes further support this conclusion. Examples include five genes that are associated primarily with anti-cancer activity (*CXCL10*, *MICA*, *FPR2*, *CASP5*, and *CASP7*), three genes that are associated with both anti-cancer and anti-microbial activity (*OAS1*, *ATF3*, and *IFIT3*), and four genes that are associated primarily with the defense response to viruses and bacteria (*CCL4L1*, *IL1B*, *ANKRD22*, and *TLR4*). This finding for genes upregulated in the TM group appears to confirm prevention or reversal of the second component of the CTRA.

This evidence for prevention or reversal of both components of the CTRA expression pattern raises another key point. Although initial evidence for the CTRA came from studies with severely stressed individuals [24,25], the results of the current study indicate a reduction in the CTRA in the TM group compared to healthy controls. This suggests that nominally healthy 65-year-olds carry a substantial load of stress effects, i.e., an allostatic overload [2,51], possibly due to accumulated effects of mild stressors. This is consistent with previous results from studies of short-term and long-term meditation practice indicating that the TM program reduces stress effects well below the level found in the general population [18,46,47].

Other evidence connecting stress effects with inflammation and disease is found in the relationship between genes grouped through ontological process term enrichment and genes grouped through disease association analysis. Using gene ontological term enrichment, 35 differentially expressed genes were classified as related to "response to stress." Of these 35 genes, 27 also were found among the 49 genes classified under inflammation by disease association analysis, and 30 were found among the 64 genes classified under CVD, consistent with known associations between stress response, inflammation, and CVD. Furthermore, consistent with a close association between inflammation and CVD, 47 of the 49 inflammation genes also were found among the CVD-associated genes. Stress response genes were highly represented in the other disease categories as well. All these stress response genes, as well as all the disease-associated genes, were downregulated in the TM group relative to the control group, a direction more likely to be associated with benefits to health.

Another important prediction from prior research concerns evidence for a stress-induced reduction in energy efficiency. Recent articles by Picard, McEwen et al. summarize the critical roles that mitochondrial energy production and other mitochondrial functions play in stress and adaptation [27,31]. As reviewed by Jevning et al. [48], evidence that practice of TM programs increases energy efficiency includes decreased oxygen consumption, decreased respiratory rate, and decreased blood lactate levels. Lactate, a product of glycolysis that is produced in the blood mainly by erythrocytes, is increased during anaerobic metabolism and decreases acutely in erythrocytes during practice of TM [52]. Two observations in the present study provide evidence for higher energy efficiency in these long-term practitioners. Both may center on the role of SOCS3 in mitochondrial energy metabolism.

SOCS3, downregulated in the TM group and prominent in Network 1, codes for a chemokine that is important in regulating energy metabolism through inhibitory effects on AMP-dependent protein kinase (AMPK) and leptin [53]. AMPK is central to energy metabolism in mitochondria, thus affecting cellular and whole-body energy levels [54,55]. Increased SOCS3 due to stress and increased inflammatory cytokines is documented to inhibit AMPK, causing insulin resistance in several tissues [56,57]. SOCS3 also can inhibit STAT3 activation [58], providing another possible route for decreased energy efficiency in mitochondria. Mitochondrial STAT3 plays a direct role in maintaining optimal function of the electron transport chain [59]. It is likely that removing inhibitory effects on AMPK by lowering SOCS3 contributes to the improved energy efficiency observed in practitioners of TM programs.

The second observation is related to this and provides confirmatory evidence for more efficient energy production in the TM group. It involves hematologic system development and function, a major theme in the pathway analyses. The top six genes upregulated in the control group are mainly found in erythrocytes and are critical to erythrocyte function. Such large differences in expression of these genes likely reflect the presence of a greater number of reticulocytes (immature erythrocytes) in the control group blood samples. When erythrocyte production is high, reticulocytes, some of which may be large, even nucleated, can enter the bloodstream and contaminate PBMC samples. If mitochondrial oxidative phosphorylation is inefficient, more oxygen is required for a given level of energy production. Even moderate exercise, the level claimed by all study participants, is likely to produce chronic intermittent hypoxia in those with the lowest energy efficiency, and chronic intermittent hypoxia is known to increase erythropoiesis [60].

Supporting the hypothesis that inefficient mitochondrial energy production causes increased erythrocyte production in the control group, both *GATA1* and *GATA2*, master regulators of erythropoiesis [61], were significantly upregulated in this group. The increased expression of *GATA* normally causes an increase in erythropoietin, the direct stimulant of erythropoiesis [61]. Furthermore, *TAL1*, a regulator of erythropoietin receptor sensitivity [62], was significantly increased in the control group, and expression of *EPOR*, coding for the erythropoietin receptor, was increased as well, though not significantly. All these data are consistent with a substantially lower energy efficiency in the control group compared with the TM group.

Another of the many potentially important observations in this study may deserve mention here. Based on the evidence that chronic stress can cause a decrease in telomere length (for review, see [63]), the increased *TAL1* expression found here in the control group is potentially a mediator of reduced telomerase activity. TAL1 inhibits the promotor of hTERT, the catalytic subunit of telomerase [64]. Elevated TAL1, therefore, could cause a reduction in telomerase activity and telomere length.

Predictably, the larger, less well-matched groups of TM and control participants in which 15 key genes were studied by qPCR showed fewer statistically significant expression differences than were found in the microarray comparison of the well-matched groups. Nevertheless, for each of the main areas discussed, differential expression of one or more key genes reached significance. Thus, results for *SOCS3* and *ITGB5* verified an anti-inflammatory state; results for *SOCS3* and *AHSP* verified a state of enhanced energy efficiency, and the result for *CXCL10* (tumor suppressor) verified a higher defense response in the meditation group. It is expected that qPCR data on a larger sample of the 200 genes from the discovery step would give greater confirmation of these outcomes.

In an associated study in preparation [65], the transcriptomic data reported here were compared with cortisol and electroencephalographic (EEG) data from these larger groups, along with similar data from younger groups Results of that study tend to confirm the significance of the present findings in relation to proposed anti-stress and anti-aging effects of this meditation program.

5. Conclusions

The results of this study are intriguing and appear to provide strong directions for future studies. Finding 200 genes that met the dual cut-off criteria, and distinctive patterns of expression that appear to align with predictions from past research, provides a plausible framework. Many of the differentially expressed genes have previously demonstrated connections to stress effects, including to specific diseases related to stress. Although the possibility exists that the group differences are due to variables other than meditation practice, none of the data collected appear to shed light on this question. In addition to a future replication using RNA-seq, a larger N, and a larger sample of genes for validation, studies will be pursued on genes such as *SOCS3*, *AHSP*, and *CXCL10* that showed robust differences and have important functional implications.

Supplementary Materials: The following are available online at https://www.mdpi.com/1010-660 X/57/3/218/s1, Table S1: Primary Sequences for qPCR Reactions, Table S2: Differentially Expressed Genes and Loci, Figure S1: Network 3 (p-score 18): Cellular movement, immune cell trafficking, hematologic system development and function, Figure S2: Network 4 (p-score 17): Cellular function and maintenance, hematologic system development and function, and infectious disease, Figure S3: Network 5 (p-score 15): Cell cycle, cancer, organ morphology.

Author Contributions: Conceptualization, S.W., K.G.W. and F.T.T.; methodology, S.W., M.S., J.F. and K.G.W.; validation, J.F., K.G.W., and M.S.; formal analysis, S.K., C.L.D., S.W., K.G.W. and J.F.; investigation, S.W., S.K., K.G.W. and J.F.; resources, F.T.T. and M.S.; data curation, C.L.D., S.W. and J.F.; writing—original draft preparation, S.W., K.G.W. and J.F.; writing—review and editing, K.G.W., S.W., J.F. and F.T.T.; visualization, K.G.W. and S.W.; supervision, J.F., K.G.W., M.S., F.T.T., R.K.W., P.M., N.K.L., G.S. and J.S.; project administration, S.W., F.T.T. and K.G.W. All authors have read and agreed to the published version of the manuscript.

Funding: This research received no external funding.

Institutional Review Board Statement: The study was conducted in accordance with the Declaration of Helsinki, and the protocol was approved by the Ethics Committee of Maharishi International University (Project Identification Code: 06012010W) completed on 1 June 2010.

Informed Consent Statement: All participants gave written informed consent for inclusion before they participated in the study.

Data Availability Statement: Processed raw data from the microarray experiment have been deposited in the ArrayExpress database at EMBL-EBI and can be accessed at the following link: https://www.ebi.ac.uk/arrayexpress/experiments/E-MTAB-10252, accessed on 23 March 2021.

Acknowledgments: This study represents partial fulfillment of doctoral degree requirements in physiology and health at Maharishi International University (S.W.). We thank the staff of the Center for Prostate Disease Research, Rockville, Maryland, and Shiv Srivastava, Scientific Director, for use of their facilities and for assistance in RNA extraction.

Conflicts of Interest: The authors declare no conflict of interest. Neither Maharishi International University nor its faculty has financial ties to Maharishi Foundation, the non-profit educational body overseeing instruction in the Transcendental Meditation technique and its related programs.

References

1. McEwen, B.S.; Akil, H. Revisiting the Stress Concept: Implications for Affective Disorders. *J. Neurosci.* **2020**, *40*, 12–21. [CrossRef] [PubMed]
2. Juster, R.P.; McEwen, B.S.; Lupien, S.J. Allostatic load biomarkers of chronic stress and impact on health and cognition. *Neurosci. Biobehav. Rev.* **2010**, *35*, 2–16. [CrossRef]
3. Bairey Merz, C.N.; Dwyer, J.; Nordstrom, C.K.; Walton, K.G.; Salerno, J.W.; Schneider, R.H. Psychosocial stress and cardiovascular disease: Pathophysiological links. *Behav. Med.* **2002**, *27*, 141–147. [CrossRef] [PubMed]
4. Karlamangla, A.S.; Singer, B.H.; Seeman, T.E. Reduction in allostatic load in older adults is associated with lower all-cause mortality risk: MacArthur studies of successful aging. *Psychosom. Med.* **2006**, *68*, 500–507. [CrossRef] [PubMed]
5. Wiley, J.F.; Gruenewald, T.L.; Karlamangla, A.S.; Seeman, T.E. Modeling multisystem physiological dysregulation. *Psychosom. Med.* **2016**, *78*, 290–301. [CrossRef]
6. Hovatta, I.; Juhila, J.; Donner, J. Oxidative stress in anxiety and comorbid disorders. *Neurosci. Res.* **2010**, *68*, 261–275. [CrossRef]
7. Palta, P.; Samuel, L.J.; Miller, E.R., 3rd; Szanton, S.L. Depression and oxidative stress: Results from a meta-analysis of observational studies. *Psychosom. Med.* **2014**, *76*, 12–19. [CrossRef]
8. Shear, J. Transcendental Meditation. In *The Experience of Meditation: Experts Introduce the Major Traditions*, 1st ed.; Shear, J., Ed.; Paragon House: St. Paul, MN, USA, 2006; pp. 23–48.
9. Forem, J. *Transcendental Meditation: The Essential Teachings of Maharishi Mahesh Yogi*; Hay House, Inc.: New York, NY, USA, 2012; p. 361.
10. Wallace, R.K. Physiological effects of transcendental meditation. *Science* **1970**, *167*, 1751–1754. [CrossRef] [PubMed]
11. Rees, B.; Travis, F.; Shapiro, D.; Chant, R. Reduction in posttraumatic stress symptoms in Congolese refugees practicing transcendental meditation. *J. Trauma. Stress* **2013**, *26*, 295–298. [CrossRef] [PubMed]

12. Nidich, S.; Mills, P.J.; Rainforth, M.; Heppner, P.; Schneider, R.H.; Rosenthal, N.E.; Salerno, J.; Gaylord-King, C.; Rutledge, T. Non-trauma-focused meditation versus exposure therapy in veterans with post-traumatic stress disorder: A randomised controlled trial. *Lancet Psychiatry* **2018**, *5*, 975–986. [CrossRef]
13. Bandy, C.L.; Dillbeck, M.C.; Sezibera, V.; Taljaard, L.; Wilks, M.; Shapiro, D.; de Reuck, J.; Peycke, R. Reduction of PTSD in South African university students using Transcendental Meditation practice. *Psychol. Rep.* **2019**. [CrossRef]
14. Orme-Johnson, D.W.; Barnes, V.A. Effects of the transcendental meditation technique on trait anxiety: A meta-analysis of randomized controlled trials. *J. Altern. Complement. Med.* **2013**, *20*, 330–341. [CrossRef]
15. Barnes, V.A.; Orme-Johnson, D.W. Prevention and treatment of cardiovascular disease in adolescents and adults through the Transcendental Meditation((R)) Program: A research review update. *Curr. Hypertens. Rev.* **2012**, *8*, 227–242. [CrossRef]
16. Schneider, R.H.; Grim, C.E.; Rainforth, M.V.; Kotchen, T.; Nidich, S.I.; Gaylord-King, C.; Salerno, J.W.; Kotchen, J.M.; Alexander, C.N. Stress reduction in the secondary prevention of cardiovascular disease: Randomized, controlled trial of transcendental meditation and health education in Blacks. *Circ. Cardiovasc. Qual. Outcomes* **2012**, *5*, 750–758. [CrossRef] [PubMed]
17. Walton, K.G.; Schneider, R.H.; Nidich, S.I.; Salerno, J.W.; Nordstrom, C.K.; Bairey Merz, C.N. Psychosocial stress and cardiovascular disease Part 2: Effectiveness of the Transcendental Meditation program in treatment and prevention. *Behav. Med.* **2002**, *28*, 106–123. [CrossRef] [PubMed]
18. Nidich, S.I.; Rainforth, M.V.; Haaga, D.A.; Hagelin, J.; Salerno, J.W.; Travis, F.; Tanner, M.; Gaylord-King, C.; Grosswald, S.; Schneider, R.H. A randomized controlled trial on effects of the Transcendental Meditation program on blood pressure, psychological distress, and coping in young adults. *Am. J. Hypertens.* **2009**, *22*, 1326–1331. [CrossRef]
19. Orme-Johnson, D. Medical care utilization and the transcendental meditation program. *Psychosom. Med.* **1987**, *49*, 493–507. [CrossRef]
20. Herron, R.E. Changes in physician costs among high-cost transcendental meditation practitioners compared with high-cost nonpractitioners over 5 years. *Am. J. Health Promot.* **2011**, *26*, 56–60. [CrossRef] [PubMed]
21. Travis, F.; Shear, J. Focused attention, open monitoring and automatic self-transcending: Categories to organize meditations from Vedic, Buddhist and Chinese traditions. *Conscious. Cogn.* **2010**, *19*, 1110–1118. [CrossRef]
22. Mahone, M.C.; Travis, F.; Gevirtz, R.; Hubbard, D. fMRI during Transcendental Meditation practice. *Brain Cogn.* **2018**, *123*, 30–33. [CrossRef]
23. Miller, G.E.; Murphy, M.L.; Cashman, R.; Ma, R.; Ma, J.; Arevalo, J.M.; Kobor, M.S.; Cole, S.W. Greater inflammatory activity and blunted glucocorticoid signaling in monocytes of chronically stressed caregivers. *Brain Behav. Immun.* **2014**, *41*, 191–199. [CrossRef]
24. Cole, S.W. Elevating the perspective on human stress genomics. *Psychoneuroendocrinology* **2010**, *35*, 955–962. [CrossRef]
25. Powell, N.D.; Sloan, E.K.; Bailey, M.T.; Arevalo, J.M.; Miller, G.E.; Chen, E.; Kobor, M.S.; Reader, B.F.; Sheridan, J.F.; Cole, S.W. Social stress up-regulates inflammatory gene expression in the leukocyte transcriptome via beta-adrenergic induction of myelopoiesis. *Proc. Natl. Acad. Sci. USA* **2013**, *110*, 16574–16579. [CrossRef]
26. Cole, S.W. Human social genomics. *PLoS Genet.* **2014**, *10*, e1004601. [CrossRef] [PubMed]
27. Picard, M.; McEwen, B.S.; Epel, E.S.; Sandi, C. An energetic view of stress: Focus on mitochondria. *Front. Neuroendocrinol.* **2018**. [CrossRef] [PubMed]
28. Picard, M.; McManus, M.J.; Gray, J.D.; Nasca, C.; Moffat, C.; Kopinski, P.K.; Seifert, E.L.; McEwen, B.S.; Wallace, D.C. Mitochondrial functions modulate neuroendocrine, metabolic, inflammatory, and transcriptional responses to acute psychological stress. *Proc. Natl. Acad. Sci. USA* **2015**, *112*, E6614–E6623. [CrossRef]
29. Picard, M.; Prather, A.A.; Puterman, E.; Cuillerier, A.; Coccia, M.; Aschbacher, K.; Burelle, Y.; Epel, E.S. A Mitochondrial Health Index Sensitive to Mood and Caregiving Stress. *Biol. Psychiatry* **2018**. [CrossRef] [PubMed]
30. Kauppila, T.E.S.; Kauppila, J.H.K.; Larsson, N.G. Mammalian Mitochondria and Aging: An Update. *Cell Metab.* **2017**, *25*, 57–71. [CrossRef] [PubMed]
31. Picard, M.; McEwen, B.S. Psychological Stress and Mitochondria: A Systematic Review. *Psychosom. Med.* **2018**, *80*, 141–153. [CrossRef]
32. Black, D.S.; Cole, S.W.; Irwin, M.R.; Breen, E.; St Cyr, N.M.; Nazarian, N.; Khalsa, D.S.; Lavretsky, H. Yogic meditation reverses NF-kappaB and IRF-related transcriptome dynamics in leukocytes of family dementia caregivers in a randomized controlled trial. *Psychoneuroendocrinology* **2013**, *38*, 348–355. [CrossRef]
33. Epel, E.S.; Puterman, E.; Lin, J.; Blackburn, E.H.; Lum, P.Y.; Beckmann, N.D.; Zhu, J.; Lee, E.; Gilbert, A.; Rissman, R.A.; et al. Meditation and vacation effects have an impact on disease-associated molecular phenotypes. *Transl. Psychiatry* **2016**, *6*, e880. [CrossRef] [PubMed]
34. Bhasin, M.K.; Denninger, J.W.; Huffman, J.C.; Joseph, M.G.; Niles, H.; Chad-Friedman, E.; Goldman, R.; Buczynski-Kelley, B.; Mahoney, B.A.; Fricchione, G.L.; et al. Specific Transcriptome Changes Associated with Blood Pressure Reduction in Hypertensive Patients After Relaxation Response Training. *J. Altern. Complement. Med.* **2018**, *24*, 486–504. [CrossRef]
35. Chaix, R.; Alvarez-Lopez, M.J.; Fagny, M.; Lemee, L.; Regnault, B.; Davidson, R.J.; Lutz, A.; Kaliman, P. Epigenetic clock analysis in long-term meditators. *Psychoneuroendocrinology* **2017**, *85*, 210–214. [CrossRef] [PubMed]
36. Buric, I.; Farian, M.; Jong, J.; Mee, C.; Brazil, I.A. What is the molecular signature of mind-body interventions? A systematic review of gene expression changes induced by meditation and related practices. *Front. Immunol.* **2017**, *8*, 1–17. [CrossRef]
37. Kaliman, P. Epigenetics and meditation. *Curr. Opin. Psychol.* **2019**, *28*, 76–80. [CrossRef]

38. Jaksik, R.; Iwanaszko, M.; Rzeszowska-Wolny, J.; Kimmel, M. Microarray experiments and factors which affect their reliability. *Biol. Direct.* **2015**, *10*, 46. [CrossRef]
39. Okamoto, T.; Okabe, S. Ultraviolet absorbance at 260 and 280 nm in RNA measurement is dependent on measurement solution. *Int. J. Mol. Med.* **2000**, *5*, 657–659. [CrossRef]
40. Du, P.; Kibbe, W.A.; Lin, S.M. lumi: A pipeline for processing Illumina microarray. *Bioinformatics* **2008**, *24*, 1547–1548. [CrossRef] [PubMed]
41. Galili, T. dendextend: An R package for visualizing, adjusting and comparing trees of hierarchical clustering. *Bioinformatics* **2015**, *31*, 3718–3720. [CrossRef] [PubMed]
42. Kramer, A.; Green, J.; Pollard, J., Jr.; Tugendreich, S. Causal analysis approaches in Ingenuity Pathway Analysis. *Bioinformatics* **2014**, *30*, 523–530. [CrossRef]
43. Da Huang, W.; Sherman, B.T.; Lempicki, R.A. Systematic and integrative analysis of large gene lists using DAVID bioinformatics resources. *Nat. Protoc.* **2009**, *4*, 44–57. [CrossRef]
44. Schmittgen, T.D.; Livak, K.J. Analyzing real-time PCR data by the comparative C(T) method. *Nat. Protoc.* **2008**, *3*, 1101–1108. [CrossRef] [PubMed]
45. Miller, G.E.; Chen, E.; Sze, J.; Marin, T.; Arevalo, J.M.; Doll, R.; Ma, R.; Cole, S.W. A functional genomic fingerprint of chronic stress in humans: Blunted glucocorticoid and increased NF-kappaB signaling. *Biol. Psychiatry* **2008**, *64*, 266–272. [CrossRef]
46. MacLean, C.R.; Walton, K.G.; Wenneberg, S.R.; Levitsky, D.K.; Mandarino, J.P.; Waziri, R.; Hillis, S.L.; Schneider, R.H. Effects of the Transcendental Meditation program on adaptive mechanisms: Changes in hormone levels and responses to stress after 4 months of practice. *Psychoneuroendocrinology* **1997**, *22*, 277–295. [CrossRef]
47. Walton, K.G.; Pugh, N.D.; Gelderloos, P.; Macrae, P. Stress reduction and preventing hypertension: Preliminary support for a psychoneuroendocrine mechanism. *J. Altern. Complement. Med.* **1995**, *1*, 263–283. [CrossRef] [PubMed]
48. Jevning, R.; Wallace, R.K.; Beidebach, M. The physiology of meditation: A review. A wakeful hypometabolic integrated response. *Neurosci. Biobehav. Rev.* **1992**, *16*, 415–424. [CrossRef]
49. Chaves de Souza, J.A.; Nogueira, A.V.; Chaves de Souza, P.P.; Kim, Y.J.; Silva Lobo, C.; Pimentel Lopes de Oliveira, G.J.; Cirelli, J.A.; Garlet, G.P.; Rossa, C., Jr. SOCS3 expression correlates with severity of inflammation, expression of proinflammatory cytokines, and activation of STAT3 and p38 MAPK in LPS-induced inflammation in vivo. *Mediators Inflamm.* **2013**, *2013*, 650812. [CrossRef]
50. Kuparinen, T.; Marttila, S.; Jylhava, J.; Tserel, L.; Peterson, P.; Jylha, M.; Hervonen, A.; Hurme, M. Cytomegalovirus (CMV)-dependent and -independent changes in the aging of the human immune system: A transcriptomic analysis. *Exp. Gerontol.* **2013**, *48*, 305–312. [CrossRef]
51. McEwen, B.S.; Stellar, E. Stress and the individual. Mechanisms leading to disease. *Arch. Intern. Med.* **1993**, *153*, 2093–2101. [CrossRef]
52. Jevning, R.; Wilson, A.F.; Pirkle, H.; O'Halloran, J.P.; Walsh, R.N. Metabolic control in a state of decreased activation: Modulation of red cell metabolism. *Am. J. Physiol.* **1983**, *245*, C457–C461. [CrossRef]
53. Steinberg, G.R.; McAinch, A.J.; Chen, M.B.; O'Brien, P.E.; Dixon, J.B.; Cameron-Smith, D.; Kemp, B.E. The suppressor of cytokine signaling 3 inhibits leptin activation of AMP-kinase in cultured skeletal muscle of obese humans. *J. Clin. Endocrinol. Metab.* **2006**, *91*, 3592–3597. [CrossRef]
54. Dzamko, N.L.; Steinberg, G.R. AMPK-dependent hormonal regulation of whole-body energy metabolism. *Acta Physiol.* **2009**, *196*, 115–127. [CrossRef]
55. Herzig, S.; Shaw, R.J. AMPK: Guardian of metabolism and mitochondrial homeostasis. *Nat. Rev. Mol. Cell Biol.* **2018**, *19*, 121–135. [CrossRef]
56. Yang, Z.; Hulver, M.; McMillan, R.P.; Cai, L.; Kershaw, E.E.; Yu, L.; Xue, B.; Shi, H. Regulation of insulin and leptin signaling by muscle suppressor of cytokine signaling 3 (SOCS3). *PLoS ONE* **2012**, *7*, e47493. [CrossRef]
57. Cao, L.; Wang, Z.; Wan, W. Suppressor of Cytokine Signaling 3: Emerging role linking central insulin resistance and Alzheimer's disease. *Front. Neurosci.* **2018**, *12*, 417. [CrossRef]
58. Carow, B.; Rottenberg, M.E. SOCS3, a Major Regulator of Infection and Inflammation. *Front. Immunol.* **2014**, *5*, 58. [CrossRef]
59. Wegrzyn, J.; Potla, R.; Chwae, Y.J.; Sepuri, N.B.; Zhang, Q.; Koeck, T.; Derecka, M.; Szczepanek, K.; Szelag, M.; Gornicka, A.; et al. Function of mitochondrial Stat3 in cellular respiration. *Science* **2009**, *323*, 793–797. [CrossRef] [PubMed]
60. Park, H.Y.; Hwang, H.; Park, J.; Lee, S.; Lim, K. The effects of altitude/hypoxic training on oxygen delivery capacity of the blood and aerobic exercise capacity in elite athletes—A meta-analysis. *J. Exerc. Nutrition Biochem.* **2016**, *20*, 15–22. [CrossRef] [PubMed]
61. Nogueira-Pedro, A.; dos Santos, G.G.; Oliveira, D.C.; Hastreiter, A.A.; Fock, R.A. Erythropoiesis in vertebrates: From ontogeny to clinical relevance. *Front. Biosci.* **2016**, *8*, 100–112.
62. Rogers, H.; Wang, L.; Yu, X.; Alnaeeli, M.; Cui, K.; Zhao, K.; Bieker, J.J.; Prchal, J.; Huang, S.; Weksler, B.; et al. T-cell acute leukemia 1 (TAL1) regulation of erythropoietin receptor and association with excessive erythrocytosis. *J. Biol. Chem.* **2012**, *287*, 36720–36731. [CrossRef]

63. De Punder, K.; Heim, C.; Wadhwa, P.D.; Entringer, S. Stress and immunosenescence: The role of telomerase. *Psychoneuroendocrinology* **2019**, *101*, 87–100. [CrossRef] [PubMed]
64. Terme, J.M.; Mocquet, V.; Kuhlmann, A.S.; Zane, L.; Mortreux, F.; Wattel, E.; Duc Dodon, M.; Jalinot, P. Inhibition of the hTERT promoter by the proto-oncogenic protein TAL1. *Leukemia* **2009**, *23*, 2081–2089. [CrossRef] [PubMed]
65. Wenuganen, S.; Walton, K.G.; Travis, F.; Wallace, R.K.; Fagan, J. (Maharishi International University, Fairfield, IA, USA); Stalder, T.; Kirschbaum, C. (Technical University of Dresden, Dresden, Germany); Shrivastava, M. (Uniformed Services University of the Health Sciences, Bethesda, MD, USA). Personal communication, 2020.

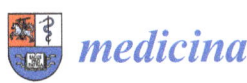

Review

On the Neurobiology of Meditation: Comparison of Three Organizing Strategies to Investigate Brain Patterns during Meditation Practice

Frederick Travis

Center for Brain, Consciousness and Cognition, Maharishi International University, Fairfield, IA 52557, USA; ftravis@miu.edu; Tel.: +1-641-472-1209

Received: 14 October 2020; Accepted: 16 December 2020; Published: 18 December 2020

Abstract: Three broad organizing strategies have been used to study meditation practices: (1) consider meditation practices as using similar processes and so combine neural images across a wide range of practices to identify the common underlying brain patterns of meditation practice, (2) consider meditation practices as unique and so investigate individual practices, or (3) consider meditation practices as fitting into larger categories and explore brain patterns within and between categories. The first organizing strategy combines meditation practices defined as deep concentration, attention to external and internal stimuli, and letting go of thoughts. Brain patterns of different procedures would all contribute to the final averages, which may not be representative of any practice. The second organizing strategy generates a multitude of brain patterns as each practice is studied individually. The rich detail of individual differences within each practice makes it difficult to identify reliable patterns between practices. The third organizing principle has been applied in three ways: (1) grouping meditations by their origin—Indian or Buddhist practices, (2) grouping meditations by the procedures of each practice, or (3) grouping meditations by brain wave frequencies reported during each practice. Grouping meditations by their origin mixes practices whose procedures include concentration, mindfulness, or effortless awareness, again resulting in a confounded pattern. Grouping meditations by their described procedures yields defining neural imaging patterns within each category, and clear differences between categories. Grouping meditations by the EEG frequencies associated with their procedures yields an objective system to group meditations and allows practices to "move" into different categories as subjects' meditation experiences change over time, which would be associated with different brain patterns. Exploring meditations within theoretically meaningful categories appears to yield the most reliable picture of meditation practices.

Keywords: meditation; focused attention; open monitoring; Transcendental Meditation

1. Introduction

Meditation practices have become part of the business, education and self-help cultures in the West [1]. A search on Pubmed with "meditation" as the key word yielded 7340 hits. To understand the nature of meditation practices, different strategies have been used to group individual studies into larger categories for analysis. This paper compares three strategies to organize meditation research. These three strategies are: (1) consider meditation as using similar cognitive process and so research the common underlying brain patterns of meditation, (2) consider each meditation practice as unique and so investigate individual practices and report patterns of each practice, or (3) consider that meditations fit into larger categories and compare brain patterns within and between categories.

This paper is not an exhaustive review of all papers on meditation practices. Rather, it compares the conclusions from these three strategies to group the data. It is written to alert researchers to the impact of different organizing strategies on their conclusions from meditation research.

2. First Strategy: Identify Underlying Brain Patterns of Meditation Practices

If a common brain pattern underlies most meditation practices, then combining many trials through principal components analysis or averaging should bring out the assumed underlying pattern. This strategy has been used in psychological and EEG (electroencephalography) research. In psychometric studies of intelligence, the first unrotated factor in a principal components analysis of intelligence tests is considered to indicate a broad mental capacity that influences performance across a range of reasoning and problem solving tests, called "g" or general intelligence [2,3]. In the EEG domain, EEG signals from successive stimulus presentations are time locked to the stimulus onset and then averaged. The averaging reduces the noise and brings out, through constructive interference, the brain components common in that task [4]. In each of these examples, a common, underlying pattern emerges from the analysis.

Table 1 lists a sampling of studies that used the "underlying-pattern" organizing principle. Notice the range of meditation practices included in each study and the lack of convergence of the results they report. The studies are listed chronologically.

Table 1. Sample of research combining neural images recorded in different meditation traditions in the final averages.

Reference	Design	Result
Luders [5]	22 meditation and 22 age-matched controls. Meditations included Zazen, Shamatha, Vipassana, and Others: 63% used deep concentration, 36% control of breath, 32% visualization, 32% attention to external and internal stimuli, 14% withdrawal of sensory perceptions and 18% letting go of thoughts.	Total grey matter volumes were similar in both groups (meditator and control). There were local differences. Meditators had thicker: • Right orbito-frontal cortex; • Right thalamus; • Left inferior temporal; • Right hippocampus.
Luders [6]	27 meditation and 27 age-matched controls. Average age: 52 years. 55% practiced: Shamatha, Vipassana, or Zazen.	Fractional anisotropy (FA) (integrity of white matter) was higher in meditators compared to controls within major projection pathways, commissural pathways, and association pathways.
Luders [7]	50 long-term meditators and 50 age-matched controls. Age range: 27–71 years. Meditations included Zazen, Shamatha, Vipassana.	Negative correlation of global and local gray matter with age for both meditators and controls. However, the group-by-age interaction was highly significant ($p = 0.003$) with lower grey matter by age for controls.
Fox [8]	Meta-analysis of 21 neuroimaging studies with N = 300 meditation practitioners: Insight, Zen, Tibetan, Buddhist, Mindfulness Based Stress Reduction, Integrative Mind-Body Training, Soham, Loving-Kindness meditation, and "Various".	Five regions were thicker in meditators: • Meta-awareness (frontopolar cortex); • Exteroceptive and interoceptive body awareness (sensory cortices and insula); • Memory consolidation and reconsolidation (hippocampus); • Self and emotion regulation (anterior and mid cingulate; orbitofrontal cortex); • Intra- and interhemispheric communication (superior longitudinal fasciculus; corpus callosum). There was, however, a negative correlation with effect size differences and length of meditation practice.
Lomas [9]	Meta-analysis of 54 studies of EEG from Mindfulness Based Cognitive Training (2), Mindfulness (13), Vipassana (6), mind/body training (2), Zen (13), various (5).	• Delta EEG power (5 total): Significantly higher in 1 study, lower in four. • Theta EEG power (19 total): Significantly higher in 10 studies, lower in three, and no differences in six others. • Posterior Alpha EEG power (20 total): Significantly higher in 13 studies, lower in one, and no differences in six others. • Beta EEG power (12 total): Significantly higher in four studies, lower in one, and no differences in seven others. • Gamma EEG power (7 total): Significantly higher in three studies, lower in one, and no differences in three others.

Table 1. Cont.

Reference	Design	Result
Boccio [10]	Meta-analysis with Mindfulness practices (5), Vipassana (12), Kundalini (11), Integrative Body Mind Training (3), MBSR (11), Zen (4).	Areas activated included the medial prefrontal cortex, motor cortex gyrus, anterior cingulate cortex, insula, claustrum, precuneus, parahippocampal gyrus, middle occipital gyrus, inferior parietal lobule, lentiform nucleus and thalamus.
Luders [11]	50 long-term meditators and 50 age-matched controls. Meditations included Zazen, Shamatha, Vipassana, as in the first study.	Estimating brain ages. • At age fifty, brains of meditators were estimated to be 7.5 years younger than those of controls; • For every additional year over fifty, meditators' brains were estimated to be an additional 1 month and 22 days younger than their chronological age.
Luders [12]	Meta-analysis of 9 studies: Dzogchen, Loving-kindness meditation, Sahaja yoga meditation, Shamatha, Vipassana, Zen.	Long term meditators (10 years or more) vs. controls had: • Higher whole brain grey matter; • Thicker cortices overall; • High white matter integrity—Higher fractional anisotropy.
Van Aalst [13]	Meta-analysis of 34 studies of Yoga practice: Ashtanga, Iyengar, Vinyasa, Kripalu, Kundalini, Nidra, Sahaja, Sivananda and Hatha yoga.	Yoga practitioners had increased gray matter volume in the insula and hippocampus and increased activation of prefrontal cortical regions. There was, however, high variability in the neuroimaging findings

2.1. Changes in Gray Matter Volumes

Luders and colleagues reported no group differences in total cortical thickness, but higher grey matter volumes in right sub-cortical areas in the meditation group [5]. In contrast, their 2019 research reported higher grey matter volume and thicker cortices overall in the meditation group [12]. These contradictory findings could reflect different contributions of different practices in each meditation study.

Fox and colleagues reviewed 21 neuroimaging studies and found thicker cortices in brain areas supporting a wide range of cognitive processes including meta-awareness (frontopolar cortex), body awareness (sensory cortices and insula), memory consolidation and reconsolidation (hippocampus), self and emotion regulation (anterior and mid cingulate; orbitofrontal cortex) and intra- and interhemispheric communication [8]. This wide range of meditation effects could reflect the contributions of different meditation practices. Unexpectedly, Fox and colleagues reported a *negative* correlation with magnitude of brain differences and length of meditation practice. This suggests that other factors besides meditation practice may be influencing these findings.

Grey matter volume decreased with age with all subjects, though the decrease was less in the meditating subjects [7]. At age 50, brains of meditators were estimated to be 7.5 years younger than those of controls [11]. This finding could be a characteristic of most meditation practices since experience is reported to affect grey matter volumes across the lifespan [14]. In addition, yoga practices with and without meditation and with and without postures reported higher insula and hippocampal grey matter volumes.

2.2. Changes in White Matter Volumes

Two studies reported that fractional anisotropy, an indicator of white matter fiber integrity, was higher in the meditating population. One was a study of 27 meditating and control subjects [6]. The second was a meta-analysis of nine studies [12]. White matter changes may also be common to all meditations, different meditation procedures would be expected to affect different brain networks since different kinds of experiences change white matter networks in different ways. For instance, studying for the Law School Administration Test increased white matter tract integrity in frontal executive areas [15], while juggling increases white matter integrity in the right posterior parietal cortex, related to detecting motion [16].

2.3. Summary of this Section

The assumption that a common brain marker would emerge by combining different meditation practices together in one analysis is flawed. Meditation procedures differ. Some meditations involve deep concentration, others prescribe attention to external and internal stimuli [17], and others are inwardly directed towards nondual states [18]. Thus, brain patterns from different practices would not be expected to converge to a common pattern. Looking at brain areas reported active during meditation practices in the above table, we find all brain areas—except for primary sensory cortices—were reported to be activated by meditation practices.

3. Second Strategy: Researching Individual Meditation Practices

Research has investigated shorter term (state) and long term (trait) brain patterns during individual meditation practices.

- Buddhist Shamatha meditation, a concentrative technique, is associated with activation in the fronto-parietal attention network and deactivation of regions related to conceptual thought and emotions [19,20].
- Loving-kindness/compassion meditation in expert meditators activated limbic areas and a network associated with Theory of Mind—right temporal lobes, temporo-parietal junction, medial prefrontal and posterior cingulate cortices [21–23]. A meta-analysis of 16 fMRI studies of compassion meditation revealed patterns of activation in four brain areas: periaqueductal grey, anterior insula, anterior cingulate, and inferior frontal gyrus. This meta-analysis replicated earlier findings but did not find activation in areas typically connected with compassion including the dorsolateral prefrontal cortex, orbital prefrontal cortex and the amygdala [24].
- Mindfulness meditation was marked by deactivation of medial prefrontal cortices but activation of lateral prefrontal cortices, the secondary somatosensory cortex, the inferior parietal lobule and the insula [25–28]. A meta-analysis of 21 fMRI studies of mindful practices used activation likelihood estimate methods to compare mindfulness with control conditions. Loci of activation were found in the frontal regions including the medial prefrontal gyrus, anterior cingulate, insula, and globus pallidus [29].
- Vipassana expert meditators had bilateral activation in the rostral anterior cingulate cortex and in the dorsal medial prefrontal cortex [30–32].
- Zen meditation is reported to lead to increased alpha and theta activity in many brain regions, including the frontal cortex, and decreases in the Default Mode Network [33–35].
- Network analysis of imaging data from 12 experienced Zen meditators and 12 controls during an attention to breathing protocol reported extensive connections of frontoparietal circuits with early visual and executive control areas [36].
- Relaxation meditation (Yoga Nidra) activated the hippocampus and posterior mental imagery areas, and deactivated the frontal executive control network system, in a positron emission tomography study [37,38].
- Kundalini yoga activated left fronto-temporal regions and deactivated the left posterior parietal lobe in a PET study [39,40].
- Mantra recitation with meaning activated the hippocampi/parahippocampal area, middle cingulate cortex and the precentral cortex bilaterally [41].
- Kirtan Kriya activated the medial prefrontal cortex and left caudate nuclei and deactivated the left superior occipital and inferior parietal cortex, as well as the right inferior occipital cortex [42,43].
- Ashtanga yoga deactivated the medial prefrontal cortex, anterior cingulate gyrus, and inferior parietal cortices [42,44].

- Transcendental Meditation practice is marked by frontal alpha1 coherence (8–10 Hz) [45–47], and ventral medial and anterior cingulate sources of alpha activity, in an magnetoencephalography study [48], and higher frontal and lower brainstem blood flow in an fMRI study [49].

Summary of this Section

This overview demonstrates that meditation practices have pervasive effects on brain functioning, activating and deactivating different brain networks. For instance, mindfulness, Vipassana and TM activate the dorsolateral prefrontal cortex, but only TM also activates the medial prefrontal cortex, part of the emotional regulation network in the brain [38]. Loving kindness and Kirtan Yoga also activate the medial prefrontal cortex but do not affect dorsolateral prefrontal cortex functioning. Mindfulness practices activate the inferior parietal cortices, as does Yoga Nidra, but Yoga Nidra deactivates dorsolateral prefrontal cortex.

This organizing strategy generates a multitude of brain patterns as each practice is studied individually. Research should be done to understand the details of each practice. However, the rich detail of individual differences within each practice makes it difficult to identify reliable patterns between practices.

4. Third Strategy: Organizing Meditations into Larger Classes

A third organizing strategy is to group practices based on theoretical frameworks and identify neural patterns within and between each group. This should reduce the variability within and between groups and so lead to a more reliable picture of brain patterns during meditation. We will review the impact of three grouping strategies: grouping meditations by their traditions—Indian or Buddhism traditions, grouping meditations by their procedures, and grouping meditations by EEG frequencies associated with the cognitive processes used in each practice.

4.1. Grouping Meditations by Their Source: Indian or Buddhist Traditions

Most eastern meditation practices were developed within the Indian and Buddhist traditions. Meditations in the Buddhist tradition are dynamic cognitive practices [50]. They include mindfulness as a central aspect, i.e., sustained attention and mental presence on breathing, on the contemplation of the body and on the observation of the contents of the mind [51]. During mindfulness practices one attends to " ... whatever predominates in awareness, moment to moment. The intention is not to choose a single object of focus, but rather to explore changing experience" [52]. This cognitive process—attending nonjudgmentally to the unfolding of experience moment by moment—has been applied to eating [53], walking [54], awareness of breathing [55] and awareness of thoughts and emotions [56].

In contrast, meditations in the Indian tradition are structured to reach a state of content-free awareness—the state of Yoga or Samadhi [57]. The procedures in these meditations involve less cognitive control and recommend: "We simply need to be what we are." ([58] or "Step out of the process of experiencing and arrive at the state of Being." [59].

Chiesa and colleagues conducted a meta-analysis of eighteen neural imaging studies: ten Buddhist meditations and eight Indian meditations [57]. The practices from the Buddhist tradition included Vipassana, Zen, Loving-kindness/compassion, and Mindfulness-Based Stress Reduction. The practices from the Indian tradition included Yoga Nidra (guided relaxation), Kundalini yoga (chanting, singing, breathing exercises, and repetitive poses to move kundalini energy up the spine), chanting of "OM", Kirtan Kriya (singing of mantras) and Shabdha Kriya Yoga (singing of mantras and breath control used before going to sleep).

Comparing meditations in these two groups, Buddhist meditations were characterized by bilateral activation in the frontal superior medial gyrus, activation in the right parietal supramarginal gyrus (associated with language processing) and the supplementary motor area. Indian meditations were associated with left lateralized activation of the post-central gyrus (touch), the superior parietal lobe (touch), the hippocampus (memory and spatial planning), the left superior temporal gyrus (phonological word processing), and the right middle cingulate cortex (attention) [57].

The Buddhist meditations in this study enhanced brain areas associated with language processing and motor areas. Indian meditations in this study enhanced brain areas associated with sensory processing, language processing, attention, and memory areas.

Buddhist and Indian traditions include practices that involve minimal cognitive control such as Dzogchen meditation in the Tibetan Buddhist tradition, Zazen in the Buddhist tradition and Transcendental Meditation in the Indian tradition. These were not included in this meta-analysis. Dzogchen describes meditation as " ... the state of relaxation—a means by which we can be what we are, without tension, tyranny or anxiety ... .We simply need to be what we are." ([58], p. 14). Zazen is described as "the practice of being what we are, of allowing, permitting, opening ourselves to ourselves. In doing that we enter directly the depth of our living—a depth that goes beyond our individual life and touches all lives." ([60], p. 26). Transcending during Transcendental Meditation practice is described as "When we have transcended the field of the experience of the subtlest object, the experiencer is left by himself ... the experiencer steps out of the process of experiencing and arrives at the state of Being. The mind is then found in the state of Being." ([59], p. 29).

Combining cognitively active meditations involving sustained attention, mental presence on breathing, contemplation of the body or observation of the contents of the mind with meditation described as only needing "to be what we are" is mixing meditations with very different procedures. This could lead to distorted conclusions about meditation practices.

4.2. Grouping Meditations by their Procedures: Four Categories of Meditation

Fox and colleagues started with the assumption that meditation practices with different procedures would be associated with different neural imaging patterns [17]. They defined four categories of meditation based on their procedures: *Focused Attention, Mantra Recitation, Open Monitoring, and Loving Kindness. Focused Attention* is directing attention to one specific object while monitoring and disengaging from extraneous thoughts or stimuli; *Mantra Recitation* is repetition of a sound with the goals of calming the mind and avoiding mind-wandering; *Open-Monitoring* is bringing attention to the present moment and impartially observing all mental contents as they naturally arise and subside; and *Loving-kindness* is deepening feelings of sympathetic joy for all living beings, as well as promoting altruistic [56,61].

The authors reviewed 78 functional neuroimaging (fMRI and PET) meditation studies involving 527 participants and placed the studies into these four categories [17]. In this meta-analysis, *Focused Attention* meditations included Tibetan Buddhism, Vipassana, Theravada Buddhism and Zen, *Mantra Recitation Meditation* included kundalini, ACEM, SOHAM and Pure Land Buddhist meditations, *Open Monitoring* included Yoga Nidra and Mindfulness practices, and *Loving kindness* included Tibetan Buddhist meditations.

The meditations within each category had similar activation patterns, but there was little convergence between the categories. During *Focused Attention* meditations, activations were observed in two brain areas associated with voluntary regulation of thought and action, the premotor cortex and dorsal anterior cingulate cortex. During *Mantra Recitation* meditations, areas of activations included the posterior dorsolateral prefrontal cortex, motor cortex, and putamen/lateral globus pallidus. During *Open Monitoring* meditations, significant clusters of activation were observed: the insula, left inferior frontal and motor cortices. During *Loving kindness* meditations, higher brain activation as observed in the right anterior insula/frontal operculum, and anterior inferior parietal lobule.

These four categories of meditation differed on the level of description of their procedures and on the level of brain activation patterns [17]. This supports the value of assigning meditations to meaningful categories before combining neural imaging data.

The categories could have been further refined. *Focused Attention* and *Open Monitoring* refer to the procedures used during meditation practice. *Mantra recitation meditation* and *Loving-kindness/compassion* refer to the content of the meditation. These are distinctly different groupings—"procedures used" versus "content of the meditation." The authors discussed this contradiction. In addition, they noted that *Mantra Recitation Meditation* could reasonably be placed within the *Focused Attention* category since most mantra meditations involve directing attention to the mantra while disengaging from extraneous thoughts [17]. Similarly, *Loving-kindness/Compassion* meditations could be considered a form of *Focused Attention* since one focuses intensively on the target of loving-kindness, while cultivating a consistent emotional tone to the exclusion of other [17].

4.3. Grouping Meditations by EEG Activation Patterns: Three Categories of Meditation

Travis and Shear started with descriptions of meditation procedures, as Fox and colleagues did, and then assigned frequency bands to the cognitive processes reflected in those descriptions [62]. Then, based on these EEG frequency bands, meditations were grouped into categories. These categories are procedural categories as defined by EEG frequencies and are not limited by the domain of the meditation practice, such as perceptual, cognitive, affective, or nondual domains [50].

Two categories of meditation procedures, *Focused Attention* and *Open Monitoring*, had been earlier defined by Lutz and colleagues [61] and were used by Fox. These two categories were the starting point for this three-category classification of meditations.

4.3.1. Focused Attention

Focused Attention meditation " ... entails voluntary focusing attention on a chosen object in a sustained fashion. "([61], p. 1). Voluntary focused attention is associated with gamma activity (30–50 Hz). Gamma is seen in any task that involves effortful thinking and control of the mind [63]. Gamma EEG is driven by local processing within short-range connections responsible for perceptual awareness [64], selective attention [65], neuronal processing and communication between regions [66]. In a study of experienced Buddhist practitioners, higher gamma EEG was seen in the posterior cingulate cortex, a major posterior hub in the default mode network [67].

4.3.2. Open monitoring

Open monitoring meditations " ... involve nonreactive monitoring of the content of experience from moment to moment, primarily as a means to recognize the nature of emotional and cognitive patterns" ([61], p. 1). Nonreactive monitoring is associated with midline frontal theta. Theta is produced whenever one attends to internal mental processing [32]. Frontal midline theta is a marker of working memory tasks, and episodic memory encoding and retrieval processes [68]. Brandmeyer and Delorme compared EEG correlates of novice mindfulness subjects, whose minds wandered frequently during the practice to EEG from experienced mindfulness subjects whose minds wandered less. They found higher midline theta EEG and somatosensory alpha in the experienced subjects [69]. A recent meta-analyses of EEG patterns [9] also reported that alpha was found in posterior, parietal or central areas during open monitoring practices [46].

4.3.3. Automatic Self-Transcending

Travis and Shear added a third category, *Automatic Self-Transcending*, for meditations that transcend their steps of practice [62]. This would include meditation practices such as Dzogchen "We simply need to be what we are." ([58], p. 14), and Transcendental Meditation practice " ... the experiencer steps out of the process of experiencing and arrives at the state of Being. The mind is then found in the state of Being." ([59] p. 29).

Frontal alpha EEG is predicted to characterize meditations with these procedures. Alpha oscillations have been found to play an active role in the suppression of task-irrelevant processing [66], being negatively correlated with local cortical excitability [70]. Frontal alpha could indicate that frontal executive processing is being inhibited.

4.3.4. Application of this Model

Travis and Shear used these EEG frequency bands to assign meditations to categories [62]. Meditations that were characterized by gamma EEG were placed in the *Focused Attention* category. They included Compassion [61], Qigong [71], Zen [35,60] and Vipassana meditations [32,72]. The essence-of-mind technique, a Tibetan Buddhist technique aimed at experiencing a brilliantly awake, limitless, a non-dual state of awareness, is also characterized by higher gamma and beta-2 EEG [73] and would be placed in this category.

Meditations that were characterized by midline theta and posterior alpha EEG were placed in the *Open Monitoring* category. They included Mindfulness practices [28,69], Zazen [74], and Sahaja [75,76].

Meditations that were characterized by frontal alpha1 EEG were placed in the *Automatic Self-Transcending* category. They included Transcendental Meditation [45,47], a case study of a Qigong master [77] and a study of 25 Zen-Buddhist priests [78].

Automaticity: Why Zen Buddhism and Qigong Might Be in This Category

Gamma EEG is most often reported during Zen Buddhism and Qigong practice [79]. This is understandable since these practices require focus and control of mental processes. However, even highly complex, controlled cognitive processes can become automatic with extensive practice—the task is performed without attention to each step and performance is not affected by increasing task loads [80]. Experienced Vipassana practitioners reported "effortless doing," a calm, tranquil, relaxed, and effortless way of acting [81]. Expert Buddhist practitioners report "effortless concentration" characterized by reduced need to consciously direct, sustain and orient attention [61]. These are examples of automaticity resulting from long-term practice.

The TM technique is designed to be automatic. One learns how to use the "natural tendency" of the mind to transcend [82]. The movement of the mind to more interesting experiences is what is intended by the phrase the "natural tendency" of the mind. When the object of experience is rated as being highly interesting, it is associated with greater positive emotional tone than when the person is on-task [83]. The mind transcends because one's attention is pulled by the inherent pleasure of the state of inner silence devoid of changing thoughts, feelings or perceptions [49,84]. This claim is supported by high activation levels in the default mode network during Transcendental Meditation practice.

Default Mode Network Activation—A Marker of Automaticity

Activation/deactivation patterns of the default mode network (DMN) are an objective marker of cognitive control used in a task [84,85]. The DMN includes medial and lateral parietal cortices, and the precuneus and medial prefrontal cortex [86,87]. The DMN is deactivated during goal-directed behaviors requiring executive control and activated during self-referential mental activity, when envisioning the future and when envisioning the actions of others [88].

All meditations in the *Focused Attention* and *Open Monitoring* categories are reported to lead to decreased activity of the default mode network [89,90] including Zen [35], Vipassana [91], mindfulness practices [92,93], and Loving-Kindness [94]. Decrease in default activation is expected since these meditation practices involve voluntary attention to a specific object or attending to moment-by-moment changing experiences. In contrast, default mode network activation remains high during Transcendental Meditation practice [84].

Default Mode Network and Mind Wandering

High DMN activity has also been reported during rumination and is associated with depression. Zhou and colleagues conducted a meta-analysis of 14 fMRI studies with 286 participants. High depression was marked by activation of four sub-systems of the default network: the anterior prefrontal cortex, dorsal medial prefrontal cortex, posterior cingulate cortex and posterior inferior parietal lobe [95]. This finding can be interpreted as high DMN activation causing or indicating rumination and depression. This conclusion is an example of the logical fallacy of affirming the consequent. Namely: if depression is associated with high DMN activity, then high DMN activity indicates depression in all populations.

Mind-wandering often involves negative content such as guilty daydreaming, ruminating thoughts and unpleasant emotions [96,97]. However, mind-wandering more often involves positive content rather than negative content [98]. This positive content includes future-focused, autobiographical planning [99] oriented toward personal goal resolution [100]. Positive mind-wandering allows attentional cycling between personally meaningful values and external goals [101].

Previous studies reporting a relationship between mind-wandering and depression combined positive mind-wandering, rumination, and worry under the single term "repetitive thinking" [102,103]. The negative effects of "mind-wandering" vanished when "negative" mind-wandering (perseverative cognition) is differentiated from "positive" mind-wandering. Research reports that *positive* mind-wandering and depression symptoms are not correlated at baseline or at one-year [104]. When compared to positive mind-wandering, perseverative cognition was associated with higher levels of cognitive inflexibility (slower reaction times, higher levels of intrusiveness), autonomic rigidity (lower heart rate variability), and worsening mood (more symptoms of depression) compared to positive mind-wandering [105]. (See this book chapter for a discussion of negative and positive mind wandering [106]).

4.4. Summary of this Section

Grouping meditations by theoretically meaningful categories resulted in models in which brain patterns (neural imaging patterns or EEG frequencies) were similar within categories but different between categories. An examination of the four-category model brought up two questions. First, two categories were procedural categories (*Focused Attention* and *Open Monitoring*) while the other two were defined by the contents of meditation practice (*Mantra recitation* or *Loving-kindness/compassion*). These are distinctly different groupings—"procedures used" versus "meditation content". Second, two of the categories, *Mantra Recitation* and *Loving-kindness/Compassion* could arguably be placed within the *Focused Attention* category since they both involve focusing on a specific target—voluntary verbal-motor production, or a consistent emotional tone—to the exclusion of others. Fox and colleagues discussed this last issue [17].

The three-category model uses EEG patterns associated with three distinct meditation procedures—focused attention, open monitoring, and automatic self- transcending—to objectively assign meditation practices to categories. This creates categories with similar content—procedure related EEG frequencies—and allows meditation practices to move between categories as procedures change with long-term practice, such as from focused concentration to "effortless concentration" [61].

Figure 1a–c display brain areas activated by meditations in each category. The findings of Fox's meta-analysis of 78 studies were used to identify brain areas active during *Focused Attention* and *Open Monitoring* meditations [8]. Mahone's fMRI research on Transcendental Meditation practice was used to identify brain areas active during *Automatic Self-Transcending* meditations [49]. This figure includes cortical and sagittal sections of the brain. Brain areas active during *Focused Attention* meditations are colored blue in Figure 1a, are colored yellow during *Open Monitoring* meditations in Figure 1b, and colored red during *Automatic Self-Transcending* meditations in Figure 1c. In addition, the insula was active during *Open Monitoring* meditations, and the pons and cerebellum were *deactivated* during *Automatic Self-Transcending* meditations. The brain's areas are distinct for each category, engaging different frontal, motor, parietal, and anterior cingulate cortices. The Brodmann areas are in the background of this figure to help the reader locate the areas that were active. More brain areas may be indicated for *Focused Attention* since this category includes brain areas during Mantra Recitation and Compassion meditation. They were included since they are both characterized by gamma EEG.

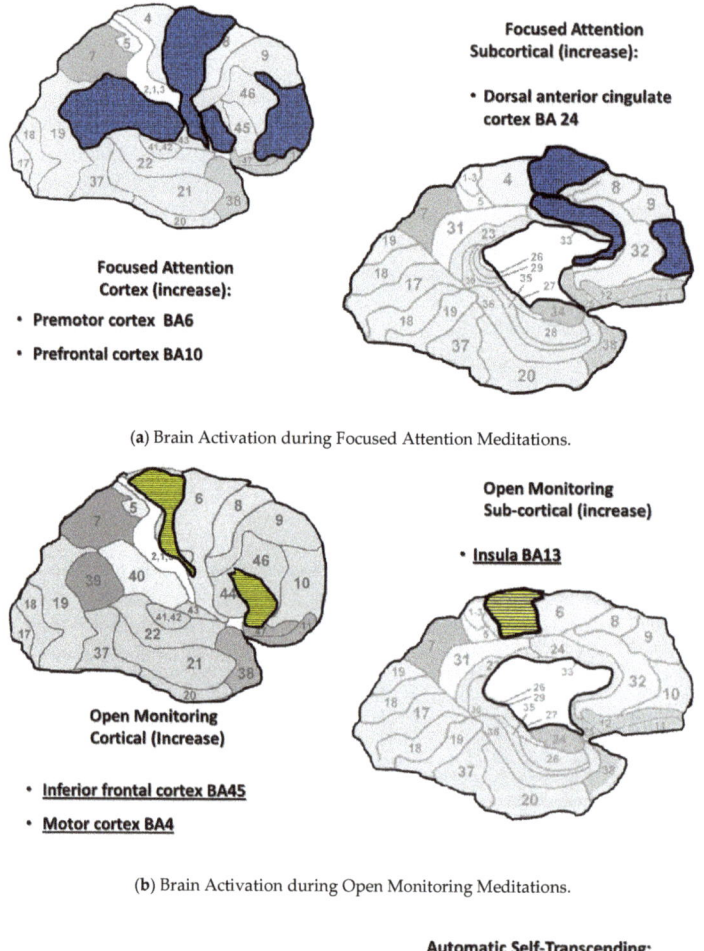

(a) Brain Activation during Focused Attention Meditations.

(b) Brain Activation during Open Monitoring Meditations.

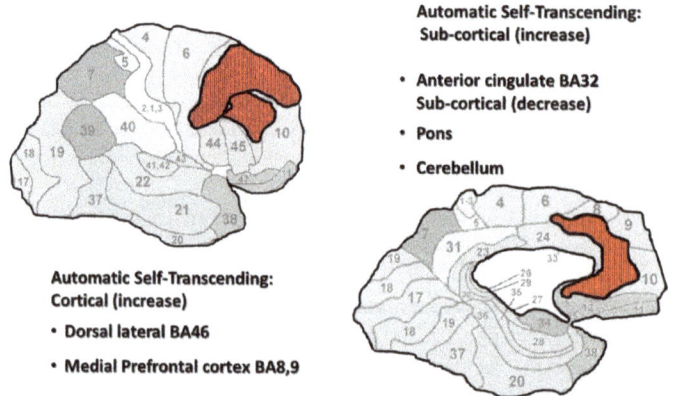

(c) Brain Activation during Automatic Self-Transcending Meditations.

Figure 1. (a–c). Neural imaging research shows distinct cortical and subcortical activation/deactivation patterns in three categories of meditation. Cortical and subcortical areas active during *Focused Attention* meditations (**a**), *Open Monitoring* meditations (**b**), and *Automatic Self-Transcending* meditations (**c**).

In addition, these three categories were marked by distinct EEG patterns. *Focused Attention* meditations were marked by posterior gamma. *Open Monitoring* meditations were marked by frontal midline theta and posterior alpha2. *Automatic Self-Transcending* meditations were marked by frontal alpha1.

5. Recommended Grouping Strategy

Grouping meditations by theoretically meaningful categories appears to be the best strategy to define the neurobiology of meditation. This strategy controls for the fatal flaw of combining, into a single average, meditation practices involving outward directed attention to objects or the senses, and inner-directed attention to cognitive and affective processes or nondual states (1st strategy). These different procedures would necessarily involve different brain patterns, and, when averaged together, would define a brain pattern unlike any meditation practice.

Two examples of combining meditations into meaningful categories were discussed. The four-category model of meditation created by descriptions of the procedures [17] yielded distinct neural patterns within each category with few similarities between categories. The three-category model defined by EEG frequencies associated with meditation procedures yielded distinct EEG patterns within each category with few similarities between categories. In addition, using EEG frequencies to assign meditations to categories allows practices to "move" into different categories as subjects' meditation experiences change over time, which would be associated with different brain patterns.

Funding: This research received no external funding.

Acknowledgments: We thank Abe Bornstein for his input on the figures.

Conflicts of Interest: The author reports no conflict of interests.

References

1. Stulberg, B.; Magness, S. *Peak Performance: Elevate Your Game, Avoid Burnout, and Thrive with the New Science of Success*; Rodale Books: New York, NY, USA, 2017.
2. Spearman, C. General intelligence: Objectively determined and measured. *Am. J. Psychol.* **1904**, *15*, 201–292. [CrossRef]
3. Undheim, J.O. On intelligence II: A neo-Spearman model to replace Cattell's theory of fluid and crystallized intelligence. *Scand. J. Psychol.* **1981**, *22*, 181–187. [CrossRef]
4. Helfrich, R.F.; Knight, R.T. Cognitive neurophysiology: Event-related potentials. *Handb. Clin. Neurol.* **2019**, *160*, 543–558. [CrossRef] [PubMed]
5. Luders, E.; Toga, A.W.; Lepore, N.; Gaser, C. The underlying anatomical correlates of long-term meditation: Larger hippocampal and frontal volumes of gray matter. *Neuroimage* **2009**, *45*, 672–678. [CrossRef]
6. Luders, E.; Clark, K.; Narr, K.L.; Toga, A.W. Enhanced brain connectivity in long-term meditation practitioners. *Neuroimage* **2011**, *57*, 1308–1316. [CrossRef]
7. Luders, E.; Cherbuin, N.; Kurth, F. Forever Young(er): Potential age-defying effects of long-term meditation on gray matter atrophy. *Front. Psychol.* **2014**, *5*, 1551. [CrossRef]
8. Fox, K.C.; Nijeboer, S.; Dixon, M.L.; Floman, J.L.; Ellamil, M.; Rumak, S.P.; Sedlmeier, P.; Christoff, K. Is meditation associated with altered brain structure? A systematic review and meta-analysis of morphometric neuroimaging in meditation practitioners. *Neurosci. Biobehav. Rev.* **2014**, *43*, 48–73. [CrossRef]
9. Lomas, T.; Ivtzan, I.; Fu, C.H. A systematic review of the neurophysiology of mindfulness on EEG oscillations. *Neurosci. Biobehav. Rev.* **2015**, *57*, 401–410. [CrossRef]
10. Boccia, M.; Piccardi, L.; Guariglia, P. The Meditative Mind: A Comprehensive Meta-Analysis of MRI Studies. *Biomed. Res. Int.* **2015**, *2015*, 419808. [CrossRef]
11. Luders, E.; Cherbuin, N.; Gaser, C. Estimating brain age using high-resolution pattern recognition: Younger brains in long-term meditation practitioners. *Neuroimage* **2016**, *134*, 508–513. [CrossRef]
12. Luders, E.; Kurth, F. The neuroanatomy of long-term meditators. *Curr. Opin. Psychol.* **2019**, *28*, 172–178. [CrossRef]

13. van Aalst, J.; Ceccarini, J.; Demyttenaere, K.; Sunaert, S.; Van Laere, K. What Has Neuroimaging Taught Us on the Neurobiology of Yoga? A Review. *Front. Integr. Neurosci.* **2020**, *14*, 34. [CrossRef] [PubMed]
14. Hubener, M.; Bonhoeffer, T. Neuronal plasticity: Beyond the critical period. *Cell* **2014**, *159*, 727–737. [CrossRef] [PubMed]
15. Mackey, A.P.; Whitaker, K.J.; Bunge, S.A. Experience-dependent plasticity in white matter microstructure: Reasoning training alters structural connectivity. *Front. Neuroanat.* **2012**, *6*, 32. [CrossRef]
16. Scholz, J.; Klein, M.C.; Behrens, T.E.; Johansen-Berg, H. Training induces changes in white-matter architecture. *Nat. Neurosci.* **2009**, *12*, 1370–1371. [CrossRef]
17. Fox, K.C.; Dixon, M.L.; Nijeboer, S.; Girn, M.; Floman, J.L.; Lifshitz, M.; Ellamil, M.; Sedlmeier, P.; Christoff, K. Functional neuroanatomy of meditation: A review and meta-analysis of 78 functional neuroimaging investigations. *Neurosci. Biobehav. Rev.* **2016**, *65*, 208–228. [CrossRef]
18. Ponlop, R.D. *Wild Awakening: The Heart of Mahamudra and Dzogchen*; Shambhala Publications: Boston, MA, USA, 2013.
19. Brefczynski-Lewis, J.A.; Lutz, A.; Schaefer, H.S.; Levinson, D.B.; Davidson, R.J. Neural correlates of attentional expertise in long-term meditation practitioners. *Proc. Natl. Acad. Sci. USA* **2007**, *104*, 11483–11488. [CrossRef] [PubMed]
20. Blase, K.L.; van Waning, A. Heart Rate Variability, Cortisol and Attention Focus During Shamatha Quiescence Meditation. *Appl. Psychophysiol. Biofeedback* **2019**, *44*, 331–342. [CrossRef] [PubMed]
21. Lutz, A.; Greischar, L.L.; Perlman, D.M.; Davidson, R.J. BOLD signal in insula is differentially related to cardiac function during compassion meditation in experts vs. novices. *Neuroimage* **2009**, *47*, 1038–1046. [CrossRef]
22. Le Nguyen, K.D.; Lin, J.; Algoe, S.B.; Brantley, M.M.; Kim, S.L.; Brantley, J.; Salzberg, S.; Fredrickson, B.L. Loving-kindness meditation slows biological aging in novices: Evidence from a 12-week randomized controlled trial. *Psychoneuroendocrinology* **2019**, *108*, 20–27. [CrossRef]
23. Leung, M.K.; Chan, C.C.; Yin, J.; Lee, C.F.; So, K.F.; Lee, T.M. Increased gray matter volume in the right angular and posterior parahippocampal gyri in loving-kindness meditators. *Soc. Cogn. Affect. Neurosci.* **2013**, *8*, 34–39. [CrossRef] [PubMed]
24. Kim, J.J.; Cunnington, R.; Kirby, J.N. The neurophysiological basis of compassion: An fMRI meta-analysis of compassion and its related neural processes. *Neurosci. Biobehav. Rev.* **2020**, *108*, 112–123. [CrossRef] [PubMed]
25. Farb, N.A.S.; Segal, Z.V.; Mayberg, H.; Bean, J.; McKeon, D.; Fatima, Z. Attending to the present: Mindfulness meditation reveals distinct neural modes of self-reference. *Soc. Cogn. Affect. Neurosci.* **2007**, *2*, 313–322. [CrossRef] [PubMed]
26. Malinowski, P.; Moore, A.W.; Mead, B.R.; Gruber, T. Mindful Aging: The Effects of Regular Brief Mindfulness Practice on Electrophysiological Markers of Cognitive and Affective Processing in Older Adults. *Mindfulness* **2017**, *8*, 78–94. [CrossRef]
27. Singleton, O.; Holzel, B.K.; Vangel, M.; Brach, N.; Carmody, J.; Lazar, S.W. Change in Brainstem Gray Matter Concentration Following a Mindfulness-Based Intervention is Correlated with Improvement in Psychological Well-Being. *Front. Hum. Neurosci.* **2014**, *8*, 33. [CrossRef]
28. Gotink, R.A.; Meijboom, R.; Vernooij, M.W.; Smits, M.; Hunink, M.G. 8-week Mindfulness Based Stress Reduction induces brain changes similar to traditional long-term meditation practice–A systematic review. *Brain Cogn.* **2016**, *108*, 32–41. [CrossRef]
29. Falcone, G.; Jerram, M. Brain Activity in Mindfulness Depends on Experience: A Meta-Analysis of fMRI Studies. *Mindfulness* **2018**, *9*, 1319–1329. [CrossRef]
30. Holzel, B.K.; Ott, U.; Hempel, H.; Hackl, A.; Wolf, K.; Stark, R. Differential engagement of anterior cingulate and adjacent medial frontal cortex in adept meditators and non-meditators. *Neurosci. Lett.* **2007**, *421*, 16–21. [CrossRef]
31. Chiesa, A. Vipassana meditation: Systematic review of current evidence. *J. Altern. Complement. Med.* **2010**, *16*, 37–46. [CrossRef]
32. Kakumanu, R.J.; Nair, A.K.; Venugopal, R.; Sasidharan, A.; Ghosh, P.K.; John, J.P.; Mehrotra, S.; Panth, R.; Kutty, B.M. Dissociating meditation proficiency and experience dependent EEG changes during traditional Vipassana meditation practice. *Biol. Psychol.* **2018**, *135*, 65–75. [CrossRef]

33. Chiesa, A. Zen meditation: An integration of current evidence. *J. Altern. Complement. Med.* **2009**, *15*, 585–592. [CrossRef] [PubMed]
34. Lo, P.-C.; Tian, W.J.M.; Liu, F.-L. Macrostate and Microstate of EEG Spatio-Temporal Nonlinear Dynamics in Zen Meditation. *J. Behav. Brain Sci.* **2017**, *7*, 705–721. [CrossRef]
35. Pagnoni, G.; Cekic, M.; Guo, Y. "Thinking about not-thinking": Neural correlates of conceptual processing during Zen meditation. *PLoS ONE* **2008**, *3*, e3083. [CrossRef] [PubMed]
36. Kemmer, P.B.; Guo, Y.; Wang, Y.; Pagnoni, G. Network-based characterization of brain functional connectivity in Zen practitioners. *Front. Psychol.* **2015**, *6*, 603. [CrossRef] [PubMed]
37. Lou, H.C.; Kjaer, T.W.; Friberg, L.; Wildschiodtz, G.; Holm, S.; Nowak, M. A 15O–H$_2$O PET study of meditation and the resting state of normal consciousness. *Hum. Brain Mapp.* **1999**, *7*, 98–105. [CrossRef]
38. Parker, S. Training attention for conscious non-REM sleep: The yogic practice of yoga-nidra and its implications for neuroscience research. *Prog. Brain Res.* **2019**, *244*, 255–272. [CrossRef]
39. Khalsa, D.S.; Amen, D.; Hanks, C.; Money, N.; Newberg, A. Cerebral blood flow changes during chanting meditation. *Nucl. Med. Commun.* **2009**, *30*, 956–961. [CrossRef]
40. Arambula, P.; Peper, E.; Kawakami, M.; Gibney, K.H. The physiological correlates of Kundalini Yoga meditation: A study of a yoga master. *Appl. Psychophysiol. Biofeedback* **2001**, *26*, 147–153. [CrossRef]
41. Engstrom, M.; Pihlsgard, J.; Lundberg, P.; Soderfeldt, B. Functional magnetic resonance imaging of hippocampal activation during silent mantra meditation. *J. Altern. Complement. Med.* **2010**, *16*, 1253–1258. [CrossRef]
42. Wang, D.J.; Rao, H.; Korczykowski, M.; Wintering, N.; Pluta, J.; Khalsa, D.S. Cerebral blood flow changes associated with different meditation practices and perceived depth of meditation. *Psychiatry Res.* **2011**, *191*, 60–67. [CrossRef]
43. Moss, A.S.; Wintering, N.; Roggenkamp, H.; Khalsa, D.S.; Waldman, M.R.; Monti, D.; Newberg, A.B. Effects of an 8-week meditation program on mood and anxiety in patients with memory loss. *J. Altern. Complement. Med.* **2012**, *18*, 48–53. [CrossRef] [PubMed]
44. van Aalst, J.; Ceccarini, J.; Schramm, G.; Van Weehaeghe, D.; Rezaei, A.; Demyttenaere, K.; Sunaert, S.; Van Laere, K. Long-term Ashtanga yoga practice decreases medial temporal and brainstem glucose metabolism in relation to years of experience. *EJNMMI Res.* **2020**, *10*, 50. [CrossRef] [PubMed]
45. Travis, F.; Haaga, D.A.; Hagelin, J.; Tanner, M.; Arenander, A.; Nidich, S.; Gaylord-King, C.; Grosswald, S.; Rainforth, M.; Schneider, R.H. A self-referential default brain state: Patterns of coherence, power, and eLORETA sources during eyes-closed rest and Transcendental Meditation practice. *Cogn. Process.* **2010**, *11*, 21–30. [CrossRef]
46. Travis, F. Temporal and spatial characteristics of meditation EEG. *Psychol. Trauma* **2019**, *12*, 111–115. [CrossRef] [PubMed]
47. Travis, F.T.; Tecce, J.; Arenander, A.; Wallace, R.K. Patterns of EEG Coherence, Power, and Contingent Negative Variation Characterize the Integration of Transcendental and Waking States. *Biol. Psychol.* **2002**, *61*, 293–319. [CrossRef]
48. Yamamoto, S.; Kitamura, Y.; Yamada, N.; Nakashima, Y.; Kuroda, S. Medial prefrontal cortex and anterior cingulate cortex in the generation of alpha activity induced by transcendental meditation: A magnetoencephalographic study. *Acta Med. Okayama* **2006**, *60*, 51–58. [CrossRef]
49. Mahone, M.C.; Travis, F.; Gevirtz, R.; Hubbard, D. fMRI during Transcendental Meditation practice. *Brain Cogn.* **2018**, *123*, 30–33. [CrossRef]
50. Nash, J.D.; Newberg, A.; Awasthi, B. Toward a unifying taxonomy and definition for meditation. *Front. Psychol.* **2013**, *4*, 806. [CrossRef]
51. Wynne, A. *The Origin of Buddhist Meditation*; Routledge: London, UK, 2009.
52. Siegel, R.D.; Germer, C.K.; Olendzki, A. *Mindfulness: What Is It? Where Did It Come from*; Springer: New York, NY, USA, 2009.
53. Nelson, J.B. Mindful Eating: The Art of Presence While You Eat. *Diabetes Spectr.* **2017**, *3*, 171–174. [CrossRef]
54. Teut, M.; Roesner, E.J.; Ortiz, M.; Reese, F.; Binting, S.; Roll, S.; Fischer, H.F.; Michalsen, A.; Willich, S.N.; Brinkhaus, B. Mindful walking in psychologically distressed individuals: A randomized controlled trial. *Evid. Based Complement. Altern. Med.* **2013**, *2013*, 9–16. [CrossRef]
55. Cho, H.; Ryu, S.; Noh, J.; Lee, J. The Effectiveness of Daily Mindful Breathing Practices on Test Anxiety of Students. *PLoS ONE* **2016**, *11*, e0164822. [CrossRef] [PubMed]

56. Kabat-Zinn, J. Mindfulness-Based Interventions in Context: Past, Present, and Future. *Clin. Psychol. Sci. Pract.* **2003**, *10*, 144–156. [CrossRef]
57. Tomasino, B.; Chiesa, A.; Fabbro, F. Disentangling the neural mechanisms involved in Hinduism- and Buddhism-related meditations. *Brain Cogn.* **2014**, *90*, 32–40. [CrossRef] [PubMed]
58. Chogyam, N.; Dechen, K. *Roaring Silence: Discovering the Mind of Dozgchen*; Shambhalam Publications: Boston, MA, USA, 2002.
59. Maharishi, M.Y. *Science of Being and Art of Living*; Plume: New York, NY, USA, 2001.
60. Tanahasi, K. *Beyond THinking: A Guide to Zen Meidtation*; Shambhala: Boston, MA, USA, 2004.
61. Lutz, A.; Slagter, H.A.; Dunne, J.D.; Davidson, R.J. Attention regulation and monitoring in meditation. *Trends Cogn. Sci.* **2008**, *12*, 163–169. [CrossRef] [PubMed]
62. Travis, F.; Shear, J. Focused attention, open monitoring and automatic self-transcending: Categories to organize meditations from Vedic, Buddhist and Chinese traditions. *Conscious. Cogn.* **2010**, *19*, 1110–1118. [CrossRef] [PubMed]
63. Braboszcz, C.; Cahn, B.R.; Levy, J.; Fernandez, M.; Delorme, A. Increased Gamma Brainwave Amplitude Compared to Control in Three Different Meditation Traditions. *PLoS ONE* **2017**, *12*, e0170647. [CrossRef]
64. Fries, P.; Womelsdorf, T.; Oostenveld, R.; Desimone, R. The effects of visual stimulation and selective visual attention on rhythmic neuronal synchronization in macaque area V4. *J. Neurosci.* **2008**, *28*, 4823–4835. [CrossRef]
65. Fell, J.; Fernandez, G.; Klaver, P.; Elger, C.E.; Fries, P. Is synchronized neuronal gamma activity relevant for selective attention? *Brain Res. Brain Res. Rev.* **2003**, *42*, 265–272. [CrossRef]
66. Jensen, O.; Mazaheri, A. Shaping functional architecture by oscillatory alpha activity: Gating by inhibition. *Front. Hum. Neurosci.* **2010**, *4*, 186. [CrossRef]
67. van Lutterveld, R.; Houlihan, S.D.; Pal, P.; Sacchet, M.D.; McFarlane-Blake, C.; Patel, P.R.; Sullivan, J.S.; Ossadtchi, A.; Druker, S.; Bauer, C.; et al. Source-space EEG neurofeedback links subjective experience with brain activity during effortless awareness meditation. *Neuroimage* **2017**, *151*, 117–127. [CrossRef]
68. Hsieh, L.T.; Ranganath, C. Frontal midline theta oscillations during working memory maintenance and episodic encoding and retrieval. *Neuroimage* **2014**, *85 Pt 2*, 721–729. [CrossRef]
69. Brandmeyer, T.; Delorme, A. Reduced mind wandering in experienced meditators and associated EEG correlates. *Exp. Brain Res.* **2018**, *236*, 2519–2528. [CrossRef]
70. Palva, S.; Palva, J.M. Functional roles of alpha-band phase synchronization in local and large-scale cortical networks. *Front. Psychol.* **2011**, *2*, 204. [CrossRef] [PubMed]
71. Litscher, G.; Wenzel, G.; Niederwieser, G.; Schwarz, G. Effects of QiGong on brain function. *Neurol. Res.* **2001**, *23*, 501–505. [CrossRef] [PubMed]
72. Cahn, B.R.; Delorme, A.; Polich, J. Occipital gamma activation during Vipassana meditation. *Cogn. Process.* **2010**, *11*, 39–56. [CrossRef]
73. Schoenberg, P.L.A.; Ruf, A.; Churchill, J.; Brown, D.P.; Brewer, J.A. Mapping complex mind states: EEG neural substrates of meditative unified compassionate awareness. *Conscious. Cogn.* **2018**, *57*, 41–53. [CrossRef] [PubMed]
74. Pagnoni, G. The contemplative exercise through the lenses of predictive processing: A promising approach. *Prog. Brain Res.* **2019**, *244*, 299–322. [CrossRef] [PubMed]
75. Aftanas, L.I.; Golocheikine, S.A. Human anterior and frontal midline theta and lower alpha reflect emotionally positive state and internalized attention: High-resolution EEG investigation of meditation. *Neurosci. Lett.* **2001**, *310*, 57–60. [CrossRef]
76. Baijal, S.; Srinivasan, N. Theta activity and meditative states: Spectral changes during concentrative meditation. *Cogn. Process.* **2010**, *11*, 31–38. [CrossRef] [PubMed]
77. Qin, Z.; Jin, Y.; Lin, S.; Hermanowicz, N.S. A forty-five year follow-up EEG study of Qigong practice. *Int. J. Neurosci.* **2009**, *119*, 538–552. [CrossRef]
78. Huang, H.Y.; Lo, P.C. EEG dynamics of experienced Zen meditation practitioners probed by complexity index and spectral measure. *J. Med. Eng. Technol.* **2009**, *33*, 314–321. [CrossRef] [PubMed]
79. Brandmeyer, T.; Delorme, A.; Wahbeh, H. The neuroscience of meditation: Classification, phenomenology, correlates, and mechanisms. In *Progress in Brain Research*; Elsevier: Amsterdam, The Netherlands, 2019; Volume 244, pp. 1–29.

80. Schneider, W.; Pimm-Smith, M.; Worden, M. Neurobiology of attention and automaticity. *Curr. Opin. Neurobiol.* **1994**, *4*, 177–182. [CrossRef]
81. Garrison, K.A.; Santoyo, J.F.; Davis, J.H.; Thornhill, T.A.T.; Kerr, C.E.; Brewer, J.A. Effortless awareness: Using real time neurofeedback to investigate correlates of posterior cingulate cortex activity in meditators' self-report. *Front. Hum. Neurosci.* **2013**, *7*, 440. [CrossRef] [PubMed]
82. Maharishi, M.Y. *Maharishi Mahesh Yogi on the Bhagavad Gita*; Penguin Books: New York, NY, USA, 1969.
83. Franklin, M.S.; Mrazek, M.D.; Anderson, C.L.; Smallwood, J.; Kingstone, A.; Schooler, J.W. The silver lining of a mind in the clouds: Interesting musings are associated with positive mood while mind-wandering. *Front. Psychol.* **2013**, *4*, 583. [CrossRef] [PubMed]
84. Travis, F.; Parim, N. Default mode network activation and Transcendental Meditation practice: Focused Attention or Automatic Self-transcending? *Brain Cogn.* **2017**, *111*, 86–94. [CrossRef]
85. Fox, M.D.; Raichle, M.E. Spontaneous fluctuations in brain activity observed with functional magnetic resonance imaging. *Nat. Rev. Neurosci.* **2007**, *8*, 700–711. [CrossRef]
86. Raichle, M.E. The brain's default mode network. *Annu. Rev. Neurosci.* **2015**, *38*, 433–447. [CrossRef]
87. Raichle, M.E.; Macleod, A.M.; Snyder, A.Z.; Powers, W.J.; Gusnard, D.A.; Shulman, G.L. A default mode of brain function. *Proc. Natl. Acad. Sci. USA* **2001**, *98*, 676–682. [CrossRef]
88. Buckner, R.L.; Vincent, J.L. Unrest at rest: Default activity and spontaneous network correlations. *Neuroimage* **2007**, *37*, 1091–1096. [CrossRef]
89. Garrison, K.A.; Zeffiro, T.A.; Scheinost, D.; Constable, R.T.; Brewer, J.A. Meditation leads to reduced default mode network activity beyond an active task. *Cogn. Affect. Behav. Neurosci.* **2015**, *15*, 712–720. [CrossRef]
90. Simon, R.; Engstrom, M. The default mode network as a biomarker for monitoring the therapeutic effects of meditation. *Front. Psychol.* **2015**, *6*, 776. [CrossRef] [PubMed]
91. Bærentsen, K.B.; Stødkilde-Jørgensen, H.; Sommerlund, B.; Hartmann, T.; Damsgaard-Madsen, J.; Fosnæs, M. An investigation of brain processes supporting meditation. *Cogn. Process.* **2010**, *11*, 57–84. [CrossRef] [PubMed]
92. Ives-Deliperi, V.L.; Solms, M.; Meintjes, E.M. The neural substrates of mindfulness: An fMRI investigation. *Soc. Neurosci.* **2011**, *6*, 231–242. [CrossRef] [PubMed]
93. Taylor, V.A.; Grant, J.; Daneault, V.; Scavone, G.; Breton, E.; Roffe-Vidal, S. Impact of mindfulness on the neural responses to emotional pictures in experienced and beginner meditators. *Neuroimage* **2011**, *57*, 1524–1533. [CrossRef]
94. Brewer, J.A.; Worhunsky, P.D.; Gray, J.R.; Tang, Y.Y.; Weber, J.; Kober, H. Meditation experience is associated with differences in default mode network activity and connectivity. *Proc. Natl. Acad. Sci. USA* **2011**, *108*, 20254–20259. [CrossRef]
95. Zhou, H.X.; Chen, X.; Shen, Y.Q.; Li, L.; Chen, N.X.; Zhu, Z.C.; Castellanos, F.X.; Yan, C.G. Rumination and the default mode network: Meta-analysis of brain imaging studies and implications for depression. *Neuroimage* **2020**, *206*, 116287. [CrossRef]
96. Antrobus, J.S.; Singer, J.L.; Goldstein, S.; Fortgang, M.S. Mind wandering and cognitive structure. *Trans. N. Y. Acad. Sci.* **1970**, *32*, 242–252. [CrossRef]
97. Singer, J.L. Navigating the stream of consciousness: Research in daydreaming and related inner experiences. *Am. Psychol.* **1975**, *30*, 727–738. [CrossRef]
98. Killingsworth, M.A.; Gilbert, D.T. A wandering mind is an unhappy mind. *Science* **2010**, *330*, 932. [CrossRef]
99. Stawarczyk, D.; Majerus, S.; Maj, M.; Van der Linden, M.; D'Argembeau, A. Mind-wandering: Phenomenology and function as assessed with a novel experience sampling method. *Acta Psychol.* **2011**, *136*, 370–381. [CrossRef]
100. Baird, B.; Smallwood, J.; Schooler, J.W. Back to the future: Autobiographical planning and the functionality of mind-wandering. *Conscious. Cogn.* **2011**, *20*, 1604–1611. [CrossRef] [PubMed]
101. Baird, B.; Smallwood, J.; Mrazek, M.D.; Kam, J.W.; Franklin, M.S.; Schooler, J.W. Inspired by distraction: Mind wandering facilitates creative incubation. *Psychol. Sci.* **2012**, *23*, 1117–1122. [CrossRef] [PubMed]
102. Vess, M.; Leal, S.A.; Hoeldtke, R.T.; Schlegel, R.J.; Hicks, J.A. True self-alienation positively predicts reports of mindwandering. *Conscious. Cogn.* **2016**, *45*, 89–99. [CrossRef] [PubMed]
103. Hobbiss, M.H.; Fairnie, J.; Jafari, K.; Lavie, N. Attention, mindwandering, and mood. *Conscious. Cogn.* **2019**, *72*, 1–18. [CrossRef]

104. Ottaviani, C.; Shapiro, D.; Couyoumdjian, A. Flexibility as the key for somatic health: From mind wandering to perseverative cognition. *Biol. Psychol.* **2013**, *94*, 38–43. [CrossRef]
105. Ottaviani, C.; Couyoumdjian, A. Pros and cons of a wandering mind: A prospective study. *Front. Psychol.* **2013**, *4*, 524. [CrossRef]
106. Travis, F. *Negative and Positive Mindwandering*; IGI Global: Hershey, PA, USA, 2020.

Publisher's Note: MDPI stays neutral with regard to jurisdictional claims in published maps and institutional affiliations.

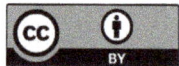

© 2020 by the author. Licensee MDPI, Basel, Switzerland. This article is an open access article distributed under the terms and conditions of the Creative Commons Attribution (CC BY) license (http://creativecommons.org/licenses/by/4.0/).

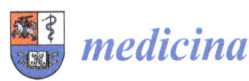

Review

Ayurgenomics and Modern Medicine

Robert Keith Wallace

Department of Physiology and Health, Maharishi International University, Fairfield, IA 52556, USA; kwallace@miu.edu

Received: 7 October 2020; Accepted: 27 November 2020; Published: 30 November 2020

Abstract: Within the disciplines of modern medicine, P4 medicine is emerging as a new field which focuses on the whole patient. The development of Ayurgenomics could greatly enrich P4 medicine by providing a clear theoretical understanding of the whole patient and a practical application of ancient and modern preventative and therapeutic practices to improve mental and physical health. One of the most difficult challenges today is understanding the ancient concepts of Ayurveda in terms of modern science. To date, a number of researchers have attempted this task, of which one of the most successful outcomes is the creation of the new field of Ayurgenomics. Ayurgenomics integrates concepts in Ayurveda, such as Prakriti, with modern genetics research. It correlates the combination of three doshas, Vata, Pitta and Kapha, with the expression of specific genes and physiological characteristics. It also helps to interpret Ayurveda as an ancient science of epigenetics which assesses the current state of the doshas, and uses specific personalized diet and lifestyle recommendations to improve a patient's health. This review provides a current update of this emerging field.

Keywords: Ayurgenomics; Ayurveda; genomics; P4 medicine; diet; lifestyle; disease; prevention; personalized medicine

---

1. Introduction

Ayurveda is the ancient system of traditional medicine in India. The term Ayurveda comes from two Sanskrit words, "ayus", meaning life or lifespan, and "Veda", meaning knowledge or science. Ayurveda may be translated as "the science of life", or more specifically, "the science of lifespan". Ayurveda was originally an oral tradition of natural health, and it was much later that this knowledge was written down in books [1]. Some of the knowledge became fragmented and lost due to many years of foreign rule in India.

The Tridosha theory of Ayurveda explains that there are three fundamental principles or forces, called doshas, which govern the physiology of each individual. Vata is the dosha involved in transportation in the body; from the transportation of molecules to the transportation of nervous impulses. It arises from the elements of ether and air. Pitta is the dosha that governs the process of digestion, as well as all metabolic pathways inside each cell. It is formed from fire and water. Kapha is the dosha that governs structure and cohesion in the body. It is an expression of earth and water. Each individual is born with a particular combination of these three doshas; this is called Prakriti. There are seven basic types of Prakriti: Vata; Pitta; Kapha; Vata/Pitta; Pitta/Kapha; Vata/Kapha; and Vata/Pitta/Kapha.

Is there a scientific explanation for Prakriti? The best description so far has come from the new field of Ayurgenomics, which attempts to describe Prakriti types in terms of modern genetics and physiology.

2. Studies on the Genetic Basis of Prakriti

A number of studies have correlated Prakriti with specific genetic and physiological measures. One early study in 2005 evaluated 76 subjects both for their Prakriti and human leucocyte antigen

(HLA) DRB1 types. The researchers observed a correlation between HLA type and Prakriti type, with a complete absence of the *HLA DRB1*02* allele in the Vata type and of *HLA DRB1*13* in the Kapha type. Furthermore, HLA DRB1*10 had higher allele frequency in the Kapha type compared to the Pitta and Vata types [2].

In 2008, a comprehensive study was done correlating biochemical and genome wide expression levels in subjects from the three main Prakriti groups. There were many distinct differences in the regulation of genes in each of the main Prakriti groups. In Pitta types, for example, there was an over-expression of genes in the immune response pathways. In Vata males, there was an over-expression of genes related to cell cycles, particularly in the regulation of cyclin-dependent protein kinase activity and the regulation of enzyme activity. In Kapha males, there was a down-regulation of genes involved in fibrinolysis and an up-regulation of genes involved in ATP and cofactor biosynthesis. In addition, the researchers observed certain physiological differences such as Kapha types having higher levels of triglycerides, total cholesterol, high low-density lipoprotein (LDL) and low high-DL (HDL), compared to Pitta and Vata types. In Pitta types, they found hemoglobin and the red blood count were higher, whereas serum prolactin was higher in Vata types [3].

A study in 2010 studied high-altitude adaptation and common variations rs479200 (C/T) and rs480902 (T/C) in the EGLN1 gene. They found that the TT genotype of rs479200 was more frequent in Kapha types, and was correlated with a higher expression of EGLN1. In contrast, it was present at a significantly lower frequency in Pitta, and nearly absent in natives of high altitude. One of their interpretation is that Pitta types are more protected at high altitudes (see Table 1) [4].

Table 1. Example of Prakriti and gene expression.

Prakriti Type	Gene Expression	Disease
Kapha/Vata	EGLN 1 higher	High Altitude Pulmonary Edema
Pitta	EGLN 1 lower	more adaptive for higher altitudes

Furthermore, a 2010 study showed that within Kapha types, there was a down-regulation of CYP2C19 genotypes, a family of genes that is involved in the detoxification and metabolism of certain drugs and an up-regulated in Pitta types [5]. In 2012, a paper appeared indicating that CD25 (activated B cells) and CD56 (natural killer cells) were higher in Kapha types [6].

A paper in 2012 studied rheumatoid arthritis patients and found that inflammatory genes were up-regulated in Vata types, while in Pitta and Kapha types there was an up-regulation of oxidative stress pathway genes [7]. In 2015, one of the most extensive and rigorous studies found that 52 SNPs (single nucleotide polymorphism) were significantly different in the three main types of Prakritis. Research also showed that the SNP (rs11208257) in PGM1 gene is correlated with energy production and is more homogenous and constant in Pitta than with Vata and Kapha types [8].

Another study done in 2015 identified DNA methylation signatures that distinguish the three major Prakriti types. The authors suggest that DNA methylation is probably coupled to chromatin regulation as a contributor to different Prakriti phenotypes, and that this research provides insight into the epigenetic mechanisms of the Ayurvedic personalized system of medicine [9].

One final paper in 2015 extended an earlier study, and found the combination of derived EGLN1 allele (HAPE associated) and ancestral VWF allele (thrombosis associated) was significantly high in the Kapha Prakriti group compared to the Pitta Prakriti group. They also showed a genetic link between EGLN1 and VWF, which could modify thrombosis/bleeding susceptibility and outcomes of hypoxia [10].

3. Studies on Physiology, Disease and Prakriti

A paper in 2003 showed that the Kapha Prakriti groups had a number of biochemical differences from Pittas or Vatas. They showed higher digoxin levels, increased glycoconjugate levels, increased free radical production and reduced scavenging, as well as increased tryptophan catabolites and reduced tyrosine catabolites [11]. In 2011, researchers found a significant decrease in the diastolic blood pressure immediately after isotonic exercise for five minutes in Vata-Kapha types, in contrast to Pitta-Kapha and Vata-Pitta types [12]. In another study, it was found that ADP-induced maximal platelet aggregation (MPA) was maximum among Vata-Pitta-type individuals [13].

Research reported in 2014 found a correlation between body mass index (BMI) and Prakriti type. It was reported that Kapha Prakriti subjects had a higher BMI than those with a Vata Prakriti [14]. A paper in 2015 found that Kapha types have higher parasympathetic activity and lower sympathetic activity in terms of cardiovascular reactivity, compared to Pitta or Vata types [15].

Several papers have also correlated disease conditions with Prakriti. A 2012 paper reported that Vata-Kapha types had significantly higher triglyceride, VLDL and LDL levels, as well as lower HDL cholesterol when compared with other constitution types. The researchers also found that Vata-Kapha Prakriti individuals had higher risk for diabetes mellitus, hypertension and dyslipidemia. In addition, Vata-Kapha types had higher levels of biochemical markers such as IL6, TNF alpha, hsCRP and HOMA IR. The Vata-Kapha and Kapha Prakriti groups were both correlated with higher levels of the inflammatory markers. The conclusion of the authors was that there is a high correlation of risk factors associated with the Vata-Kapha and Kapha Prakriti groups [16].

Another paper in 2012 looked at diabetic patients and studied the effects of walking (isotonic exercise). There was a significant decrease in systolic blood pressure in Vata-Pitta, Pitta-Kapha and Vata-Kapha types after walking. There was also a significant decrease in mean diastolic blood pressure in Vata-Pitta types [17]. Another paper found that the incidence of Parkinson's disease was highest in patients with a Vata Prakriti [18]. In a 2015 study of patients with irritable bowel syndrome, it was found that most of the Vata type patients had developed IBS-C, or irritable bowel syndrome associated with constipation. The patients who were Pitta dominant developed IBS-D, or irritable bowel syndrome associated with diarrhea. The quality of life was found to be better in in Pitta-type patients [19]. Finally, several papers have focused on the connection between the microbiome composition and Prakriti, and found a significant correlation between specific bacteria groups and Prakriti [20–22].

4. Theoretical Papers

In addition to the research papers, there have been a number of theoretical and review papers. In 2008 and 2010, papers began promoting the idea of the connection between Ayurveda and genomics [23,24]. In 2011, a review and theoretical papers appeared in which the term Ayurgenomics was presented [25–28]. Since 2012, there have been many theoretical and review papers on Ayurgenomics from different angles [29–41]. In a few of these papers, the focus is also on related fields such as Pharmacogenetics and Ayurnutrigenomics [31,32]. In one 2016 paper, Ayurveda is described as an ancient science of epigenetics [42].

5. Modern Medicine and Ayurgenomics

Modern medicine uses a highly reductionist system to describe the fundamental basis of our physiology and health, using terms like genome, gene expression and epigenetics. Ayurveda uses an entirely different holistic system, which includes terms such as dosha and Prakriti.

Unfortunately, modern medicine has not recognized many of the useful preventative approaches of Ayurveda, due to a cognitive bias against folk or traditional medicine. Even though traditional systems of medicine are still widely used in many countries around the world, more research on their preventative and therapeutic treatment programs is necessary [43].

Up to now, the research has been primarily on specific herbal preparations, with the main outcome being an attempt to isolate one active ingredient which can then be used by a pharmaceutical company. Ayurgenomics offers a new bridge between traditional medicine and modern medicine by providing a rigorous scientific understanding of basic concepts, and at the same time incorporating the practical preventative approaches of Ayurveda into modern medicine.

Over the last ten years, a new field has arisen in modern medicine, which is known as P4 medicine. The four Ps are: predictive; preventive; personalized; and participatory [44–47]. This new system attempts to switch the emphasis from a disease-oriented system to a wellness-oriented system centered around the patient. It is closely related to other new fields such as Integrative Medicine, Functional Medicine, Lifestyle Medicine, Personalized Medicine and Preventive Medicine.

Ayurveda and other systems of traditional medicine have been patient-oriented and predictive, preventive, personalized and participatory for many thousands of years.

Long before the advent of epigenetic and other fields such as nutrigenetics, Ayurveda understood how diet and other lifestyle factors could affect our health. They recognized what modern medicine is only beginning to comprehend, that prevention is key to health. Improvements in diet, sleep, exercise and stress management are crucial for an effectively preventative system of medicine.

The development of Ayurgenomics, as we have said, helps give credibility to Ayurveda and other systems of traditional medicine by describing their ancient concepts in terms of modern science. New approaches in Ayurgenomics, which use big data analysis and machine learning, may greatly facilitate this whole process [36,37,39]. Of course, the therapeutic programs of these system will ultimately have to be tested through carefully controlled clinical trials.

Ayurveda and genomics can contribute to each other. Modern science can help Ayurveda as an evidence-based system of medicine, and Ayurveda can help modern medicine, particularly through its preventative approaches. This is especially true with P4 medicine, which is based on many of the same principles of Ayurveda. Having time-tested personalized preventative lifestyle recommendations would make it easy for each individual to participate in their own self-care (see Figure 1).

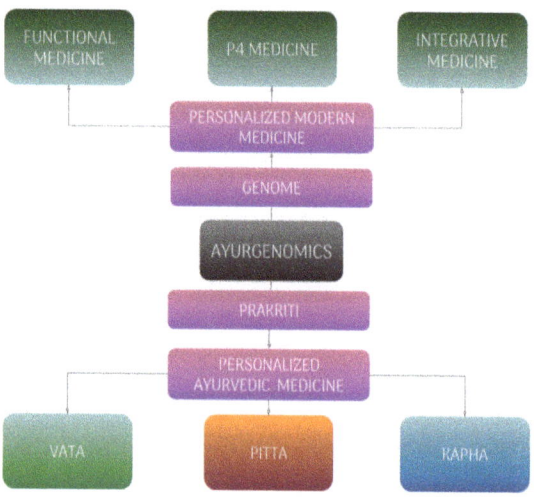

Figure 1. Ayurgenomics and its Relationship to Modern Medicine.

Ayurveda could also contribute to modern medicine in terms of the diagnosis of disease. Many believed that the enormous progress in the field of genomics would quickly bring a personalized system of medicine that could predict and prevent disease. Progress has been made, but researchers now realize that this may take longer than expected due to the highly complex nature of gene expression in the development of disease conditions. Ayurveda could help by stratifying individuals into broader categories using the Prakriti system of classification, along with modern genomics. Can we consider Prakriti as being our Ayurvedic genome? Can Ayurgenomics be used to diagnose and treat diseases?

These and many other questions will need to be answered by future research. We can only hope that a massive research effort is undertaken as soon as possible. The combination of Ayurveda and genomics promises to markedly improve many areas of healthcare throughout the world.

Funding: This research did not receive any specific grant from funding agencies in the public, commercial or not-for-profit sectors. A grant from the Wege Foundation helped pay for publication costs.

Acknowledgments: Thanks to Roxanne Medeiros for creating the graphic.

Conflicts of Interest: The author declares no conflict of interest.

References

1. Dash, B.; Sharma, R.K. *Charaka Samhita*; Caukhambha Orientalia: Varanasi, India, 1995.
2. Patwardhan, B.; Joshi, K.; Chopra, A. Classification of Human population based on HLA Gene Polymorphism and the Concept of Prakriti in Ayurveda. *J. Altern. Complementary Med.* **2005**, *11*, 349–353.
3. Prasher, B.; Negi, S.; Aggarwal, S.; Mandal, A.K.; Sethi, T.P.; Deshmukh, S.R.; Purohit, S.G.; Sengupta, S.; Khanna, S.; Mohammad, F.; et al. Whole Genome Expression and Biochemical Correlates of Extreme Constitutional Types Defined in Ayurveda. *J. Transl. Med.* **2008**, *6*, 48. [CrossRef] [PubMed]
4. Aggarwal, S.; Negi, S.; Jha, P.; Singh, P.K.; Stobdan, T.; Pasha, M.A. Indian genome variation consortium. EGLN1 involvement in high-altitude adaptation revealed through genetic analysis of extreme constitution types defined in Ayurveda. *Proc. Natl. Acad. Sci. USA* **2010**, *107*, 18961–18966. [CrossRef]
5. Ghodke, Y.; Joshi, K.; Patwardhan, B. Traditional medicine to modern pharmacogenomics: Ayurveda Prakriti type and CYP2C19 gene polymorphism associated with the metabolic variability. *Evid. Based Complementary Alternat. Med.* **2011**, 249528.
6. Rotti, H.; Guruprasad, K.P.; Nayak, J.; Kabekkodu, S.P.; Kukreja, H.; Mallya, S.; Nayak, J.; Bhradwaj, R.C.; Gangadharan, G.G.; Prasanna, B.V.; et al. Immunophenotyping of normal individuals classified on the basis of human dosha prakriti. *J. Ayurveda Integr. Med.* **2014**, *5*, 43–49. [CrossRef] [PubMed]
7. Juyal, R.C.; Negi, S.; Wakhode, P.; Bhat, S.; Bhat, B.; Thelma, B.K. Potential of ayurgenomics approach in complex trait research: Leads from a pilot study on rheumatoid arthritis. *PLoS ONE* **2012**, *7*, e45752. [CrossRef] [PubMed]
8. Govindaraj, P.; Nizamuddin, S.; Sharath, A.; Jyothi, V.; Rotti, H.; Raval, R.; Nayak, J.; Bhat, B.K.; Prasanna, B.V.; Shintre, P.; et al. Genome-wide analysis correlates Ayurveda Prakriti. *Sci. Rep.* **2015**, *5*, 15786. [CrossRef]
9. Rotti, H.; Mallya, S.; Kabekkodu, S.P.; Chakrabarty, S.; Bhale, S.; Bharadwaj, R.; Bhat, B.K.; Dedge, A.P.; Dhumal, V.R.; Gangadharan, G.G.; et al. DNA methylation analysis of phenotype specific stratified Indian population. *J. Transl. Med.* **2015**, *13*, 151. [CrossRef]
10. Aggarwal, S.; Gheware, A.; Agrawal, A.; Ghosh, S.; Prasher, B.; Mukerji, M.; Indian Genome Variation Consortium. Combined genetic effects of EGLN1 and VWF modulate thrombotic outcome in hypoxia revealed by Ayurgenomics approach. *J. Transl. Med.* **2015**, *13*, 184. [CrossRef]
11. Kurup, R.K.; Kurup, P.A. Hypothalamic digoxin, hemispheric chemical dominance, and the tridosha theory. *Int. J. Neurosci.* **2003**, *113*, 657–681. [CrossRef]
12. Tiwari, S.; Gehlot, S.; Tiwari, S.K.; Singh, G. Effect of walking (aerobic isotonic exercise) on physiological variants with special reference to Prameha (diabetes mellitus) as per Prakriti. *Ayu* **2012**, *33*, 44–49. [CrossRef] [PubMed]
13. Bhalerao, S.; Deshpande, T.; Thatte, U. Prakriti (Ayurvedic concept of constitution) and variations in Platelet aggregation. *BMC Complementary Altern. Med.* **2012**, *12*, 248–256. [CrossRef] [PubMed]
14. Rotti, H.; Raval, R.; Anchan, S.; Bellampalli, R.; Bhale, S.; Bharadwaj, R.; Bhat, B.K.; Dedge, A.P.; Dhumal, V.R.; Gangadharan, G.G.; et al. Determinants of prakriti, the human constitution types of Indian traditional medicine and its correlation with contemporary science. *J. Ayurveda Integr. Med.* **2014**, *5*, 167e75.
15. Rapolu, S.B.; Kumar, M.; Singh, G.; Patwardhan, K. Physiological variations in the autonomic responses may be related to the constitutional types defined in Ayurveda. *J. Humanitas Med.* **2015**, *5*, e7. [CrossRef]
16. Mahalle, N.P.; Kulkarni, M.V.; Pendse, N.M.; Naik, S.S. Association of constitutional type of Ayurveda with cardiovascular risk factors, inflammatory markers and insulin resistance. *J. Ayurveda Integr. Med.* **2012**, *3*, 150–157. [CrossRef]

17. Tripathi, P.K.; Patwardhan, K.; Singh, G. The basic cardiovascular responses to postural changes, exercise and cold pressor test: Do they vary in accordance with the dual constitutional types of Ayurveda? *Evid. Based Complementary Altern. Med.* **2011**, *201*, 251–259. [CrossRef]
18. Manyam, B.V.; Kumar, A. Ayurvedic constitution (prakruti) identifies risk factor of developing Parkinson's disease. *J. Altern. Complementary Med.* **2013**, *19*, 644–649. [CrossRef]
19. Shirolkar, S.G.; Tripathi, R.K.; Rege, N.N. Evaluation of prakṛti and quality-of-life in patients with irritable bowel syndrome. Ancient science of life. *J. Altern. Complementary Med.* **2015**, *34*, 210–215. [CrossRef]
20. Chauhan, N.S.; Pandey, R.; Mondal, A.K.; Gupta, S.; Verma, M.K.; Jain, S.; Ahmed, V.; Patil, R.; Agarwal, D.; Girase, B.; et al. Western Indian Rural Gut Microbial Diversity in Extreme Prakriti Endo-Phenotypes Reveals Signature Microbes. *Front. Microbiol.* **2018**, *9*, 118. [CrossRef]
21. Jnana, A.; Murali, T.S.; Guruprasad, K.P.; Satyamoorthy, K. Prakriti phenotypes as a stratifier of gut microbiome: A new frontier in personalized medicine? *J. Ayurveda Integr. Med.* **2020**, *11*, 360–365. [CrossRef]
22. Wallace, R.K. The Microbiome in Health and Disease from the Perspective of Modern Medicine and Ayurveda. *Medicina* **2020**, *56*, 462. [CrossRef] [PubMed]
23. Patwardhan, B.; Bodeker, G. Ayurvedic genomics: Establishing a genetic basis for mind-body typologies. *J. Altern. Complementary Med.* **2008**, *14*, 571–576. [CrossRef]
24. Joshi, K.; Ghodke, Y.; Shintre, P. Traditional medicine and genomics. *J. Ayurveda Integr. Med.* **2010**, *1*, 26–32. [CrossRef] [PubMed]
25. Rizzo-Sierra, C.V. Ayurvedic genomics, constitutional psychology, and endocrinology: The missing connection. *J. Altern. Complementary Med.* **2011**, *17*, 465–468. [CrossRef] [PubMed]
26. Chatterjee, B.; Pancholi, J. Prakriti-based medicine: A step towards personalized medicine. *Ayu* **2011**, *32*, 141–146. [CrossRef] [PubMed]
27. Mukerji, M.; Prasher, B. Ayurgenomics: A New Approach in Personalized and Preventive Medicine. *Sci. Cult.* **2011**, *77*, 10–17.
28. Sethi, T.P.; Prasher, B.; Mukerji, M. Ayurgenomics: A New Way of Threading Molecular Variability for Stratified Medicine. *ACS Chem. Biol.* **2011**, *6*, 875–880. [CrossRef]
29. Nayak, J. Ayurveda research: Ontological challenges. *J. Altern. Complementary Med.* **2012**, *3*, 17–20. [CrossRef]
30. Dey, S.; Pahwa, P. Prakriti and its associations with metabolism, chronic diseases, and genotypes: Possibilities of new born screening and a lifetime of personalized prevention. *J. Ayurveda Integr. Med.* **2014**, *5*, 15–24. [CrossRef]
31. Gupta, P.D. Pharmacogenetics, pharmacogenomics and Ayurgenomics for personalized medicine: A paradigm shift. *Indian J. Pharm. Sci.* **2015**, *77*, 135–141. [CrossRef]
32. Banerjee, S.; Debnath, P.; Debnath, P.K. Ayurnutrigenomics: Ayurveda-inspired personalized nutrition from inception to evidence. *J. Tradit. Complementary Med.* **2015**, *5*, 228–233. [CrossRef] [PubMed]
33. Prasher, B.; Gibson, G.; Mukerji, M. Genomic insights into ayurvedic and western approaches to personalized medicine. *J. Genet.* **2016**, *95*, 209–228. [CrossRef] [PubMed]
34. Mukerji, M.; Prasher, B. Genomics and traditional Indian ayurvedic medicine. In *Genomics and Society: Ethical, Legal, Cultural and Socioeconomic Implications*; Kumar, D., Chadwick, R., Eds.; Academic Press: Cambridge, MA, USA, 2016; pp. 271–292.
35. Prasher, B.; Varma, B.; Kumar, A.; Khuntia, B.K.; Pandey, R.; Narang, A.; Tiwari, P.; Kutum, R.; Guin, D.; Kukreti, R.; et al. Ayurgenomics for stratified medicine: TRISUTRA consortium initiative across ethnically and geographically diverse Indian populations. *J. Ethnopharmacol.* **2017**, *197*, 274–293. [CrossRef] [PubMed]
36. Mukerji, M.; Sagner, M. Genomics and Big Data Analytics in Ayurvedic Medicine. *Prog. Prev. Med.* **2019**, *4*, e0021. [CrossRef]
37. Tiwari, P.; Kutum, R.; Sethi, T.; Shrivastava, A.; Girase, B.; Aggarwal, S.; Patil, R.; Agarwal, D.; Gautam, P.; Agrawal, A.; et al. Recapitulation of Ayurveda constitution types by machine learning of phenotypic traits. *PLoS ONE* **2017**, *12*, e0185380. [CrossRef]
38. Jayasundar, R. If systems approach is the way forward, what can the Ayurvedic theory of Tridosha teach us? *Curr. Sci.* **2017**, *112*. [CrossRef]
39. Singh, H.; Bhargava, S.; Ganeshan, S.; Kaur, R.; Sethi, T.; Sharma, M.; Chauhan, M.; Chauhan, N.; Chauhan, R.; Chauhan, P.; et al. Big Data Analysis of Traditional Knowledge-based Ayurveda Medicine. *Prog. Prev. Med.* **2018**, *3*, e0020. [CrossRef]
40. Dhande, S.; Salunkhe, P. Ayurgenomics. *Inter. J. Res. Sci. Innov.* **2018**, *V*, 322–326.

41. Singh, S.; Gehlot, S.; Agrawal, N.K. Basis of Disease Manifestation: A Molecular and Ayurvedic Approach with an Integrated Concept of Ayurgenomics. *J. Nat. Remedies* **2019**, *19*. [CrossRef]
42. Sharma, H. Ayurveda: Science of life, genetics, and epigenetics. *Ayu* **2016**, *37*, 87–91. [CrossRef]
43. Lemonnier, N.; Zhou, G.B.; Prasher, B.; Mukerji, M.; Chen, Z.; Brahmachari, S.K.; Noble, D.; Auffray, C.; Sagner, M. Traditional knowledge-basedmedicine: A review of history, principles, and relevance in the present context of P4 systems medicine. *Prog. Prev. Med.* **2017**, *7*, e0011. [CrossRef]
44. Hood, L.; Heath, J.R.; Phelps, M.E.; Lin, B. Systems biology and new technologies enable predictive and preventative medicine. *Science* **2004**, *306*, 640–643. [CrossRef] [PubMed]
45. Weston, A.D.; Hood, L. Systems biology, proteomics, and the future of healthcare: Toward predictive, preventative, and personalized medicine. *J. Proteome Res.* **2004**, *3*, 179–196. [CrossRef] [PubMed]
46. Hood, L.; Balling, R.; Auffray, C. Revolutionizing medicine in the 21st century through systems approaches. *Biotechnol. J.* **2012**, *7*, 992–1001. [CrossRef] [PubMed]
47. Flores, M.; Glusman, G.; Brogaard, K.; Price, N.D.; Hood, L. P4 medicine: How systems medicine will transform the healthcare sector and society. *Pers. Med.* **2013**, *10*, 565–576. [CrossRef]

Publisher's Note: MDPI stays neutral with regard to jurisdictional claims in published maps and institutional affiliations.

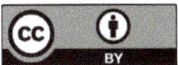

© 2020 by the author. Licensee MDPI, Basel, Switzerland. This article is an open access article distributed under the terms and conditions of the Creative Commons Attribution (CC BY) license (http://creativecommons.org/licenses/by/4.0/).

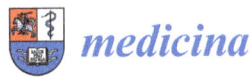

Systematic Review

A Systematic Review and Meta-Analysis of Ayurvedic Herbal Preparations for Hypercholesterolemia

Dinesh Gyawali [1,*], Rini Vohra [2], David Orme-Johnson [3], Sridharan Ramaratnam [4] and Robert H. Schneider [1,*]

1. College of Integrative Medicine, Maharishi International University, Fairfield, IA 52557, USA
2. School of Science of Consciousness, Maharishi University of Information Technology, Noida 201304, India; rinievohra@gmail.com
3. Maharishi International University, Fairfield, IA 52557, USA; davidoj@earthlink.net
4. Apollo Hospital, Greams Lane, Chennai, Tamil Nadu 600006, India; rsridharan52@gmail.com
* Correspondence: dgyawali@miu.edu (D.G.); RSchneider@miu.edu (R.H.S.)

Abstract: *Background and Objectives:* Cardiovascular disease (CVD) is the leading cause of death globally and hypercholesterolemia is one of the major risk factors associated with CVD. Due to a growing body of research on side effects and long-term impacts of conventional CVD treatments, focus is shifting towards exploring alternative treatment approaches such as Ayurveda. However, because of a lack of strong scientific evidence, the safety and efficacy profiles of such interventions have not been well established. The current study aims to conduct a systematic review and meta-analyses to explore the strength of evidence on efficacy and safety of Ayurvedic herbs for hypercholesterolemia. *Methods*: Literature searches were conducted using databases including Medline, Cochrane Database, AMED, Embase, AYUSH research portal, and many others. All randomized controlled trials on individuals with hypercholesterolemia using Ayurvedic herbs (alone or in combination) with an exposure period of $\geq$ 3 weeks were included, with primary outcomes being total cholesterol levels, adverse events, and other cardiovascular events. The search strategy was determined with the help of the Cochrane Metabolic and Endocrine Disorders Group. Two researchers assessed the risk of each study individually and discrepancies were resolved by consensus or consultation with a third researcher. Meta-analysis was conducted using the inverse variance method and results are presented as forest plots and data summary tables using Revman v5.3. *Results:* A systematic review of 32 studies with 1386 participants found randomized controlled trials of three Ayurvedic herbs, *Allium sativum* (garlic), *Commiphora mukul* (guggulu), and *Nigella sativa* (black cumin) on hypercholesterolemia that met inclusion criteria. The average duration of intervention was 12 weeks. Meta-analysis of the trials showed that guggulu reduced total cholesterol and low-density lipoprotein levels by 16.78 mg/dL (95% C.I. 13.96 to 2.61; *p*-value = 0.02) and 18.78 mg/dL (95% C.I. 34.07 to 3.48; *p* = 0.02), respectively. Garlic reduced LDL-C by 10.37 mg/dL (95% C.I. $-$17.58 to $-$3.16; *p*-value = 0.005). Black cumin lowered total cholesterol by 9.28 mg/dL (95% C.I. $-$17.36, to $-$1.19, *p*-value = 0.02). Reported adverse side effects were minimal. *Conclusion:* There is moderate to high level of evidence from randomized controlled trials that the Ayurvedic herbs guggulu, garlic, and black cumin are moderately effective for reducing hypercholesterolemia. In addition, minimal evidence was found for any side effects associated with these herbs, positioning them as safe adjuvants to conventional treatments.

Keywords: hypercholesterolemia; ayurveda; ayurvedic herbs; systematic review; meta-analysis

Citation: Gyawali, D.; Vohra, R.; Orme-Johnson, D.; Ramaratnam, S.; Schneider, R.H. A Systematic Review and Meta-Analysis of Ayurvedic Herbal Preparations for Hypercholesterolemia. *Medicina* **2021**, *57*, 546. https://doi.org/10.3390/medicina57060546

Academic Editor: Jimmy T. Efird

Received: 31 March 2021
Accepted: 18 May 2021
Published: 28 May 2021

Publisher's Note: MDPI stays neutral with regard to jurisdictional claims in published maps and institutional affiliations.

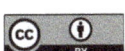

Copyright: © 2021 by the authors. Licensee MDPI, Basel, Switzerland. This article is an open access article distributed under the terms and conditions of the Creative Commons Attribution (CC BY) license (https://creativecommons.org/licenses/by/4.0/).

1. Introduction

Cardiovascular disease (CVD) is the number one cause of death globally [1]. High blood pressure, high LDL cholesterol, and smoking are the key risk factors for CVD and about 49% of Americans have at least one of the three [2]. Hypercholesterolemia (hyperlipidemia/hyperlipoproteinemia/or dyslipidemia) is a condition characterized by an elevation of any or all parameters of lipid profile or lipoprotein levels in the blood [3]. Hypercholesterolemia generally means high levels of total cholesterol or LDL-C with normal or low levels of HDL-C. The guidelines of National Cholesterol Education Program (NCEP) Adult Treatment Panel III (ATP III) suggests LDL-C level < 100 mg/dL, (100–129) mg/dL, (130–159) mg/dL, and >160 as optimal, above optimal, borderline high, and high, respectively. It also suggests that the LDL-C should be the primary target of any cholesterol reducing therapy [4]. As with other types of CVD, genetics, age, and gender are some of the non-modifiable risk factors for hypercholesterolemia. Hypercholesterolemia is one of the most significant contributors to the development of CVD, and if managed properly, is directly responsible for reducing risk of morbidity and mortality associated with CVD [5,6] (The Lipid Research Clinics Coronary Primary Prevention Trial results I and II). The burden of hypercholesterolemia is also reflected by recurring acute cardiovascular events [7] and higher healthcare costs [8]. Hypercholesterolemia is one of the top 10 costliest medical conditions in 2008 in the US adult population [9].

1.1. Treatment Approaches

Diet and lifestyle modifications with or before starting the cholesterol-lowering drugs are the primary line of treatment for hypercholesterolemia [4]. Although emphasis is given to lifestyle modifications, a majority of people are required to take drugs to have an adequate reduction in LDL-C levels [10]. At present, the main drug class of choice for hypercholesterolemia is statins. Studies have suggested that statins can reduce the chance of heart attack and prevent consequent death by 30–40% and reduce LDL-C levels by 25–40%. Other alternatives to statins are fibrates, nicotinic acids, and cholesterol absorption inhibitors such as ezetimibe [4,10]. While these cholesterol-reducing drugs are generally considered safe, they are not free from side effects [10]. It is well established now that statin use is highly associated with adverse events and their manifestations such as myositis, myalgia, rhabdomyolysis, cognitive loss, neuropathy, pancreatic and hepatic dysfunction, and sexual dysfunction [11]. In fact, statin use is also known to increase the risk of new-onset diabetes from anywhere between 28–43% [12]. Many times, drugs such as statins and ezetimibe do not even reach the desired reduction in LDL levels, with residual CVD risk still persisting [13]. Adverse events associated with conventional treatments is also one of the reasons why a large percentage of the US population does not treat hypercholesterolemia despite being aware of the condition [14]. Such issues have prompted researchers to explore alternative/integrative treatment approaches and multiple new therapies are emerging in that area [13]. Complementary and alternative medicine (CAM) treatments have shown significant benefits among individuals with hypercholesterolemia [15]. One of the CAM therapies that has shown promising results for hypercholesterolemia is Ayurveda [16].

1.2. Ayurveda

Ayurveda (translated as "the science of life") is one of the oldest medical systems in the world. Its origins date back to thousands of years ago in the Vedic era in the Indian subcontinent. Ayurveda defines life, "ayu", as a union of mind, body, spirit, and senses and health as the balanced state of these factors [17]. The wisdom of Ayurveda is based on three major classical texts, namely Charaka Samhita, Sushruta Samhita, and Ashtanga Hridaya, plus six minor texts. These ancient texts give detailed descriptions of over 700 herbs and 6000 formulations in addition to descriptions of various diseases, diagnostic methods, and dietary and lifestyle recommendations [18]. Ayurvedic treatment focuses on restoring the balance of the disturbed body–mind matrix through diet and behavioral modifications, administration of drugs, and detoxification and rejuvenation therapies. The branch of Ayurvedic science that deals with herbs and their qualities is called Dravyaguna vigyan. Ayurvedic formulations are prepared based on this knowledge and largely comprise herbs. Classical and proprietary Ayurvedic formulations may consist of a single herb or mixtures of many herbs in any form, viz., juice, extract, powder, tablet, or decoction.

Although there is no direct correlate for hypercholesterolemia in Ayurveda, dyslipidemia can be considered close to the Ayurvedic terms "medovriddhi" or "medodushti". The main herbs used in Ayurveda to reduce cholesterol are garlic (*Allium sativum*), guggulu

(*Commiphora mukul*), and arjuna (*Terminalia arjuna*) [19–21]. The authors of this paper looked into the most common Ayurvedic products used for high cholesterol. Either used alone or in combination with other herbs, these three herbs are found in most of the Ayurvedic formulations with some additional ingredients. The list of additional ingredients used in combination with the above-mentioned herbs may include pushkarmoola (*Inula racemosa*), ginger, turmeric, shilajit, punarnawa (*Boerrhavia diffusa*), triphala, *Nigella Sativa*, garcinia, *Cyperus rotundus*, and licorice. Many published clinical trials on Ayurvedic herbs for hypercholesterolemia have presented some evidence that these formulations are effective in reducing cholesterol [19–21]. However, many times, such RCTs are often limited by their study designs, sample sizes, or lack of validity and/or generalizability [22]. Recently, researchers have also been encouraged to apply principles of evidence-based medicine to Ayurveda [17,23].

1.3. Need for Study

Although there are many reviews for individual Ayurvedic herbs [20,24–27], there is a strong need to conduct a review to systematically summarize the available evidence as well as identify the strength of this evidence. Our preliminary search yielded one systematic review on the use of Ayurvedic herbs for Hyperlipidemia. Singh et al. (2007) [16] conducted a systematic review on Ayurvedic herbs and collateral treatments for hyperlipidemia and concluded that a significant number of researches show strong efficacy of Ayurvedic herbs for hyperlipidemia, with minimal reports of side effects. Despite its comprehensiveness, the review was limited by the use of randomized and quasi-randomized studies, arbitrary scoring methods to categorize studies, and a lack of systematic summarization of results using meta-analyses. With the current study, we aim to critically analyze the available evidence on potential benefits and harms of Ayurvedic herbs for hypercholesterolemia using Cochrane guidelines for conducting systematic reviews and meta-analyses. The current study adds on the systematic review of Singh et al. (2007) by providing strong conclusions using statistically accurate methods to establish unambiguous evidence.

2. Materials and Methods

The current review was conducted in accordance with the Preferred Reporting Items for Systematic Reviews and Meta-Analyses (PRISMA) guidelines [28], and a protocol was previously published with the Cochrane database [29] for systematic reviews and meta-analysis [30].

2.1. Search Strategy

A systematic literature review of all studies published and accessible through December 2020 was performed by two authors (DG and RS) using the following databases:

i. The Cochrane Library, Cochrane Database of Systematic Reviews (CDSR), Cochrane Controlled Trials Register (CENTRAL), Database of Abstracts of Reviews of Effectiveness (DARE), Health Technology Assessment Database (HTA), MEDLINE, EMBASE, AMED (Allied and Complementary Medicine Database), World Health Organization (WHO) ICTRP (International Clinical Trials Registry Platform-http://apps.who.int/trialsearch/, accessed on 1 December 2020), ClinicalTrials.gov, EU Clinical Trials Register, and Europe PubMed Central. A MEDLINE (via Ovid platform) email alert service was continuously applied to identify newly published studies using the same search strategy as described for MEDLINE. If any additional relevant key words were detected during any of the electronic or other searches, the electronic search strategies were modified to incorporate these terms and document the changes.

ii. Clinical Trial Registry India, AYUSH research portal (Evidence Based Research Data of AYUSH Systems at Global Level, Department of AYUSH, Ministry of Health & Family Welfare, Government of India), *Journal of Research in Ayurveda and Siddha, The Journal of Research & Education in Indian Medicine* (JERIM), *AYU* (publication of Gujarat Ayurveda University, India), *The International Journal for Ayurveda Research, Journal of Drug Research in Ayurveda, Journal of Ayurveda and Integrative Medicine, Ancient Science of Life, International Journal of Ayurveda and Pharma Research,* A Bibliography of Indian Medicine (ABIM), Digital Helpline for Ayurveda Research Articles (DHARA), *Indian Heart Journal.*

iii. Other resources. Every effort was made to identify other potentially eligible trials or ancillary publications by searching the reference lists of retrieved included trials, systematic reviews, meta-analyses, and health technology assessment reports. In addition, study authors of included trials were contacted to identify any further studies that may have been missed.

Selection of studies: Abstract, title, or both of every record retrieved was scanned to determine which studies should be assessed further. All potentially relevant articles were investigated as full text. In case of any discrepancy, consensus was made with a discussion between all authors. An adapted PRISMA (Preferred Reporting Items for Systematic Reviews and Meta-Analyses) flow diagram was presented showing the process of study selection [28]. For studies fulfilling inclusion criteria, key participant and intervention characteristics were abstracted and data on efficacy outcomes and adverse events were reported using standard data extraction templates as supplied by the Cochrane Metabolic and Endocrine Disorders Group and Cochrane Hypertension Group. Efforts were made to find the protocol of each included study, and primary, secondary, and other outcomes are reported in comparison with data in publications in a joint appendix, "Matrix of study endpoint (publications and trial documents)". Duplicate studies, companion documents or multiple reports of a primary study, and yield of information was maximized by collating all available data, and the most complete dataset aggregated across all known publications was used. In case of doubt, priority was given to the publication reporting the longest follow-up associated with primary or secondary outcomes of these studies.

Types of studies: All relevant randomized controlled trials (RCTs) irrespective of publication status, blinding, and language were included. The original authors were contacted to confirm the details on random list generation and allocation concealment when possible. Quasi-randomized or non-randomized and studies shorter than 3 weeks in duration were not included. However, those studies were separately analyzed to document the available evidence. Trials that studied non-pharmacological approaches of Ayurveda (for example, Panchakarma) as a single intervention were excluded. Where participants were given some other treatments such as statins, in addition to Ayurvedic herbal preparations, the studies were included if the treatment was evenly distributed between groups and it was only Ayurvedic treatment that was randomized.

Participants: All studies where participants have high blood cholesterol levels (diagnosed as per the standard laboratory tools) without restrictions of age, gender, ethnicity, and other medical conditions were included. Study participants were considered eligible irrespective of the duration and chronicity of the condition and/or treatment duration. Studies with participants having a mean total cholesterol level greater than 200 mg/dL (5.2 mmol/L) or LDL cholesterol > 130 mg/dL were included. ATP III suggests above readings are the levels of borderline high risk (NCEP, 2001). Studies where participants are not subject to standard laboratory tests to diagnose hypercholesterolemia were not included.

Interventions: The following comparisons of intervention versus control/comparator were carried out.

(a) Ayurvedic herbal preparations. These include extracts from mixtures of herbs, single herbs, Ayurvedic proprietary medicines, or a compound of herbs that are prescribed by an Ayurvedic practitioner. All the available interventions under this category, regardless of their mechanism of action, were included;

(b) Ayurvedic herbal preparations in addition to standard care. Studies with Ayurvedic herbal medicines and conventional treatment for cholesterol (for example statins) as an intervention were also included as long as both the arms of the randomized trials received the conventional treatment.

2.1.1. Comparison Groups
- Placebo compared with (a) or (b);
- Usual care compared with (a) or (b);
- Non-pharmacological intervention (for example diet, exercise, or both);
- No intervention.

2.1.2. Outcomes

Primary Outcomes
- Total cholesterol levels;
- Adverse events;
- Major adverse cardiovascular events such as MI, stroke.

Secondary Outcomes
- Serum triglyceride levels;
- High-density lipoprotein (HDL) levels;
- Low-density lipoprotein (LDL) levels;
- Changes in body mass index (BMI) and body weight;
- Morbidity and or mortality;
- Health-related quality of life;
- Socioeconomic effects.

Method and timing of outcome measurement: A systematic method was applied to measure outcomes both method wise and timing wise. Regarding methods, standardized measurement instruments were used for those outcomes which can be measured objectively, such as lipid levels, BMI, and body weight. For other outcome measures such as health-related quality of life and socioeconomic effects, standardized/valid scales of measurements were used when available, or widely acceptable definitions of the outcomes were followed.

All the studies were categorized in two broad groups based on timing of outcome measurement "short-term" group with timing of at least 3 weeks and "long-term" group of more than 6 months. Outcomes including lipid levels, BMI, and body weight were considered in the short-term group whereas other outcomes such as health-related quality of life, adverse events, morbidity, and mortality, along with lipid levels, BMI, and body weight, were considered in the long-term group.

Data collection, analysis, and calculation of treatment effects: We used pre-designed standard data abstraction forms to collect data and software Revman, Version 5.3 (The Cochrane Collaboration, The Nordic Cochrane Centre, Copenhagen, Denmark) to enter, analyze, and synthesize the data. Results were presented in forest plots and data summary tables. Dichotomous data were calculated in risk ratio or odds ratio with a 95% confidence interval (CI) whereas the continuous data were calculated in mean difference with a 95% CI and standardized mean difference with a 95% CI.

Meta-analysis method: Inverse variance method was used for meta-analysis. Dichotomous data were expressed as odds ratios (ORs) or risk ratios (RRs) with 95% confidence intervals (CIs). Continuous data were expressed as mean differences (MDs) with 95% CIs. Time-to-event data were expressed as hazard ratios (HRs) with 95% CIs. The formulas for meta-analysis were used as described by Deeks and Higgins in the supplementary statistical guidelines for the software Revman 5.3 [31]. The level at which randomization occurred was closely monitored, such as cross-over trials, cluster-randomized trials, and multiple observations for the same outcome.

2.1.3. Assessment of Risk of Bias in Included Studies

DG and RS assessed risk in individual studies independently. Disagreements were resolved by consensus, or by consultation with SR. The Cochrane Collaboration's tool was used to assess the risk of bias [29,32]. The following criteria were assessed for this purpose:

- Random sequence generation (selection bias);
- Allocation concealment (selection bias);
- Blinding of participants and personnel (performance bias);
- Blinding of outcome assessment (detection bias);
- Incomplete outcome data (attrition bias).

Risk of bias criteria was judged as "low risk", "high risk", or "unclear risk" and individual bias items were evaluated as described in the *Cochrane Handbook for Systematic Reviews of Interventions* [29].

Missing Data: Missing data were obtained from authors where possible, and reasons for missing data (attrition rates, e.g., drop-outs, losses to follow-up and withdrawals, issues of missing data and imputation methods (e.g., last observation carried forward [LOCF])) were investigated and critically appraised. Missing standard deviations (SD) were imputed (average of SD of studies where reported) and the impact of imputation on meta-analyses was investigated by sensitivity analyses.

Assessment of Heterogeneity: Causes of any significant clinical, methodological, or statistical heterogeneity were explored but the pooled effect estimate in a meta-analysis was still presented. Heterogeneity was identified through visual inspection of the forest plots and by using a standard chi-square test α and the I^2 statistic < 75% [33]. If 10 or more studies were included investigating a particular outcome, funnel plots were used to assess small study effects. Several explanations can be offered for the asymmetry of a funnel plot, including true heterogeneity of effect with respect to trial size, poor methodological design (and hence bias of small trials), and publication bias. Therefore, results were interpreted carefully [34].

2.1.4. Data Analyses

Revman (Version 5.3) was used to compute effect sizes as well as other statistical information such as *p*-values, t-scores, Q statistics, and confidence intervals. Forest plots, funnel plots, and data summary tables were created utilizing this software. Unless there was good evidence for homogeneous effects across studies, primarily low risk of bias data was summarized using a random-effects model [35]. Random-effects meta-analyses were interpreted with due consideration of the whole distribution of effects by presenting a prediction interval [36]. A prediction interval specifies a predicted range for the true treatment effect in an individual study [37]. Statistical analyses were performed according to the statistical guidelines in the latest version of the *Cochrane Handbook for Systematic Reviews of Interventions* [29].

2.2. Subgroup Analysis and Investigation of Heterogeneity

The following characteristics were expected to introduce clinical heterogeneity and, when possible, subgroup analyses were conducted:

- Age;
- Ethnicity;
- Geographical location;
- Diet pattern (Indian diet and Western diet, salt-restricted diet and salt-unrestricted diet, etc.)

2.3. Sensitivity Analysis

Sensitivity analyses was performed in order to explore the influence of the following factors (when applicable) on effect sizes:

- Restricting the analysis to published studies;
- Restricting the analysis by considering risk of bias, as specified in Section 2.1.3 (Assessment of Risk of Bias in Included Studies);
- Restricting the analysis to very long or large studies to establish the extent to which they dominate the results;

- Restricting the analysis to studies using the following filters: diagnostic criteria, imputation, language of publication, source of funding (industry versus other), and country.

The robustness of the results was tested by repeating the analysis using different measures of effect size (RR, odds ratio (OR), etc.) and different statistical models (fixed-effect and random-effects models).

2.4. Including Non-Randomized Studies

When there were only a small number of randomized studies identified for systematic review and meta-analysis, non-randomized studies were also included. These non-randomized studies may be quasi-randomized, controlled clinical trials, or simply before-after clinical trials.

However, data from both randomized and non-randomized studies were not combined together in the same analysis as this may affect the strength of the evidence. The guidelines from *Cochrane Handbook of Systematic Reviews and Meta-Analysis* says that "where randomized trial evidence is desired but unlikely to be available, eligibility criteria could only be structured to say that nonrandomized studies would only be included where randomized trials are found not to be available. In time, as such a review is updated the non-randomized studies may be dropped when randomized trials become available" [29] (p. 397).

3. Results

A total of 1756 potentially relevant studies were found by searching the databases MEDLINE, CENTRAL, AMED, EMBASE, WHO ICTRP, Dhara online, AYUSH research portal, Clinicaltrials.gov, and INDMED. Through hand searches, 18 more studies were identified. After duplication and screening of the titles of obtained records, a total of 447 studies were considered for further screening. After perusal of the titles and abstracts, 387 studies were excluded due to the following reasons: focusing on herbs not part of Ayurveda (Western and Chinese herbs), reviews, observational studies, and not meeting the inclusion criteria. Sixty studies were found potentially eligible at this stage and the full papers were obtained. Among these, 14 studies were non-randomized, 8 studies did not fulfill initial inclusion criteria, 4 were either incomplete or potentially ongoing, and the full text of 2 studies could not be obtained. Hence, only 32 studies were ultimately included in the systematic review, of which 24 studies were qualified to be included in the meta-analysis. The characteristics of the included studies are included in Table 1. An adapted PRISMA [28] flow-chart of the study selection appears in Figure 1.

Excluded studies: Among potentially relevant studies, 28 were excluded for the following reasons. Two studies were of short duration, fourteen were non-randomized, and two could not be included as their full text could not be retrieved. Ten studies did not meet the minimum inclusion criteria. Studies investigating the use of Western herbal preparations that are not used in Ayurveda and pharmacological studies were excluded. Studies of garlic using garlic oil or aged garlic were also excluded because these are not described in classical Ayurvedic literature.

Table 1. Characteristics of included studies.

Study ID	Intervention & Comparator	Duration of Intervention	Description of Participants	Trial Period	Country, Place	Setting	Ethnic Groups (%)
Prakash 2016 [38]	I: T. arjuna	12 weeks	Age < 20 years, total cholesterol ≥ 200 mg/dL, LDL-C ≥ 130 mg/dL	-	India	Outpatient clinic of university hospital	-
	C: Rosuvastatin						-
Farzaneh 2014 [39]	I: N. sativa	8 weeks	Adult overweight females with sedentary lifestyle and total cholesterol > 200 mg/dL	-	Iran	University clinic	-
	C: Placebo						-
Rathi 2013 [40]	I: Rasonadi leha + Hridroghar churna + Usual care	3 months	Patients of post MI attending private hospital of Betul, Madhya Pradesh, India	-	India	Hospital	-
	C: Usual care						
Devra 2012 [41]	I: Tulsi extract	3 months	Patients of metabolic syndrome	-	India	Hospital	-
	C: Placebo						-
Huseini 2012 [42]	I: Aloe	2 months	Patients with type 2 diabetes and hyperlipidemia	-	Iran	Outpatient clinic	-
	C: Placebo						-
Joseph 2012 [43]	I: Amla + Fenugreek	12 weeks	Patients of hypercholesterolemia with total cholesterol > 220 mg/dL	-	-	Outpatient department of tertiary teaching hospital	-
	C: Atorvastatin						
Sabzghabaee 2012 [44]	I: N. sativa	4 weeks	Patients with toral cholesterol > 200 mg/dL	July 2010–June 2011	Iran	Outpatient clinics of University hospital	-
	C: Placebp						
Sharma 2012 [45]	I: Lashunadi guggulu	45 days	Clinically diagnosed and confirmed patients of stable angina from out and in-patient departments of two hospitals of Jaipur, India	2002–2004	India	University hospital	-
	C: Placebo						
Sobenin 2010 [46]	I: Allicor	12 months	Patients with documented CHD, 40–65 years age and s. cholesterol level > 200 mg/dL	-	Russia	Probably research center	-
	C: Placebo						-
Nohr 2009 [47]	I: Guggulu formula	12 (weeks)	Patients from Norwegian general practice who are not taking any prescriptions for hypercholesterolemia, CHD, DM	Feb–May 2003	Oppland and Hedemark counties of Norway	General practice	Native Norwegians
	C: Placebo						Native Norwegians

Table 1. Cont.

Study ID	Intervention & Comparator	Duration of Intervention	Description of Participants	Trial Period	Country, Place	Setting	Ethnic Groups (%)
Qidwai 2009 [48]	I: N. sativa	6 weeks	Patients with total cholesterol level > 180 to 250 mg/dL	Feb 2006–Jan 2007	Pakistan	Outpatient clinics at university hospital	Pakistani
	C: Placebo						Pakistani
Alizadeh-Navaei 2008 [49]	I: Ginger	45 days	Patients of hyperlipidemia with cholesterol > 200 mg/dL or Triglyceride > 200 mg/dL	April 2004–May 2005	Babol, Iran	Cardiac clinic	-
	C: Placebo						-
Sobenin 2008 [50]	I: Allicor	12 weeks	Men with mild hypercholesterolemia	-	Moscow, Russia	Research center	-
	C: Placebo						-
Gardner 2007 a [51]	I: Raw Garlic	6 months	Adults with LDL-C 130–190 mg/dL	Nov 2002–June 2005	USA	University hospital clinic	White (73) Black (4) Asian (18) Hispanic (2)
	C: Placebo						White (64) Asian (14) Hispanic (4)
Gardner 2007 b [51]	I: Garlic in tablets	6 months	Adults with LDL-C 130–190 mg/dL	Nov 2002–June 2005	USA	University hospital clinic	White (66) Black (4) Asian (21) Hispanic (6)
	C: Placebo						White (64) Asian (14) Hispanic (4)
Ashraf 2005 [52]	I: Garlic	12 weeks	Type 2 diabetes mellitus patients with newly diagnosed hyperlipidaemia	-	Karachi, Pakistan	University hospital	-
	C: Placebo						-
Tanannai 2004 [53]	I: Garlic	9 months	Hypercholesterolemia	-	Bangkok, Thailand	Hospital	Thai
	C: Placebo						Thai
Satitvipawee 2003 [54]	I: Garlic	12 weeks	Hypercholesterolemia	-	Thailand	Study center	-
	C: Placebo						-
Szapary 2003 [21]	I: Guggulipid	8 (weeks)	Ambulatory, community-dwelling, healthy adults with hypercholesterolaemia	March 2000–August 2001	Philadelphia, Pa, metropolitan area	University hospital	White (85)
	C: Placebo						White (75)

Table 1. Cont.

Study ID	Intervention & Comparator	Duration of Intervention	Description of Participants	Trial Period	Country, Place	Setting	Ethnic Groups (%)
Venkataramaiah 2002 [55]	I: Abana C: Simvastatin	8 weeks	Patients with total cholesterol > 200 mg/dL or triglycerides > 200 mg/dL	-	-	-	-
Kannar 2001 [56]	I: Garlic C: Placebo	12 weeks	Volunteers who failed to comply with previous lipid-lowering therapies	-	Victoria, Australia	University clinic	-
Gardner 2001 [57]	I: Garlic C: Placebo	12 weeks	General public and employees of Stanford University	June–October, 1997	Stanford University, Palo Alto, CA	University hospital	-
Adler 1997 [58]	I: Garlic C: Placebo	12 weeks	Men with elevated T. cholesterol level > 5.2 mmol/L (200 mg/dL)	-	Guelph, Ontario, Canada	University hospital/clinic	-
Awasthi 1997 [59]	I: Lashunadi guggulu C: Placebo	2 months	Patients of chronic stbale angina from two hospitals in Jaipur	-	Jaipur, India	University hospital	-
Gaur 1997 [60]	I: Gugulipid and usual care C: Usual care	4/4 (weeks)	Patients of ischaemic stroke	-	India	-	-
Singh 1994 [61]	I: Guggluipid C: Placebo	24 weeks	Patients with hypercholesterolaemia with s. cholesterol level > 200 mg/dL	-	India	-	White (70) Black (30) White (68) Black (32)
Jain 1993 [62]	I: Garlic C: Placebo	12 weeks	Patients with s. total cholesterol level > 220 mg/dL	-	USA	Outpatient clinic	-
Tiwari 1991 [63]	I: Abana C: Propanlol	6 months	Diagnosed cases of hypertension and Angina pectoris	-	India	University hospital	-
Mader 1990 [64]	I: Garlic C: Placebo	4 months	Patients of hyperlipidaemia from 30 different practices in Germany	-	Germany	General practice	-
Nityanand 1989 [65]	I: Guggluipid C: Clofibrate	12 weeks	Patients with s. cholesterol levels > 220 mg/dL	-	India	-	-

Table 1. *Cont.*

Study ID	Intervention & Comparator	Duration of Intervention	Description of Participants	Trial Period	Country, Place	Setting	Ethnic Groups (%)
Verma 1988 [66]	I: Guggulu	16 weeks	Patients of hyperlipidaemia between age 40–60 years Type IIa or IIb of Frederichsons classification of hyperlipidemia	-	India	University hospital	-
	C: Placebo						-
Kotiyal 1984 [67]	I: Guggulu	12 weeks	Patients with features of obesity, 10% overweight for one's height, age, and sex	-	India	Medical OPD of a hospital	-
	C: Placebo						-
Kuppurajan 1978 [68]	I: Guggulu	3 weeks	Patients with s. cholesterol > 300 mg/dL or total lipids > 750 mg/dL	-	India	-	-
	C: Placebo						-

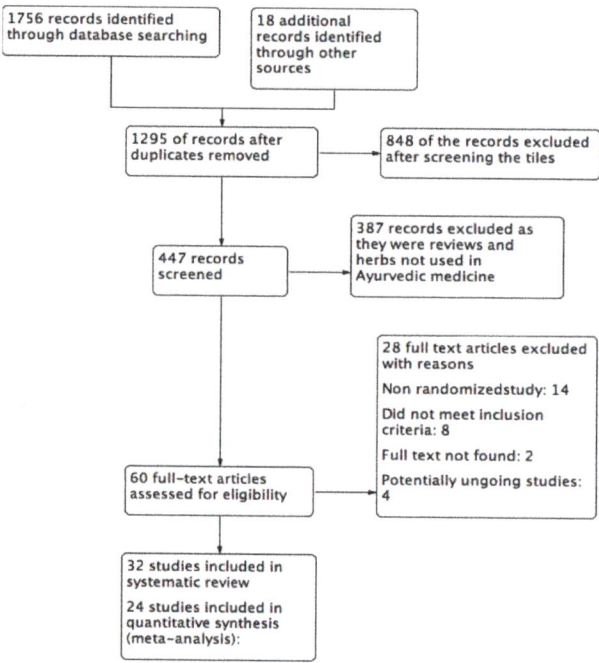

Figure 1. Study flow diagram on Ayurvedic herbal preparations for hypercholesterolemia.

Risk of bias assessment: Although the majority of the studies were randomized and double-blind, they failed to provide details of random sequence generation and allocation concealment. It was definitely inadequate in the majority of the studies. Only six studies out of 32 explained the random sequence generation. Two studies had high risk of bias in blinding whereas seven studies did not specify their blinding status. Both participants and investigators were blinded in 22 studies. In general, the blinding was achieved by using identical looking treatment and placebo tablets or capsules. However, the blinding of participants and investigators was more common than the blinding of outcome assessors. There was less information about the outcome assessment methods and personnel. Fifteen studies were prone to have attrition bias as the dropouts were not included in the final analysis. In one of the studies [59], 50% withdrawal was reported and the explanation was given as "unavoidable circumstances". In another study [48], 39 out of 64 participants in the treatment group and 34 out of 59 participants in the control group completed the study. Since many of the studies did not provide information on their protocol, it is hard to say if selective outcome reporting bias existed. However, based on the methods in the studies, all but three of the studies did not seem to have selective outcome reporting bias. A table of risk of bias assessment is given in Table 2.

Table 2. Risk of bias for included studies.

Study ID	Random Sequence Generation	Allocation Concealment	Blinding	Attrition Bias	Selective Outcome Reporting
Prakash 2016	U	U	U	U	L
Farzaneh 2014	U	U	L	H	L
Rathi 2013	U	U	U	H	L
Devra 2012	U	U	U	U	L

Table 2. *Cont.*

Study ID	Random Sequence Generation	Allocation Concealment	Blinding	Attrition Bias	Selective Outcome Reporting
Huseini 2012	L	L	L	L	L
Joseph 2012	U	U	U	U	L
Sabzghabaee 2012	U	L	U	U	L
Sharma 2012	U	U	L	H	L
Sobenin 2010	U	U	L	H	L
Nohr 2009	L	L	L	H	L
Qidwai 2009	U	U	L	H	L
Alizadeh-Navaei 2008	U	U	L	U	L
Sobenin 2008	U	U	L	U	L
Gardner 2007	L	L	L	L	L
Ashraf 2005	U	U	H	L	L
Tanamai 2004	U	U	L	H	L
Satitvipawee 2003	L	L	L	L	L
Szapary 2003	L	L	L	L	L
Venkataramaiah 2002	U	U	U	U	U
Kannar 2001	U	U	L	L	L
Gardner 2001	U	U	L	L	L
Adler 1997	U	U	L	L	L
Awasthi 1997	U	U	L	H	L
Gaur 1997	U	U	U	H	L
Singh 1994	U	U	L	H	L
Jain 1993	U	U	H	L	L
Tiwari 1991	U	U	L	H	L
Mader 1990	L	L	L	L	L
Nityanand 1989	U	U	L	H	L
Verma 1988	U	U	L	U	L
Kotiyal 1984	U	U	L	U	L
Kuppurajan 1978	U	U	L	H	L

L: low risk; H: high risk; U: unclear risk.

3.1. Effects of Ayurvedic Herbs

3.1.1. Total Cholesterol (TC) (mg/dL)

Overall, Ayurvedic herbal formulations were found to be effective in reducing total cholesterol by approximately 7.5%. A meta-analysis of 24 randomized controlled trials on four different Ayurvedic interventions, namely garlic, guggulu, *Nigella sativa*, and a combination of garlic and guggulu (*Lashunadi Guggulu*), involved a total of 1386 participants with 699 in the Ayurvedic group and 687 participants in the control group (Table 3).

Figure 2, a forest plot of the meta-analysis, shows that the most effective intervention is Lashunadi Guggulu (garlic + guggulu), with a reduction of 38.28 mg/dL in TC (95% C.I.: −55.11 to 21.14; $p < 0.00001$). The second most effective intervention was guggulu (*Commiphora mukul*), reducing TC by 16.78 mg/dL (95% C.I.: −13.96 to −2.61; $p = 0.02$) or almost 8.5% of borderline high TC levels. The third most effective intervention for reducing high TC was found to be garlic. Analysis of findings from 11 studies comparing

404 participants taking garlic with 409 participants on a placebo showed that garlic reduces TC by 12.45 mg/dL (95% C.I.: −18.68 to −6.22, p < 00001). Finally, the intervention with the least effect was found to be *Nigella sativa*, reducing TC by 9.28 mg/dL (95% C.I.: −17.36 to −1.19; p = 0.02).

Table 3. Effect of Ayurvedic herbal preparations in total cholesterol (mg/dL).

Outcome or Subgroup	Studies	Participants	Statistical Method	Effect Estimate
1.1 Total Cholesterol level	24	1386	Mean Difference (IV, Random, 95% CI)	
1.1.1 Garlic	11	813	Mean Difference (IV, Random, 95% CI)	−12.45 (−18.68, −6.22)
1.1.2 Guggulu	8	380	Mean Difference (IV, Random, 95% CI)	−16.78 (−30.96, −2.61)
1.1.3 Nigella	3	163	Mean Difference (IV, Random, 95% CI)	−9.28 (−17.36, −1.19)
1.1.5 Garlic + guggulu	2	30	Mean Difference (IV, Random, 95% CI)	−38.28 (−55.11, −21.44)

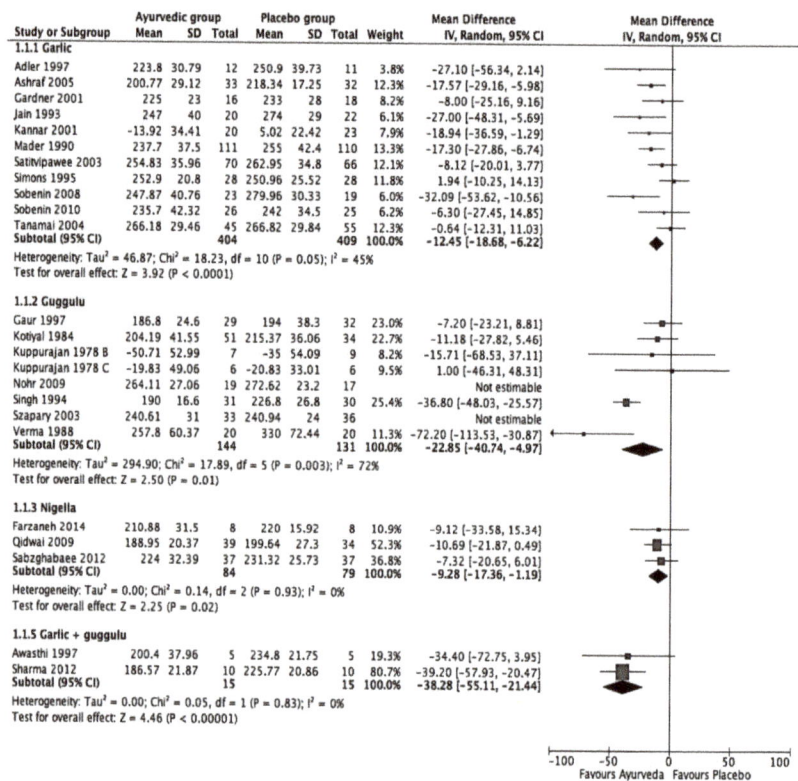

Figure 2. Forest plot on effect of Ayurvedic herbal preparations on total cholesterol (mg/dL).

3.1.2. LDL Cholesterol (mg/dL)

As shown in Table 4 and Figure 3, garlic was found to reduce LDL-C by 10.37 mg/dL (95% C.I.: −17.58 to −3.16; p = 0.005). This result is nearly 8% of the borderline LDL-C levels. The heterogeneity between garlic studies was 66%. As compared to the placebo, guggulu was found to reduce LDL-C by −18.78 mg/dL (95% C.I.: −34.07 to −3.48; p = 0.02). Unlike the results for total cholesterol, *Nigella sativa* did not have significant effects on a reduction in LDL-C (2.12 mg/dL (95% C.I.: −7.85 to 3.6; p = 0.47)), as shown in Figure 3. Altogether, these studies included 163 participants, of which 84 people were in an intervention group and the remaining 79 were in the control group.

Table 4. Effect of Ayurvedic herbal preparations on LDL-C (mg/dL).

Outcome or Subgroup	Studies	Participants	Statistical Method	Effect Estimate
1.2 LDL-Cholesterol level	21	1183	Mean Difference (IV, Random, 95% CI)	
1.2.1 Garlic	12	734	Mean Difference (IV, Random, 95% CI)	−10.37 (−17.58, −3.16)
1.2.2 Guggulu	5	266	Mean Difference (IV, Random, 95% CI)	−18.78 (−34.07, −3.48)
1.2.3 Nigella	3	163	Mean Difference (IV, Random, 95% CI)	−2.12 (−7.85, 3.60)
1.2.5 Garlic + guggulu	1	20	Mean Difference (IV, Random, 95% CI)	−51.43 (−69.87, −32.99)

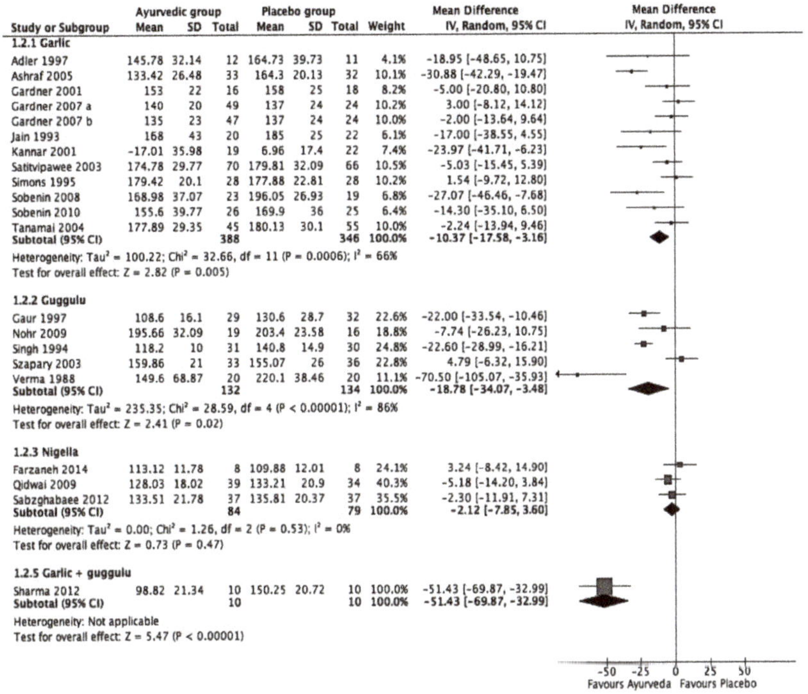

Figure 3. Forest plot on the effect of Ayurvedic herbal preparations on LDL-C (mg/dL).

3.1.3. Triglycerides (mg/dL)

Meta-analyses of the four interventions showed (Table 5 and Figure 4) garlic to be the least effective in reducing raised TG levels (3.1 mg/dL (95% C.I.: −16.63 to 10.42; p value = 0.65)), as shown in Figure 4. *N. Sativa* was found to be the most effective intervention, where the meta-analysis of three studies showed that it reduces TG by −21.09 mg/dL (95% C.I.: −44.96 to −2.77; p value = 0.08). Although the confidence interval of the effect size is wide and the p value of the final effect is 0.08, the heterogeneity among the studies was fairly low at 28%. *Lashunadi guggulu*, according to the combined results of two small studies, reduces TG levels by 13.23 mg/dL (95% C.I.: −28.53 to 2.07; p value = 0.09). Six studies on guggulu, when meta-analyzed, showed that guggulu helps to reduce TG levels by 7.35 mg/dL (95% C.I.: −23.29 to 8.59; p value = 0.0037). Here, two studies that showed positive results in other cholesterol levels are negative and opposite in one study.

Table 5. Effect of Ayurvedic herbal preparations on triglycerides (mg/dL).

Outcome or Subgroup	Studies	Participants	Statistical Method	Effect Estimate
1.3 Triglycerides level	23	1364	Mean Difference (IV, Random, 95% CI)	
1.3.1 Garlic	12	819	Mean Difference (IV, Random, 95% CI)	−3.10 (−16.63, 10.42)
1.3.2 Guggulu	6	352	Mean Difference (IV, Random, 95% CI)	−7.35 (−23.29, 8.59)
1.3.3 Nigella	3	163	Mean Difference (IV, Random, 95% CI)	−21.09 (−44.96, 2.77)
1.3.5 Garlic + guggulu	2	30	Mean Difference (IV, Random, 95% CI)	−13.23 (−28.53, 2.07)

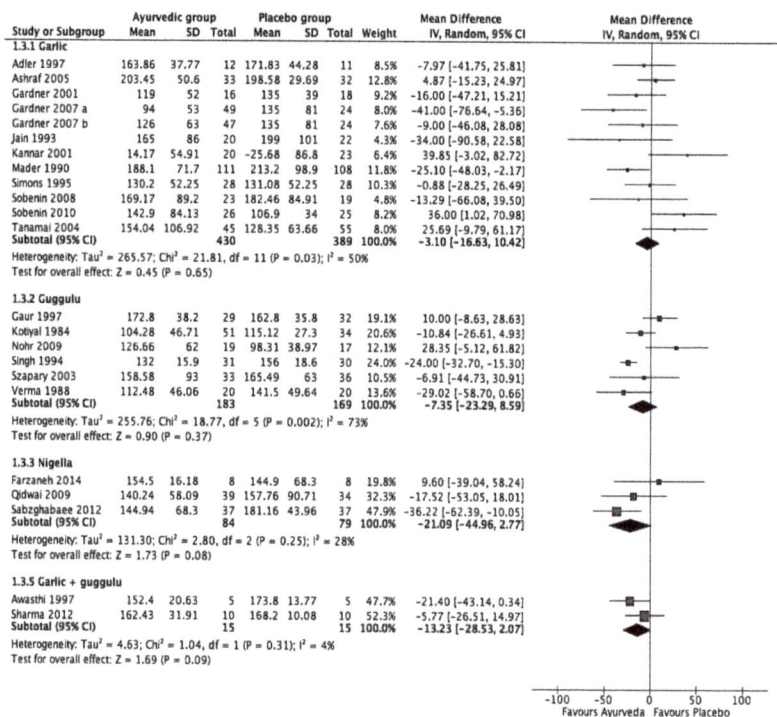

Figure 4. Forest plot on effect of Ayurvedic herbal preparations in triglycerides (mg/dL).

3.1.4. HDL (mg/dL)

The meta-analysis of 21 RCTs with 1186 participants (615 in the Ayurvedic group and 571 in the placebo group, as shown in Table 6) suggest the statistically non-significant effect of Ayurvedic interventions on HDL-C. Guggulu alone and when mixed with garlic, however, showed positive and statistically significant results in increasing HDL-C. Analysis of end results from five RCTs in guggulu involving 264 total subjects showed that, as compared to the placebo, guggulu increased HDL-C by a small but significant difference of 2.19 mg/dL (95% C.I.: 0.27 to 4.12; p value = 0.03). On the other hand, results from a single study showed that *Lashunadi guggulu* was found to be raising HDL-C levels by 10 mg/dL (95% C.I.: 5.87 to 14.13; $p < 0.00001$). *N. sativa* also did not seem to have a significant effect on HDL-C. Results of the meta-analysis of three studies showed that it raised HDL-C levels by 1.92 mg/dL (95% C.I.: −1.62 to 5.45; $p = 0.29$). These studies involved a total of 163 participants. Garlic was also found to have no significant effect on HDL-C levels. Among 12 studies involving 736 participants, five studies claimed that garlic reduces HDL-C, and one study by Gardner et al. [51] found out that garlic neither reduces nor increases HDL-C. The studies were also highly heterogeneous with a high 97%

I^2 statistic. Though it may not even be relevant to conduct a meta-analysis on the effects of garlic on HDL-C, it is presented in the forest plot to show the current evidence (Figure 5).

Table 6. Effect of Ayurvedic herbal preparations on HDL-C (mg/dL).

Outcome or Subgroup	Studies	Participants	Statistical Method	Effect Estimate
1.4 HDL-Cholesterol level	21	1186	Mean Difference (IV, Random, 95% CI)	
1.4.1 Garlic	12	736	Mean Difference (IV, Random, 95% CI)	−2.91 (−9.19, 3.37)
1.4.2 Guggulu	5	267	Mean Difference (IV, Random, 95% CI)	2.19 (0.27, 4.12)
1.4.3 Nigella	3	163	Mean Difference (IV, Random, 95% CI)	1.92 (−1.62, 5.45)
1.4.5 Garlic + guggulu	1	20	Mean Difference (IV, Random, 95% CI)	10.00 (5.87, 14.13)

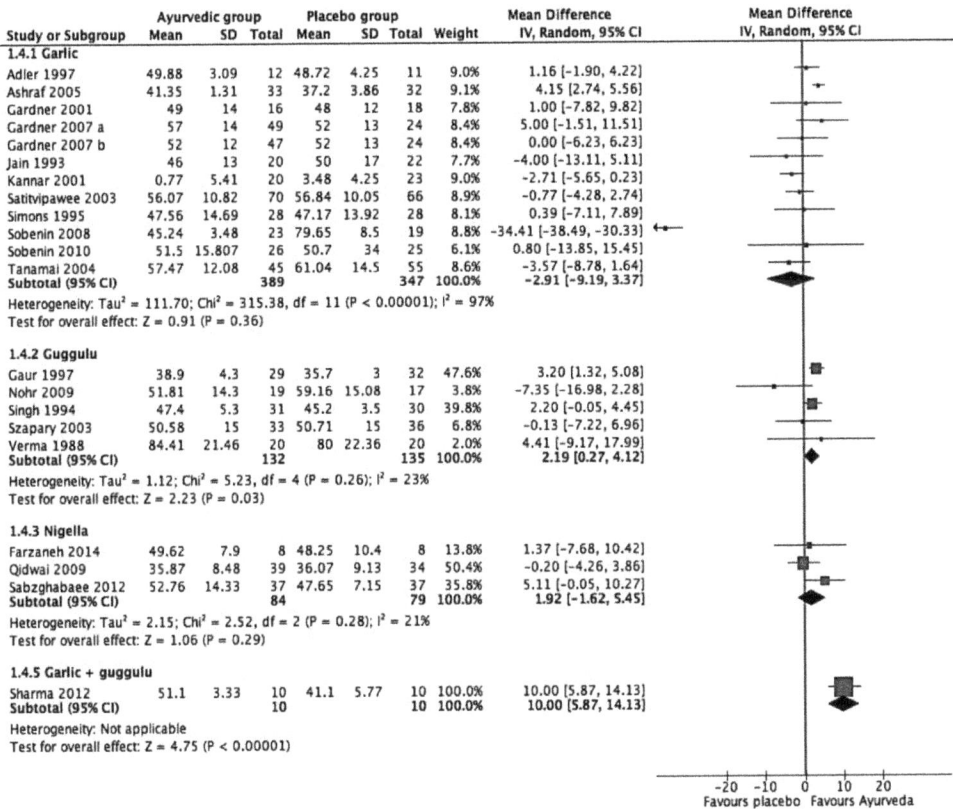

Figure 5. Forest plot on effect of Ayurvedic herbal preparations in HDL-C (mg/dL).

4. Discussion

The findings of the current meta-analyses are consistent with the clinical experiences and recommendations of traditional Ayurvedic literature. The two promising herbs for clinical improvements in hypercholesterolemia were found to be garlic and guggulu. This systematic review and meta-analysis suggested that Ayurvedic herbal preparations are safe and effective in reducing major cholesterol biomarkers. In addition to the studies conducted on these four interventions, 32 randomized controlled studies found out that there are 10 additional Ayurvedic interventions such as holy basil, ginger, fenugreek, and Indian gooseberry, which are capable of correcting hypercholesterolemia. However, a majority of studies were conducted on garlic, guggulu, *Nigella sativa*, and *Lashunadi guggulu* (a garlic and guggulu combination). It was also observed that amongst all of these Ayurvedic interventions, garlic and guggulu stood out as the most effective interventions. Although *Lashunadi guggulu* topped the list in its effectiveness, due to the lack of enough number of studies, the strength of the evidence on this finding is fairly low. Garlic and guggulu had the most consistent effects on cholesterol, except garlic did not seem to be as effective in increasing HDL-C as compared to guggulu. Both garlic and guggulu were not found to be effective in reducing TG levels, as the effect size was not statistically significant. Studies on garlic were less heterogeneous than studies conducted on guggulu. However, the overall effect size of guggulu exceeds that of garlic.

4.1. Commiphora Mukul (Guggulu)

Amongst all of the Ayurvedic interventions studied, *Commiphora mukul*, commonly known as guggul(u) was found to have the biggest effect size. Seven randomized controlled trials in eight trial arms enrolling a total of 380 participants compared guggulu with a placebo for its effect on various cholesterol levels. It was observed that guggulu reduces TC by 16.78 mg/dL (95% C.I.: 30.96 to 2.61, p value = 0.02) and LDL-C by 18.78 mg/dL (95% C.I.: 34.07 to 3.48, p value = 0.02). These findings on guggulu came from the analysis of end results from eight trial arms of seven RCTs involving 380 people (184 in the control group and 197 in the experimental group). One of the studies included in this analysis [66] seems to have had a big influence on the overall effect of this intervention. Heterogeneity among these seven studies was 75%, which still allowed the conduction of the meta-analysis. Likewise, as compared to a placebo, guggulu reduced TG levels by 7.35 mg/dL (95% C.I.: 23.29 to 8.59; p value = 0.37) and raised HDL-C by 2.19 mg/dL (95% C.I. 0.27 to 4.12; p-value = 0.03). This effect size counts for a reduction in TC and LDL-C by nearly 6.5% and 10%, respectively. This finding is of clinical significance, as it is associated with a 38% reduction in the risk of coronary events at age 50 (Law et. al, 1994) [69]. The risk of coronary events is *dependent* on other cardiovascular risk factors such as hypertension and age. In addition, it is also understood that a 10% reduction in LDL-C levels helps minimize the risk of coronary and vascular events [70]. Out of eight trial arms included in analysis, all but two studies [21,47] were conducted in the Western population with a typical Western diet. When a sensitivity analysis was performed by excluding these two studies, then the effect size was 22.85 (95% C.I.: 40.74, 4.97). Another possibility is that the discrepancies are due to the dietary habits of Indian and Western populations. Another postulation could be that this native Indian plant is better suited to natives of India—as the Vedic scriptures say, "local plants and herbs are best suited to the local people" [71].

One of the studies included in the analysis of guggulu is Verma (1988) [66] and shows a bigger effect size. However, this study included patients with a baseline total cholesterol level of 275 mg/dL or more or triglycerides levels of 200 mg/dL. Thus, there is a possibility that guggulu is more effective when the baseline cholesterol and triglyceride levels are high. Moreover, Verma (1988) describes the process of purification of guggulu. Purification of guggulu is also associated with its chances of posing any side effects. Although there were no serious adverse events posed by guggulu, a small proportion of participants did experience diarrhea, headaches, and skin rashes. These side effects are minimal when compared to the threats posed by conventional drug therapy. Purified guggulu seems to have fewer side effects. The study by Szapary et al. [21], which showed negative effects of guggulu, did not mention if the product was purified as per the Ayurvedic protocol or not. Additionally, the study included an extracted version of guggulu prepared by a commercial manufacturer. Thus, there is an inherent chance of bias despite the fact that it was the first methodologically sound randomized controlled trial conducted on guggulu in the West. When asked for further comments, no response was received from the principal author [21].

So far, the types of guggulu used for clinical trials are very diverse. Some studies used purified crude gum guggulu as recommended by Ayurvedic texts, whereas others used a guggulu extract called guggulipid. Guggulipid is extracted from the plant by using ethyl acetate and is mixed with petroleum ether to produce a product called fraction A [26]. This fraction A guggulu has been used in some trials. Extracting the active ingredient of guggulu is not an Ayurvedic practice, so it might be a plausible reason for this observation. Guggulu has been qualitatively reviewed by few several groups of researchers in the past [16,26,72]. So far, none of the reviews conducted a meta-analysis of guggulu studies. This work is first of its kind and thus cannot be compared with any previous meta-analysis. In summary, guggulu is moderately effective in terms of total cholesterol, LDL-C, and HDL-C, and there is a strong evidence to this end. Thus, it can be recommended as an adjuvant to cholesterol-lowering pharmacological therapy or as a supplement to a healthier diet and lifestyle for those who have borderline cholesterol levels.

4.1.1. Garlic

It was observed that garlic reduces total cholesterol by almost 5% and LDL-C by 6% in subjects with elevated total cholesterol levels (mean TC > 200 mg/dL), and has a statistically non-significant effect on HDL-C and triglycerides. This observed reduction in LDL and total cholesterol is clinically relevant as it is associated with a reduction in the risk of adverse coronary and vascular events [69,70].

The results also suggested that garlic was highly tolerable and does not pose any side effects, which are more common with conventional therapies. In a majority of the studies, bad smell or odor was the only major side effect of garlic. A small proportion of the population did experience some gastrointestinal issues such as belching and acid reflux, but in comparison to statins, these side effects are not serious. Statins, on the other hand, do pose some serious adverse effects including a high risk of diabetes, cognitive and muscular impairment, sexual dysfunction, mood swings, anxiety, and irritability [73].

These findings corroborate the results of previous meta-analyses and systematic reviews [74–76]. In previous literature, the effect of garlic on cholesterol levels has been a debatable topic. Time and again, many individual trials of garlic have reported diverse therapeutic effect size of garlic on cholesterol levels. The study by Stevinson et al. [76] was one of the earliest meta-analysis of garlic on hypercholesterolemia and included 13 trials, whereas the recent and most updated study, by Ried et al. [74], included 39 studies. The studies by Stevinson et al. and Ried et al. both suggest that garlic reduces TC levels by approximately 15 mg/dL, whereas the study by Reinhart et al. [75] suggests its effect size is nearly half of what was observed by previous studies, i.e., −7.34 mg/dL. They attribute this smaller effect size to including newer studies, which exhibit more modest effects than older studies. However, the recent and most updated meta-analysis on garlic by Ried et al. [74] seems to be the most comprehensive one.

Meanwhile, observed results from this study have suggested that garlic has a modest effect size of −12.45 mg/dL. One reason behind this finding may have to do with the type of included studies in this review. Because Ayurveda does not entertain the use of aged garlic, extracted garlic oil, or extracted compound of allicin from garlic, and uses whole garlic as a preparation, this work did not include any of the studies that used those various forms of garlic as an intervention. There is a common trend of using aged garlic and a lot of studies had to be excluded for using aged garlic as an intervention. However, the studies that used whole garlic or dried garlic powder were included, as it is the common practice to use whole garlic cloves in Ayurvedic pharmaceutical science [71]. From a pharmacological point of view, it is believed that the active compound called allicin, a garlic derivative, is responsible for reducing cholesterol levels and for the distinctive smell of garlic [77]. Allicin is a volatile compound and is responsible transiently for cardiovascular effects [77]. However, the exact ingredients and their mechanism of action still remains unknown. On the other hand, Ayurveda has been using garlic for treating Hridroga, an Ayurvedic term for cardiovascular diseases [71]. In Ayurveda, garlic, which possesses all five tastes except sour taste, is capable for clearing channels and all the coverings (avarana) because of its pungent and piercing qualities [71,78].

In conclusion, the findings of this review suggest that garlic is superior to placebos in reducing elevated total cholesterol and LDL-C levels. Garlic has also been shown to have additional cardiovascular benefits such as reducing high blood pressure [79]. When taken together, garlic preparations can be considered as a general heart tonic with cholesterol regulating properties. It can also be used as a preventive agent in borderline cholesterol levels, with a higher safety and tolerability profile than statins.

4.1.2. Nigella Sativa

Another intervention that showed some efficacy on cholesterol levels was *Nigella sativa*. Commonly known as black cumin and Upakunchika in Ayurveda, it is more famous for its digestive effect. Ideally, *Nigella sativa* seed powder is used in Ayurveda, so studies of its seed oil or other extracts were not included. Based on the analysis of three studies on *Nigella sativa*, it was observed that it reduces total cholesterol by 9.28 mg/dL (95% C.I.: 17.36 to 1.19, $p = 0.02$). However, it does not seem to have a statistically significant effect on other parameters such as LDL-C 2.12 mg/dL (95% C.I.: 7.85 to 3.6; $p = 0.47$), triglycerides 21.09 mg/dL (95% C.I.: to -2.77; $p = 0.08$), and HDL-C 1.92 mg/dL (95% C.I.:1.62 to 5.45; $p = 0.29$). This observation is comparable to the results of a recently published systematic review by Sahebkar et al. [80]. The difference between the current study and [80] is the inclusion criteria; the present study only included studies with whole seed powder, whereas Sahebkar et al. [80] included other versions of *Nigella sativa* such as seed oil and also had no restriction on baseline total cholesterol levels for the inclusion criteria, which limited the number of studies in this meta-analysis.

As an addition to the herbs mentioned above, we also conducted a systematic review to examine the effects of *Terminalia arjuna* on lipid parameters of hypercholesterolemic patients. Due to a lack of strict randomized controlled designs and inconsistencies in Arjuna preparations being used, the meta-analytic results are not included in our main results section. Nonetheless, the findings from such quasi-randomized studies are still worth mentioning. After analyzing data from 14 arms of 10 different studies enrolling 547 participants, it was observed that Ayurvedic herbal preparations with *Terminalia arjuna* as a main ingredient reduces total cholesterol by 19.47 mg/dL (95% C.I.:30.73, 8.20, $p = 0.0007$), LDL-C by 16.33 mg/dL (95% C.I.:23.21, 9.45, $p < 0.00001$), triglycerides by 11.24 mg/dL (95% C.I.:22.02, 0.46, $p = 0.04$), and raises HDL-C by 5.16 mg/dL (95% C.I.:2.62, 7.69, $p < 0.00001$). Overall, Arjuna may also be considered as a viable herb that can be quite beneficial for patients with hypercholesterolemia.

4.1.3. Adverse Effects

No serious adverse events were reported in the majority of the studies, except Szapary (2003) [21] reported that one patient each from experimental group and control group had serious side effects and Joseph (2012) reported that one participant in the active control group withdrew due to a five-fold increase in serum creatinine level. Other minor adverse events such as gastrointestinal upset, skin rashes, nausea, and bad odor of breath and body were also reported in few other studies [47,56].

Limitations: Although every effort was made to discover all eligible studies published through December 2020, there is a possibility of some studies still being left behind. Most of the studies that were seemingly eligible did not qualify given our inclusion criteria, but some of the studies did show consistent findings with our study [55–57]. A Pakistani study by Zeb et al. [81] examined the impact of garlic powder, coriander powder, and a mixture of the two on lipid profile as compared to a placebo. Garlic powder was found to be the most effective in reducing TC and LDL and increasing HDL, as compared to all other groups. The latest study by Iskander et al. [82] showed that a nutraceutical combination including g gugguluipid showed a significant reduction in TC and LDL levels after 8 weeks of consumption in a randomized, placebo-controlled double-blind trial. Another study by Kuchewar et al. [83] found beneficial effects of Triphala on the lipid profile of patients with dyslipidemia. Many other herbs such as Amla [84,85] have also shown promising results for controlling lipid parameters among patients with hyperlipidemia/dyslipidemia. However, these studies failed to meet the inclusion criteria of the current review.

5. Conclusions

Findings from these systematic reviews and meta-analyses indicate that there is moderate to high strength evidence that several Ayurvedic herbal preparations, i.e., guggulu, garlic, and black cumin, are safe and effective in reducing high levels of cholesterol to a moderate extent. The data suggest that these preparations may be used as first-line therapies or adjuncts to conventional care. We encourage future research to pursue randomized clinical trials with a larger sample size, longer durations, and with clinical outcomes of cardiovascular disease. In addition to the herbs studied, future randomized controlled trials are needed to investigate the efficacy of other Ayurvedic herbal preparations such as Arjuna, Triphala, and Amla in patients with hypercholesterolemia.

Author Contributions: Conceptualization, D.G. and R.H.S.; Methodology, D.G. and R.H.S.; Software, D.G.; Data Analysis, D.G.; Visualization, D.G; Resources, D.O.-J. and S.R.; Writing—Original Draft Preparation, D.G.; Writing—Review & Editing, R.V.; Supervision, R.H.S. All authors have read and agreed to the published version of the manuscript.

Funding: The study received the Cochrane Complementary Medicine bursary award for the year 2015.

Acknowledgments: The authors appreciate administrative contributions of John Salerno.

Conflicts of Interest: The authors declare no conflict of interest.

References

1. Mendis, S.; Puska, P.; Norrving, B. *Global Atlas on Cardiovascular Disease Prevention and Control*; World Health Organization: Geneva, Switzerland, 2011.
2. Centers for Disease Control and Prevention. Vital signs: Prevalence, treatment, and control of high levels of low-density lipoprotein cholesterol-United States, 1999–2002 and 2005–2008. *MMWR* **2011**, *4*, 109–114.
3. Gupta, A.; Sehgal, V.; Mehan, S. Hyperlipidemia: An updated review. *Int. J. Biopharm. Toxicol. Res.* **2011**, *1*, 81–89.
4. National Cholesterol Education Program (NCEP). Expert Panel on Detection, Evaluation, and Treatment of High Blood Cholesterol in Adults (Adult Treatment Panel III) Final Report. *Circulation* **2002**, *106*, 3143. [CrossRef]
5. The Lipid Research Clinics Coronary Primary Prevention Trial Results. *JAMA* **1984**, *251*, 351–364. [CrossRef] [PubMed]
6. The Lipid Research Clinics Coronary Primary Prevention Trial Results. II. The Relationship of Reduction in Incidence of Coronary Heart Disease to Cholesterol Lowering. *JAMA* **1984**, *251*, 365–374. [CrossRef]
7. Punekar, R.S.; Fox, K.M.; Richhariya, A.; Fisher, M.D.; Cziraky, M.; Gandra, S.R.; Toth, P.P. Burden of First and Recurrent Cardiovascular Events among Patients with Hyperlipidemia. *Clin. Cardiol.* **2015**, *38*, 483–491. [CrossRef] [PubMed]
8. Bahia, L.R.; Rosa, R.S.; Santos, R.D.; Araújo, D.V. Estimated costs of hospitalization due to coronary artery disease attributable to familial hypercholesterolemia in the Brazilian public health system. *Arch. Endocrinol. Metab.* **2018**, *62*, 303–308. [CrossRef]
9. Soni, A. Top 10 Most Costly Conditions among Men and Women, 2008: Estimates for the U.S. Civilian Noninstitutionalized Adult Population, Age 18 and Older, Med. Expend. Panel Surv. (2011) Statistical Brief #331). Available online: https://meps.ahrq.gov/data_files/publications/st331/stat331.shtml (accessed on 10 November 2020).
10. Scirica, B.M.; Cannon, C.P. Treatment of Elevated Cholesterol. *Circulation* **2005**, *111*, 360–363. [CrossRef]
11. Golomb, B.A.; Evans, M.A. Statin Adverse Effects. *Am. J. Cardiovasc. Drugs* **2008**, *8*, 373–418. [CrossRef]
12. Chrysant, S.G. New onset diabetes mellitus induced by statins: Current evidence. *Postgrad. Med.* **2017**, *129*, 430–435. [CrossRef]
13. Bove, M.; Cicero, A.F.; Borghi, C. Emerging drugs for the treatment of hypercholesterolemia. *Expert Opin. Emerg. Drugs* **2019**, *24*, 63–69. [CrossRef]
14. Arnett, D.K.; Jacobs, D.R.; Luepker, R.V.; Blackburn, H.; Armstrong, C.; Claas, S.A. Twenty-Year Trends in Serum Cholesterol, Hypercholesterolemia, and Cholesterol Medication Use: The Minnesota Heart Survey. *Circulation* **2005**, *112*, 3884–3891. [CrossRef]
15. Qidwai, W.; Jahan, F.; Nanji, K. Role of Complementary and Alternative Medicine in Controlling Dyslipidemia. *Evid. Based Complement. Altern. Med.* **2014**, *2014*, 1–2. [CrossRef]
16. Singh, B.B.; Vinjamury, S.P.; Der-Martirosian, C.; Kubik, E.; Mishra, L.C.; Shepard, N.P.; Singh, V.J.; Meier, M.; Madhu, S.G. Ayurvedic and collateral herbal treatments for hyperlipidemia: A systematic review of randomized controlled trials and qua-si-experimental designs. *Altern. Ther. Health Med.* **2007**, *13*, 22–28.
17. Patwardhan, B. Bridging Ayurveda with evidence-based scientific approaches in medicine. *EPMA J.* **2014**, *5*, 1–7. [CrossRef]
18. Kessler, C.; Wischnewsky, M.; Michalsen, A.; Eisenmann, C.; Melzer, J. Ayurveda: Between Religion, Spirituality, and Medicine. *Evid. Based Complement. Altern. Med.* **2013**, *2013*, 1–11. [CrossRef] [PubMed]

19. Gupta, R.; Singhal, S.; Goyle, A.; Sharma, V.N. Antioxidant and hypocholesterolaemic effects of Terminalia arjuna tree-bark powder: A randomised placebo-controlled trial. *J. Assoc. Physicians India* **2001**, *49*, 231–235.
20. Silagy, C.; Neil, A. Garlic as a Lipid Lowering Agent—A Meta-Analysis. *J. R. Coll. Physicians Lond.* **1994**, *28*, 39–45. [PubMed]
21. Szapary, P.O.; Wolfe, M.L.; Bloedon, L.T.; Cucchiara, A.J.; DerMarderosian, A.H.; Cirigliano, M.D.; Rader, D.J. Guggulipid for the Treatment of Hypercholesterolemia. *JAMA* **2003**, *290*, 765–772. [CrossRef] [PubMed]
22. Qidwai, W.; Yeoh, P.N.; Inem, V.; Nanji, K.; Ashfaq, T. Role of Complementary and Alternative Medicine in Cardiovascular Diseases. *Evid. Based Complement. Altern. Med.* **2013**, *2013*, 1–2. [CrossRef] [PubMed]
23. Patwardhan, K. Promoting evidence-base for Ayurveda. *J. Ayurveda Integr. Med.* **2019**. [CrossRef]
24. Dwivedi, S. Terminalia arjuna Wight & Arn.—A useful drug for cardiovascular disorders. *J. Ethnopharmacol.* **2007**, *114*, 114–129. [CrossRef] [PubMed]
25. Kaur, N.; Shafiq, N.; Negi, H.; Pandey, A.; Reddy, S.; Kaur, H.; Chadha, N.; Malhotra, S. Terminalia arjunain Chronic Stable Angina: Systematic Review and Meta-Analysis. *Cardiol. Res. Pract.* **2014**, *2014*, 1–7. [CrossRef] [PubMed]
26. Ulbricht, C.; Basch, E.; Szapary, P.; Hammerness, P.; Axentsev, S.; Boon, H.; Kroll, D.; Garraway, L.; Vora, M.; Woods, J. Guggul for hyperlipidemia: A review by the Natural Standard Research Collaboration. *Complement. Ther. Med.* **2005**, *13*, 279–290. [CrossRef] [PubMed]
27. Ahmada, A.; Husainb, A.; Mujeebc, M.; Alam Khan, S.; Najmi, A.K.; Siddique, N.A.; Damanhouri, Z.A.; Anwarh, F. A review on therapeutic potential of Nigella sativa: A miracle herb. *Asian Pac. J. Trop. Biomed.* **2013**, *3*, 337–352. [CrossRef]
28. Liberati, A.; Altman, D.G.; Tetzlaff, J.; Mulrow, C.; Gøtzsche, P.C.; Ioannidis, J.P.A.; Clarke, M.; Devereaux, P.J.; Kleijnen, J.; Moher, D. The PRISMA statement for reporting systematic reviews and meta-analyses of studies that evaluate health care interventions: Explanation and elaboration. *PLoS Med.* **2009**, *6*, e1000100. [CrossRef]
29. Higgins, J.P.T.; Green, S. Cochrane Handbook for Systematic Reviews of Interventions, Version 5.1.0. Updated March 2011. The Cochrane Collaboration, 2001. Available online: www.cochrane-handbook.org (accessed on 1 December 2020).
30. Gyawali, D.; Schneider, R.H.; Orme-Johnson, D.W.; Ramaratnam, S. Ayurvedic herbal preparations for hypercholesterolaemia. *Cochrane Database Syst. Rev.* **2016**, *3*. [CrossRef]
31. Deeks, J.; Higgins, J. Statistical algorithms in Review Manager 5. Available online: https://training.cochrane.org/handbook/statistical-methods-revman5 (accessed on 20 May 2021).
32. Higgins, J.P.T.; Altman, D.G.; Gøtzsche, P.C.; Jüni, P.; Moher, D.; Oxman, A.D.; Savović, J.; Schulz, K.F.; Weeks, L.; Sterne, J.A.C.; et al. The Cochrane Collaboration's tool for assessing risk of bias in randomised trials. *BMJ* **2011**, *343*, d5928. [CrossRef]
33. Higgins, J.P.T.; Thompson, S.G.; Deeks, J.J.; Altman, D.G. Measuring inconsistency in meta-analyses. *BMJ* **2003**, *327*, 557–560. [CrossRef]
34. Sterne, J.; Sutton, A.J.; Ioannidis, J.P.A.; Terrin, N.; Jones, D.R.; Lau, J.; Carpenter, J.; Rücker, G.; Harbord, R.M.; Schmid, C.H.; et al. Recommendations for examining and interpreting funnel plot asymmetry in meta-analyses of randomised controlled trials. *BMJ* **2011**, *343*, d4002. [CrossRef]
35. Wood, L.; Egger, M.; Gluud, L.L.; Schulz, K.F.; Jüni, P.; Altman, D.G.; Gluud, C.; Martin, R.M.; Wood, A.J.G.; Sterne, J.A.C. Empirical evidence of bias in treatment effect estimates in controlled trials with different interventions and outcomes: Meta-epidemiological study. *BMJ* **2008**, *336*, 601–605. [CrossRef] [PubMed]
36. Higgins, J.P.T.; Thompson, S.G.; Spiegelhalter, D.J. A re-evaluation of random-effects meta-analysis. *J. R. Stat. Soc. Ser. A* **2009**, *172*, 137–159. [CrossRef] [PubMed]
37. Riley, R.D.; Higgins, J.P.T.; Deeks, J.J. Interpretation of random effects meta-analyses. *BMJ* **2011**, *342*, d549. [CrossRef] [PubMed]
38. Prakash, V.; Sehgal, V.; Bajaj, V.; Singh, H. To compare the effects of Terminalia Arjuna with Rosuvastatin on total cholesterol and low-density lipoprotein cholesterol. *Int. J. Med. Dent. Sci.* **2016**, *5*, 1056–1066. [CrossRef]
39. Farzaneh, E.; Nia, F.R.; Mehrtash, M.; Mirmoeini, F.S.; Jalilvand, M. The effects of 8-week Nigella sativa supplementation and aerobic training on lipid profile and VO$_2$ max in sedentary overweight females. *Int. J. Prev. Med.* **2014**, *5*, 210–216.
40. Rathi, R.; Rathi, B.J. A clinical comparative study of rasonadi leha with hridrogadi churna in coronary artery disease. *Punarnav* **2013**, *1*, 44–54.
41. Devra, D.K.; Mathur, K.C.; Agrawal, R.P.; Bhadu, I.; Goyal, S.; Agarwal, V. Effect of Tulsi (*Ocimum sanctum* Linn.) on clinical and biochemical parameters of metabolic syndrome. *J. Nat. Remed.* **2012**, *12*, 63–67.
42. Huseini, H.F.; Kianbakht, S.; Hajiaghaee, R.; Dabaghian, F.H. Anti-hyperglycemic and anti-hypercholesterolemic effects of Aloe vera leaf gel in hyperlipidemic type 2 diabetic patients: A randomized double-blind placebo-controlled clinical trial. *Planta Med.* **2012**, *78*, 311–316. [CrossRef]
43. Joseph, S.; Santhosh, D.; Udupa, A.L.; Gupta, S.; Ojeh, N.; Rathnakar, U.P.; Benegal, D.; Benegal, A.; Shubha, H.V.; Rao, S.P.; et al. Hypolipidemic Activity of Phyllanthus Emblica Linn (Amla) & Trigonella Foenum Graecum (Fenugreek) Combination In Hypercholesterolemic Subjects–A Prospective, Randomised, Parallel, Open-Label, Positive Controlled Study. *Asian J. Bio. Pharma. Res.* **2012**, *2*, 225–230.
44. Sabzghabaee, A.M.; Dianatkhah, M.; Sarrafzadegan, N.; Asgary, S.; Ghannadi, A. Clinical evaluation of Nigella sativa seeds for the treatment of hyperlipidemia: A randomized, placebo controlled clinical trial. *Med. Arch.* **2012**, *66*, 198–200. [CrossRef]
45. Sharma, A.K.; Sharma, S.M.; Sharma, S.P.; Sharma, A.K. Management of stable angina with lashunadi guggulu- an ayurvedic formulation. *Ann. Ayurvedic. Med.* **2012**, *1*, 15–21.

46. Sobenin, I.A.; Pryanishnikov, V.V.; Kunnova, L.M.; Rabinovich, Y.A.; Martirosyan, D.M.; Orekhov, A.N. The effects of time-released garlic powder tablets on multifunctional cardiovascular risk in patients with coronary artery disease. *Lipids Health Dis.* **2010**, *9*, 1–6. [CrossRef] [PubMed]
47. Nohr, L.A.; Rasmussen, L.B.; Straand, J. Resin from the mukul myrrh tree, guggul, can it be used for treating hypercholesterolemia? A randomized, controlled study. *Complement. Ther. Med.* **2009**, *17*, 16–22. [CrossRef]
48. Qidwai, W.; Bin Hamza, H.; Qureshi, R.; Gilani, A. Effectiveness, safety, and tolerability of powdered nigella sativa (kalonji) seed in capsules on serum lipid levels, blood sugar, blood pressure, and body weight in adults: Results of a randomized, double-blind controlled trial. *J. Altern. Complement. Med.* **2009**, *15*, 639–644. [CrossRef]
49. Alizadeh-Navaei, R.; Roozbeh, F.; Saravi, M.; Pouramir, M.; Jalali, F.; Moghadamnia, A.A. Investigation of the effect of ginger on the lipid levels. A double blind controlled clinical trial. *Saudi Med. J.* **2008**, *29*, 1280–1284.
50. Sobenin, I.A.; Andrianova, I.V.; Demidova, O.N.; Gorchakova, T.; Orekhov, A.N. Lipid-lowering effects of time-released garlic powder tablets in double-blinded placebo-controlled randomized study. *J. Ather. Thromb.* **2008**, *15*, 334–338. [CrossRef]
51. Gardner, C.D.; Lawson, L.D.; Block, E.; Chatterjee, L.M.; Kiazand, A.; Balise, R.R.; Kraemer, H.C. Effect of raw garlic vs commercial garlic supplements on plasma lipid concentrations in adults with moderate hypercholesterolemia. *Arch. Intern. Med.* **2007**, *167*, 346–353. [CrossRef]
52. Ashraf, R.; Aamir, K.; Shaikh, A.R.; Ahmed, T. Effects of garlic on dyslipidemia in patients with type 2 diabetes mellitus. *J. Ayub. Med. Coll. Abbottabad.* **2005**, *17*, 60–64.
53. Tanamai, J.; Veeramanomai, S.; Indrakosas, N. The efficacy of cholesterol-lowering action and side effects of garlic enteric coated tablets in man. *J. Med. Ass. Thailand* **2004**, *87*, 1156–1161.
54. Satitvipawee, P.; Suparp, J.; Podhipak, A.; Viwatwongkasem, C. Can garlic extract supplement lower blood pressure in hypercholesterolemic subjects? *J. Public Health* **2003**, *33*, 18–26.
55. Double-Blind Comparative Clinical Trial of Abana and Simvastatin in Hyperlipidaemia. Available online: https://cdn.greensoft.mn/uploads/users/1977/files/tsakhurtumur%20sudalga/Abana%20sudalgaa.pdf (accessed on 28 May 2021).
56. Kannar, D.; Wattanapenpaiboon, N.; Savige, G.S.; Wahlqvist, M.L. Hypocholesterolemic effect of an enteric-coated garlic supplement. *J. Am. Coll. Nutr.* **2001**, *20*, 225–231. [CrossRef] [PubMed]
57. Gardner, C.D.; Chatterjee, L.M.; Carlson, J.J. The effect of a garlic preparation on plasma lipid levels in moderately hypercholesterolemic adults. *Atherosclerosis* **2001**, *154*, 213–220. [CrossRef]
58. Adler, A.J.; Holub, B.J. Effect of garlic and fish-oil supplementation on serum lipid and lipoprotein concentrations in hypercholesterolemic men. *Am. J. Clin. Nutr.* **1997**, *65*, 445–450. [CrossRef]
59. Awasthi, A.; Kothari, K.; Sharma, R. Evaluation of the effect of the indigenous herbal drug lashunadi guggulu in management of chronic stable Angina. *Aryavaidyan Xi* **1997**, *1*, 20.
60. Gaur, S.P.; Garg, R.K.; Kar, A.M. Gugulipid, a new hypolipidaemic agent, in patients of acute ischaemic stroke: Effect on clinical outcome, platelet function and serum lipids. *Asia Pacif. J. Pharm.* **1997**, *12*, 65–69.
61. Singh, R.B.; Niaz, M.A.; Ghosh, S. Hypolipidemic and antioxidant effects of Commiphora mukul as an adjunct to dietary therapy in patients with hypercholesterolemia. *Cardiovasc. Drugs. Ther.* **1994**, *8*, 659–664. [CrossRef]
62. Jain, A.K.; Vargas, R.; Gotzkowsky, S.; McMahon, F.G. Can garlic reduce levels of serum lipids? A controlled clinical study. *Am. J. Med.* **1993**, *94*, 632–635. [CrossRef]
63. Tiwari, A.K.; Agrawal, A.; Gode, J.D.; Dubey, G.P. Perspective, randomised crossover study of propranolol and Abana in hypertensive patients: Effect on lipids and lipoproteins. *Antiseptic.* **1991**, *88*, 14.
64. Mader, F.H. Treatment of hyperlipidaemia with garlic-powder tablets. Evidence from the German Association of General Practitioners' multicentric placebo-controlled double-blind study. *Arzneimittel-Forschung* **1990**, *40*, 1111–1116.
65. Nityanand, S.; Srivastava, J.S.; Asthana, O.P. Clinical trials with gugulipid. A new hypolipidaemic agent. *J. Assoc. Physicians Ind.* **1989**, *37*, 323–328.
66. Verma, S.K.; Bordia, A. Effect of Commiphora mukul (gum guggulu) in patients of hyperlipidemia with special reference to HDL-cholesterol. *Indian J. Med. Res.* **1988**, *87*, 356–360.
67. Kotiyal, J.P.; Singh, D.S.; Bisht, D.B. Gum guggulu (Commiphora mukul) fraction A in obesity—A double-blind clinical trial. *J. Res. Ayur. Siddha.* **1985**, *6*, 20–35.
68. Kuppurajan, K.; Rajagopalan, S.S.; Rao, T.K.; Sitaraman, R. Effect of guggul (Commiphora mukul–Engl.) on serum lipids in obese, hypercholesterolemic and hyperlipemic cases. *J. Assoc. Physicians India.* **1978**, *26*, 367–373. [PubMed]
69. Law, M.R.; Wald, N.J.; Thompson, S.G. By how much and how quickly does reduction in serum cholesterol concentration lower risk of ischaemic heart disease? *BMJ* **1994**, *308*, 367–372. [CrossRef] [PubMed]
70. Delahoy, P.J.; Magliano, D.J.; Webb, K.; Grobler, M.; Liew, D. The relationship between reduction in low-density lipoprotein cholesterol by statins and reduction in risk of cardiovascular outcomes: An updated meta-analysis. *Clin. Ther.* **2009**, *31*, 236–244. [CrossRef]
71. Chunekar, K.C. *Bhavprakash Nighantu of Bhavmisra*; Chaukambha Orientalia: Varanasi, India, 2009.
72. Urizar, N.L.; Moore, D.D. GUGULIPID: A Natural Cholesterol-Lowering Agent. *Annu. Rev. Nutr.* **2003**, *23*, 303–313. [CrossRef]
73. Golomb, B.A. Misinterpretation of trial evidence on statin adverse effects may harm patients. *Eur. J. Prev. Cardiol.* **2015**, *22*, 492–493. [CrossRef]
74. Ried, K.; Toben, C.; Fakler, P. Effect of garlic on serum lipids: An updated meta-analysis. *Nutr. Rev.* **2013**, *71*, 282–299. [CrossRef]

75. Reinhart, K.M.; Talati, R.; White, C.M.; Coleman, C.I. The impact of garlic on lipid parameters: A systematic review and meta-analysis. *Nutr. Res. Rev.* **2009**, *22*, 39–48. [CrossRef]
76. Stevinson, C.; Pittler, M.; Ernst, E. Garlic for treating hypercholesterolemia. *ACC Curr. J. Rev.* **2001**, *10*, 37. [CrossRef]
77. Amagase, H.; Petesch, B.L.; Matsuura, H.; Kasuga, S.; Itakura, Y. Intake of garlic and its bioactive components. *J. Nutr.* **2001**, *131*, 955S–962S. [CrossRef]
78. Shastri, K. *Sushruta Samhita of Maharshi Sushruta Part I*, 14th ed.; Chaukhamba Sanskrita Sansthana: Varanasi, India, 2001.
79. Wang, H.-P.; Yang, J.; Qin, L.-Q.; Yang, X.-J. Effect of Garlic on Blood Pressure: A Meta-Analysis. *J. Clin. Hypertens.* **2015**, *17*, 223–231. [CrossRef] [PubMed]
80. Sahebkar, A.; Beccuti, G.; Simental-Mendía, L.E.; Nobili, V.; Bo, S. Nigella sativa (black seed) effects on plasma lipid concentrations in humans: A systematic review and meta-analysis of randomized placebo-controlled trials. *Pharmacol. Res.* **2016**, *106*, 37–50. [CrossRef] [PubMed]
81. Zeb, F.; Safdar, M.; Fatima, S.; Khan, S.; Alam, S.; Muhammad, M.; Syed, A.; Habib, F.; Shakoor, H. Supplementation of garlic and coriander seed powder: Impact on body mass index, lipid profile and blood pressure of hyperlipidemic patients. *Pak. J. Pharm. Sci.* **2018**, *31*, 1935–1941. [PubMed]
82. Iskandar, I.; Harahap, Y.; Wijayanti, T.R.; Sandra, M.; Prasaja, B.; Cahyaningsih, P.; Rahayu, T. Efficacy and tolerability of a nutraceutical combination of red yeast rice, guggulipid, and chromium picolinate evaluated in a randomized, placebo-controlled, double-blind study. *Complement. Ther. Med.* **2020**, *48*, 102282. [CrossRef] [PubMed]
83. Kuchewar, V.V. Efficacy and safety study of triphala in patients of dyslipidemia: A pilot project. *Int. J. Res. Ayurveda Pharm.* **2017**, *8*, 177–180. [CrossRef]
84. Bhatt, J.; Hemavathi, K.G.; Gopa, B. A comparative clinical study of hypolipidemic efficacy of Amla (Emblica officinalis) with 3-hydroxy-3-methylglutaryl-coenzyme-A reductase inhibitor simvastatin. *Indian J. Pharmacol.* **2012**, *44*, 238–242. [CrossRef]
85. Upadya, H.; Prabhu, S.; Prasad, A.; Subramanian, D.; Gupta, S.; Goel, A. A randomized, double blind, placebo controlled, multicenter clinical trial to assess the efficacy and safety of Emblica officinalis extract in patients with dyslipidemia. *BMC Complement. Altern. Med.* **2019**, *19*, 27. [CrossRef]

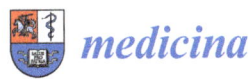

Perspective

Vegetarian Diets, Ayurveda, and the Case for an Integrative Nutrition Science

Archana Purushotham [1,*] and Alex Hankey [2]

[1] Department of Neurology, Baylor College of Medicine & Michael E. DeBakey VA Medical Center, Houston, TX 77030, USA
[2] School of Biology, Faculty of Science, MIT World Peace University, Pune 411038, Maharashtra, India; alexhankey@gmail.com
* Correspondence: archana.purushotham@bcm.edu

Abstract: Two recent studies of the health effects of vegetarian diets reported conflicting results: the EPIC-Oxford study reported a significant increase in strokes among vegetarians compared to meat-eaters among a predominantly Caucasian cohort, while another, performed on Taiwanese Buddhists, reported significantly lower incidence of strokes among vegetarians. This was doubly puzzling given the pronounced decrease in cardiovascular events among the EPIC-Oxford group. In this article, we make a detailed comparison of the actual dietary intake of various food groups by the cohorts in these studies. We then use the nutritional principles of Ayurveda—traditional Indian medicine—to show how these apparently contradictory results may be explained. Systems of traditional medicine such as Ayurveda possess profound knowledge of the effects of food on physiology. Ayurveda takes into account not just the type of food, but also multiple other factors such as taste, temperature, and time of consumption. Traditional cuisines have evolved hand in hand with such systems of medicine to optimize nutrition in the context of local climate and food availability. Harnessing the experiential wisdom of these traditional systems to create an integrative nutrition science would help fight the ongoing epidemic of chronic lifestyle diseases, and improve health and wellness.

Keywords: stroke; diet; vegetarian; vegan; Ayurveda; dosha; prakriti; integrative nutrition

Citation: Purushotham, A.; Hankey, A. Vegetarian Diets, Ayurveda, and the Case for an Integrative Nutrition Science. *Medicina* **2021**, *57*, 858. https://doi.org/10.3390/medicina57090858

Academic Editors: Robert H. Schneider and Mahadevan Seetharaman

Received: 26 May 2021
Accepted: 17 August 2021
Published: 24 August 2021

Publisher's Note: MDPI stays neutral with regard to jurisdictional claims in published maps and institutional affiliations.

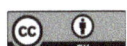

Copyright: © 2021 by the authors. Licensee MDPI, Basel, Switzerland. This article is an open access article distributed under the terms and conditions of the Creative Commons Attribution (CC BY) license (https://creativecommons.org/licenses/by/4.0/).

1. Introduction

Vegetarianism and veganism are diets growing rapidly in popularity not only because of perceived health benefits, but also because of social justice and sustainability concerns [1,2]. The EPIC-Oxford study was a longitudinal cohort study in the United Kingdom that examined the effects of diet—specifically a vegetarian diet—on cardio- and cerebro-vascular disease. Of a total of 48,188 enrollees, 16,254 were vegetarian. Over 18 years of follow-up, vegetarians had a 22% lower rate of ischemic heart disease compared to meat-eaters. This was in line with prior research: the most consistent benefits of vegetarianism have always been in cardiovascular health [3,4].

Cardiovascular and cerebrovascular disease are closely linked. They share a common pathophysiology, and have identical risk factors and principles of prevention and treatment. It was therefore rather surprising when the EPIC-Oxford study found a 20% increased risk of stroke, driven primarily by an increase in hemorrhagic stroke, in vegetarians [5]. The large size of the cohort and duration of longitudinal follow-up made this very unlikely to be an artefact.

Shortly afterward, another cohort study, this time from Taiwan, also reported on the influence of diet on stroke incidence. In two separate cohorts, one consisting of 1424/5050 vegetarians with 30,797 person-years of follow-up and another of 2719/8302 vegetarians with 76,797 person-years of follow-up, the authors found that stroke incidence was significantly lower among vegetarians. This was true in each cohort taken separately—

i.e., the result was reproducible across the two cohorts. The reduced incidence included both ischemic and hemorrhagic strokes [6].

How do we reconcile these contradictory results from large, well-planned, and well-executed studies? Lower levels of low-density lipoprotein (LDL) and lower levels of vitamin B12 were both hypothesized as possible explanations for the greater incidence of strokes in the EPIC-Oxford study [2,5]. The authors of the second study actually showed that levels of LDL and vit. B12 were significantly lower in vegetarians; yet stroke incidence was lower. In fact, it was specifically in the subgroup with inadequate vit. B12 intake that there was a significant association between vegetarian diet and lower overall stroke [6].

In this Perspective, we take a deeper look at the reported diets of the study cohorts and adopt the perspective of Ayurveda, India's traditional medical system, to try to explain these seemingly irreconcilable results.

2. Comparison of Cohort Diets

Figure 1 provides a comparison of the average nutrient intakes reported by the different diet groups in each study. Vegetarians in each study consumed fewer total calories, and a greater percentage of these was consumed as carbohydrates compared to meat-eaters. On the flip side, proteins and fats made up smaller percentages of the total caloric intake for vegetarians. Notwithstanding these commonalities, from the graph, it becomes apparent that there are fundamental differences in the patterns of nutrient intake between EPIC-Oxford's predominantly European Caucasian subjects and the Taiwanese subjects of the second study (TCHS). The latter's overall energy intake and proportion of protein and fat intake are lower, and that of carbohydrate higher, than the Oxford-EPIC subjects—so much so that the meat-eaters of TCHS consumed fewer calories, less protein and fat, and more carbohydrate than even the EPIC-Oxford vegetarians.

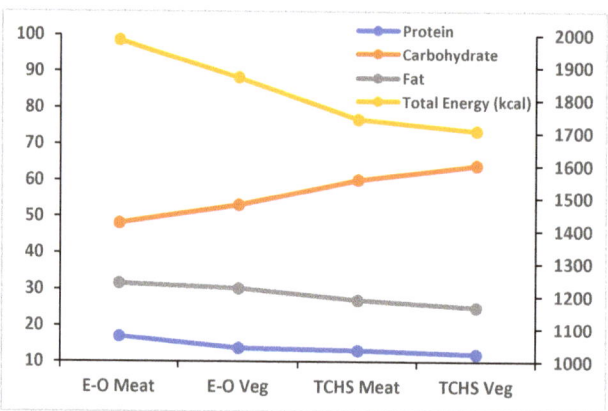

Figure 1. Comparison of the nutrient intakes in different diet groups of the EPIC-Oxford (E-O) and cohort 1 of the Taiwanese (TCHS) studies X-axis: Diet group; Y-axis (right): Total energy intake in kcal; Y-axis (left): Nutrient intake as percentage of total energy intake; Meat = Meat-eater; Veg = Vegetarian.

When the intakes of specific food groups are examined, the most striking difference between the two studies is in the consumption of soya products and legumes. TCHS vegetarians consumed 1.21 times as much plant protein, and 1.5 times as much soya-based food as TCHS meat-eaters. On the other hand, EPIC-Oxford vegetarians consumed 3.7 times as many legumes and soya-based foods as their meat-eating counterparts. In view of the aforementioned cultural propensity to eat a protein-heavy diet, this can be understood as an attempt to substitute for the missing animal protein with plant protein.

While such a simple substitution of one kind of protein for another may seem innocuous and even necessary from the perspective of Western nutrition science, Ayurveda, the system of traditional Indian medicine, believes that these foods have different effects on the body.

3. The Ayurvedic Perspective

Ayurveda is an ancient system of medicine that continues to be widely used in the Indian subcontinent today, especially for the treatment of chronic diseases such as stroke [7,8]. It uses dietary intervention as a cornerstone of therapy, both to maintain wellness and treat disease [9]. Additionally, because of the Indian subcontinent's long and popular tradition of vegetarianism stemming from the principle of *ahimsa* or non-violence, the system possesses a good deal of collective experience in maintaining the health of vegetarians. Ayurveda extensively describes the effects of different foods on the body's physiology, including meats and other non-vegetarian foods which it actively recommends in certain conditions. Looking at the dietary intakes reported above from an Ayurvedic perspective is therefore informative.

Ayurveda uses a broad, effectively systems-based three-way classification of physiological functions, called *doshas*: *vata dosha*, concerned with movement and input–output functions; *pitta dosha* concerned with turnover, i.e., digestion and metabolism; and *kapha dosha*, concerned with energy storage, growth, and lubrication [10]. Health depends on keeping *doshas* in balance [11]. Conversely, imbalances in *dosha* functions lead to disease; the pathogenesis of each disease condition is attributed to one or more *doshas* becoming progressively deranged [7,12].

In this context, each food may suppress or boost functions belonging to one or more *doshas*, thereby influencing important aspects of the overall physiology. This leads to increased or decreased susceptibility to specific medical disorders. Such effects of foods are mostly independent of the calorie–protein–carbohydrate–fat classification used in modern bioscience. Thus, while some protein-rich foods may boost a particular *dosha*, others may boost another *dosha*, or suppress the first, etc. [9]. Climate also plays a central role, since variations like windy/calm, hot/cold, and wet/dry can have deleterious effects on the *doshas*.

Revisiting the food intake of the EPIC-Oxford and TCHS dietary cohorts, the foremost difference between vegetarian and meat-inclusive diets is, of course, the absence of meat from the former. Meats overall tend to increase *kapha dosha*. Therefore, a meat-less diet, compared to a meat-eating diet, would in the long run decrease the occurrence of *kapha* disorders, which include metabolic syndrome disorders such as hypertension, diabetes, hyperlipidemia, and ischemic heart disease [13]. As previously noted, this is borne out by several research studies [3,14].

Now let us consider the effects of the much greater legume and soya-based food intake seen among the EPIC-Oxford vegetarians. In general, legumes including soya, chickpeas, and kidney beans greatly increase *vata dosha*. Indian (and other Eastern) vegetarian diets do contain quantities of legumes, but favor the less *vata*-genic ones such as the mung, highly proteinaceous urad, toor, and masoor beans. These are also prepared with special care: their effects on *doshas* are typically balanced out by liberal use of contrarily acting spices, and eating them hot and very well cooked [15]. Not adequately tempered, chronic *vata*-boosting can lead to diseases such as stroke and other neurological disorders known in Ayurveda as *Vata vyadhis* ("The Vata Diseases") [16–18].

Fermentation and some of the other processing techniques used to prepare soya products, such as soy sauce, tempeh, and soy meats, can lead to boosting of *pitta dosha*. A combined aggravation of *vata* and *pitta* is far more potent than that of either alone, especially when *pitta* is said to obstruct *vata*, and may in particular predispose to hemorrhagic strokes [19,20]. The increased stroke incidence observed in the EPIC-Oxford vegetarians, but not the TCHS vegetarians, is thus not surprising when viewed through the lens of Ayurveda.

4. Vegetarianism and Ayurveda

Traditional cuisines have evolved over millennia, informed by local medicinal knowledge to optimize health and well-being in the context of local climates and value systems. Traditional Indian cuisines, notwithstanding the wide variety across the subcontinent, are based on Ayurvedic principles, and have a common underlying theme of combining food types to promote balance of *dosha* functions in the context of local climate, season, and availability. These take into account not just the type of food, but innumerable other factors—including taste, texture, temperature, and time of consumption—that contribute to the effects of foods. For example, the *Kshemakutuhalam*, a 16th century Ayurvedic text on dietetics, describes traditional Indian cuisine, including combinations of ingredients to be used in different recipes and their health benefits, at length [21]. The three authoritative texts of Ayurveda each recommend seasonal modifications to the diet. The *Ashtanga hridayam*, one of the three, has an entire chapter devoted to *Ritucharya*—i.e., seasonal lifestyle including diet [22].

Another important Ayurvedic consideration for a meat-eater planning to turn vegetarian is the concept of *Satmya*—the importance of habituation [23]. Any change in diet from one that an individual was previously accustomed to, should be introduced gradually, in stages [24]. An abrupt change to a new diet—even if it is healthier than the prior one—can lead to ill health ("*Asatmyajanya roga*") [23]. Hence, Ayurveda would recommend that the transition to vegetarianism be a gradual one [24].

Vegetarians who do not come from a culture with a long vegetarian tradition, looking to develop their own healthy meal plans, may benefit from considering such nutritional perspectives of traditionally vegetarian cuisines.

5. Conclusions

Systems of traditional medicine such as Ayurveda possess rich knowledge of the effects of various foods on physiology, accumulated over centuries of keen observation. As evidenced above, Ayurvedic principles can shed entirely new light on an otherwise inexplicable clinical observation or outcome.

Ayurveda is a promising weapon against chronic disease [7,25,26]. Its extensive experience with holistic nutrition, together with that of other traditional systems of medicine, should be harnessed to create an integrative nutrition science to promote health and well-being.

Author Contributions: Conceptualization, data analysis, image preparation, A.P.; writing—original draft preparation, review and editing, A.P. and A.H. Both authors have read and agreed to the published version of the manuscript.

Funding: This research received no external funding.

Institutional Review Board Statement: Not applicable. This article is based only on review of previously published studies. No fresh data was collected.

Informed Consent Statement: Not applicable. The study did not directly involve any patients.

Data Availability Statement: Data was only contained in the stated references.

Acknowledgments: The authors thank Rammohan Rao, Faculty, California College of Ayurveda, Nevada City and Narendra Pendse, Medical Advisor, Institute of Ayurvedic and Integrative Medicine, Bangalore, for helpful discussions.

Conflicts of Interest: The authors declare no conflict of interest.

References

1. Segovia-Siapco, G.; Sabate, J. Health and sustainability outcomes of vegetarian dietary patterns: A revisit of the EPIC-Oxford and the Adventist Health Study-2 cohorts. *Eur. J. Clin. Nutr.* **2019**, *72*, 60–70. [CrossRef] [PubMed]
2. Lawrence, M.A.; McNaughton, S.A. Vegetarian diets and health. *BMJ* **2019**, *366*, l5272. [CrossRef] [PubMed]
3. Kahleova, H.; Levin, S.; Barnard, N.D. Vegetarian Dietary Patterns and Cardiovascular Disease. *Prog. Cardiovasc. Dis.* **2018**, *61*, 54–61. [CrossRef]

4. Dinu, M.; Abbate, R.; Gensini, G.F.; Casini, A.; Sofi, F. Vegetarian, vegan diets and multiple health outcomes: A systematic review with meta-analysis of observational studies. *Crit. Rev. Food Sci. Nutr.* **2017**, *57*, 3640–3649. [CrossRef] [PubMed]
5. Tong, T.Y.N.; Appleby, P.N.; Bradbury, K.E.; Perez-Cornago, A.; Travis, R.C.; Clarke, R.; Key, T.J. Risks of ischaemic heart disease and stroke in meat eaters, fish eaters, and vegetarians over 18 years of follow-up: Results from the prospective EPIC-Oxford study. *BMJ* **2019**, *366*, l4897. [CrossRef] [PubMed]
6. Chiu, T.H.T.; Chang, H.R.; Wang, L.Y.; Chang, C.C.; Lin, M.N.; Lin, C.L. Vegetarian diet and incidence of total, ischemic, and hemorrhagic stroke in 2 cohorts in Taiwan. *Neurology* **2020**, *94*, e1112–e1121. [CrossRef] [PubMed]
7. Harini, J.A.; Luthra, A.; Madeka, S.; Shankar, P.; Mandava, P.; Pervaje, R.; Aaron, S.; Purushotham, A. Ayurvedic Treatment of Acute Ischemic Stroke: A Prospective Observational Study. *Glob. Adv. Health Med.* **2019**, *8*. [CrossRef]
8. Pandian, J.D.; Toor, G.; Arora, R.; Kaur, P.; Dheeraj, K.V.; Bhullar, R.S.; Sylaja, P.N. Complementary and alternative medicine treatments among stroke patients in India. *Top. Stroke Rehabil.* **2012**, *19*, 384–394. [CrossRef] [PubMed]
9. Banerjee, S.; Debnath, P.; Debnath, P.K. Ayurnutrigenomics: Ayurveda-inspired personalized nutrition from inception to evidence. *J. Tradit. Complement. Med.* **2015**, *5*, 228–233. [CrossRef] [PubMed]
10. Hankey, A. Establishing the Scientific Validity of Tridosha part 1: Doshas, Subdoshas and Dosha Prakritis. *Anc. Sci. Life* **2010**, *29*, 6–18. [PubMed]
11. Acharya, J.T. *Sushruta Samhita with Nibandha Sangraha Commentary of Dalhanacharya*; Chaukhamba Orientalia: Varanasi, India, 2007.
12. Sharma, S. *Ashtanga Samgraha of Vriddha Vagbhata, Sasilekha Sanskrit Commentary by Indu*; Chaukhamba Orientalia: Varanasi, India, 2008; p. 568.
13. Mahalle, N.P.; Kulkarni, M.V.; Pendse, N.M.; Naik, S.S. Association of constitutional type of Ayurveda with cardiovascular risk factors, inflammatory markers and insulin resistance. *J. Ayurveda Integr. Med.* **2012**, *3*, 150–157. [CrossRef] [PubMed]
14. Papier, K.; Appleby, P.N.; Fensom, G.K.; Knuppel, A.; Perez-Cornago, A.; Schmidt, J.A.; Tong, T.Y.N.; Key, T.J. Vegetarian diets and risk of hospitalisation or death with diabetes in British adults: Results from the EPIC-Oxford study. *Nutr. Diabetes* **2019**, *9*, 7. [CrossRef] [PubMed]
15. Bredesen, D.E.; Rao, R.V. Ayurvedic Profiling of Alzheimer's Disease. *Altern. Ther. Health Med.* **2017**, *23*, 46–50. [PubMed]
16. Kumar, N.; Mishra, S. Critical review of Vatavyadhi in Brihattrayi. *Intl. J. Appl. Res.* **2020**, *6*, 60–62.
17. Acharya, J.T. *Charaka Samhita with Ayurveda Dipika Commentary of Chakrapanidatta*; Chaukhamba Orientalia: Varanasi, India, 2007; p. 619, Chikitsasthana Chapter 28, verse 53.
18. Murthy, K.R.S. *Madhava Nidana of Madhavakara with English translation, Critical Introduction and Appendices*; Chaukhamba Orientalia: Varanasi, India, 2009; p. 84, Chapter 22, verses 39–41.
19. Acharya, J.T. *Charaka Samhita with Ayurveda Dipika Commentary of Chakrapanidatta*; Chaukhamba Orientalia: Varanasi, India, 2007; Chikitsasthana Chapter 28, verses 61, 221–229.
20. Anoop, A.S.; Anupama, A.S.; Sagar, K. Ayurvedic understanding and management of cerebrovascular accident (stroke with ischemia and hemorrhage): A case study. *Int. J. Sci. Res.* **2020**, *9*, 75–77.
21. Kṣemaśarma. *Kṣemakutūhalam*; Foundation for Revitalization of Local Health Traditions: Bangalore, India, 2009.
22. Ashtanga Hridaya of Vagbhatta. *Ashtanga Hridaya of Vagbhatta*; Chaukhamba Orientalia: Varanasi, India, 2007; Sutrasthana 3, p. 37.
23. Ashtanga Hridaya of Vagbhatta. *Ashtanga Hridaya of Vagbhatta*; Chaukhamba Orientalia: Varanasi, India, 2007; Sutrasthana 3, verse 58.
24. Agnivesha. *Charaka Samhita*; Ayurveda Dipika by Chakrapanidatta, Chaukhamba Orientalia: Varanasi, India, 2007; Sutrasthana 7, verses 36–37.
25. Hankey, A. Ayurveda and the battle against chronic disease: An opportunity for Ayurveda to go mainstream? *J. Ayurveda Integr. Med.* **2010**, *1*, 9–12. [CrossRef] [PubMed]
26. Furst, D.E.; Venkatraman, M.M.; McGann, M.; Manohar, P.R.; Booth-LaForce, C.; Sarin, R.; Sekar, P.G.; Raveendran, K.G.; Mahapatra, A.; Gopinath, J.; et al. Double-blind, randomized, controlled, pilot study comparing classic ayurvedic medicine, methotrexate, and their combination in rheumatoid arthritis. *J. Clin. Rheumatol.* **2011**, *17*, 185–192. [CrossRef] [PubMed]

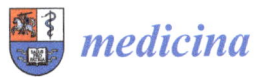

Perspective

The Future of Women and Heart Disease in a Pandemic Era: Let's Learn from the Past

Suzanne Steinbaum

Mount Sinai Hospital, New York, NY 1468, USA; drsrsteinbaum@gmail.com

Abstract: When the pandemic started in February, about 5 million women were running businesses. Just 2 months later, 25% of those businesses closed. Approximately 2.5 million women have lost their jobs or dropped out of the workforce since the pandemic, but that is just the start of the impact on women. Women have been disproportionately affected by the pandemic, as the brunt of homelife has fallen on them, and the psychosocial impact will inevitably have a physical impact. The pandemic has revealed the gender inequality that exists from the socioeconomic perspective, but soon we will see the impact from the medical perspective. Predictably, we know that the impact of stress and lack of self-care that women have had to endure heightens heart disease, already the number one killer of all women. Heart disease is 80% preventable based on the major risk factors: high cholesterol, high blood pressure, elevated sugar, obesity, smoking, sedentary lifestyle, and poor diet. But the psychological risk factors drive up biomarkers and the root causes of manifesting disease. Historically, women have been less diagnosed and treated, and less likely to receive lifesaving care in a timely fashion. The pandemic is sure to amplify these issues. Without mitigation and prevention, women's hearts will suffer. We need to be aware of this now to prepare for the future potential of a significant increase in the incidence of women and heart disease.

Keywords: pandemic and women; women and heart disease; psychological effects of pandemic; cardiac prevention; risk of heart disease in women

Citation: Steinbaum, S. The Future of Women and Heart Disease in a Pandemic Era: Let's Learn from the Past. *Medicina* **2021**, *57*, 467. https://doi.org/10.3390/medicina57050467

Academic Editors: Robert H. Schneider and Mahadevan Seetharaman

Received: 26 March 2021
Accepted: 6 May 2021
Published: 11 May 2021

Publisher's Note: MDPI stays neutral with regard to jurisdictional claims in published maps and institutional affiliations.

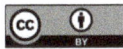

Copyright: © 2021 by the author. Licensee MDPI, Basel, Switzerland. This article is an open access article distributed under the terms and conditions of the Creative Commons Attribution (CC BY) license (https://creativecommons.org/licenses/by/4.0/).

When the pandemic started in February, about 5 million women were running businesses. Just 2 months later, 25% of those businesses closed. Approximately 2.5 million women have lost their jobs or dropped out of the workforce since the pandemic, but that is just the start of the impact on women [1]. Women have been disproportionately affected by the pandemic, as the brunt of homelife has fallen on them, and the psychosocial impact will inevitably have a physical impact. The pandemic has revealed the gender inequality that exists from the socioeconomic perspective, but soon we will see the impact from the medical perspective. As time goes on, we are going to see the impact of the stress and lack of self-care that women have had to endure, which will predictably lead to the number one killer of all women, heart disease. Heart disease is 80% preventable based on the major risk factors—high cholesterol, high blood pressure, elevated sugar, overweight, smoking, sedentary lifestyle, poor diet—but the psychological risk factors are often the reasons for driving the biomarkers up and the root cause of manifesting disease [2].

As we have identified the impact of the pandemic on the psychosocial risk factors, it becomes concerning to conceptualize what toll this will take on women's hearts. The lack of equity that has been magnified in the lives of women socially may amplify the lack of equity that women have received when it comes to heart disease. We need to be concerned that the future of medicine for women will show a more significant impact on morbidity and mortality due to the disparities in care when it comes to women and heart disease. This is a critical time to address these issues, before we feel the impact.

1. The Historical Perspective

In 1964, the American Heart Association held the first conference for women on heart disease. It was titled "Hearts and Husbands" and the objective was to learn how to keep your husband's hearts healthy. Research was done on men only at that point. Heart disease was a man's disease. Caring for women's hearts did not exist in the science, and it was not in the consciousness of the population that mattered the most: women themselves.

In 1984, more women started dying of heart disease than men, and it all directed back to the lack of science. During the 20 years prior, women were not included in the major trials on heart disease from prevention to treatment, including diagnostic strategies, pharmacologic interventions, prevention and interventional procedures. This gap in research caught up to the reality, and the outcome was an increase in women's mortality.

Then, in 1994, the Office of Women's Health was created, which was the first governmental initiative pushing the agenda of research on women and heart disease. Yet, another decade passed before Go Red for Women through the American Heart Association began promoting research, education and awareness. When Go Red for Women began in 2004, only 30% of women were aware that heart disease was even a threat. These past two decades spurred more progress and more initiatives and research. Finally, things have started to change in demonstrable ways for women's heart health, yet, still, only 38% of cardiovascular research participants are women [3].

The pervasive bias still exists. Women are less likely to be diagnosed, treated or to receive lifesaving care in a timely fashion. In fact, even when seeing their primary care doctors, cardiovascular disease is not the top concern for the women or their physicians. The primary care doctors placed a greater emphasis on weight issues and breast health over cardiovascular disease [4]. Yet, women are dying of heart disease more than all cancers combined [5].

2. The Medical Perspective

The medical community is falling short when it comes to women and their hearts. A recent global meta-analysis looked at women who had acute heart attacks to assess their outcomes. Not only did women have to wait longer for lifesaving procedures compared to male patients arriving to the hospital, but women also had increased mortality rates compared with males. In fact, there was up to a two-fold increased rate of mortality, repeat heart attack and stroke due to co-morbidities, due to delay in care and suboptimal treatment [6].

Even when looking at a younger population of women, previously considered to be immune from cardiovascular disease due to the protective effects of estrogen, there is an increase in cardiac events. The ARIC Community Surveillance Study found an increase in acute myocardial infarction hospitalizations in women less than 55 years old between 1995 and 2014. This is believed to be due to a decrease in the recognition of risk factors in this younger population, because of a lack of preventive strategies. These younger women had greater risk factors due to lifestyle choices, such as hypertension and diabetes, yet there was less likelihood for aggressive screening or treatment [7].

Other trials looked at this population of younger women and found a greater prevalence of diabetes, heart failure, chronic obstructive pulmonary disease, chronic kidney disease and obesity compared with the men.

As we are seeing what was previously considered a young healthy population, pregnant women, suffer increased rates of hypertension and diabetes, there is an increase in the risk of cardiovascular-disease-related deaths. In fact, women with obesity, hypertension and diabetes have the greatest risk of death during pregnancy [8]. The risk factors are the same risk factors that are driving the prevalence of heart disease in younger women higher and higher.

3. The Equality of Care Perspective

Women physicians are growing in numbers, and although only 13 % of cardiologists are women, more than 50% of internal medicine residents are women.

This is an important factor in women's health. One systematic review evaluated eight studies examining patient outcomes based on the physician gender. One study showed that mortality rates for patients having a heart attack were highest for female patients treated by male physicians. On the other hand, if the physician was female then the mortality rates were the same between the male and the female patients. Male physicians who had more interactions and exposure to female patients, and even with female physicians, had more success in treating female patients [9].

To be better prepared, acknowledgment of these gender roles and then training doctors about them is critical. The bias is not permanent, once it is addressed. The time has come that we pivot from the old thinking. This is not the 1950s anymore, and women in the last year have suffered in a way that has not been seen before.

4. The Psychological Perspective

My greatest concern comes down to the basics—who is suffering and who is dying from heart disease and how do we prevent it from happening in the future?

We are coming off of a time filled with changes in lifestyle and huge psychosocial implications. Coping measures for emotional upheaval impacts behavior, resulting in overeating, sedentary behavior, poor diets, increased alcohol intake and overarching stress. The implications of this reaches into our lives, and these behavioral changes affect the essence of those risk factors that lead to heart disease. Obesity, high blood pressure and high cholesterol and elevated sugars are going to affect more and more women as we get through these days of the pandemic, and hopefully soon, to the other side.

Depression itself is more common in women and doubles the risk of heart disease [10]. With stressful life events, chronic daily stressors and high levels of perceived stress, research has shown an increase in cardiovascular disease. In fact, work-related stress was associated with a 40% increased risk of cardiovascular disease, and perceived loneliness and social isolation increased the incidence by 50%. The connection between the mind and heart is significant: the more profound, the greater the burden of the psychosocial issues, like stress or depression. [11].

Not only has the emotional toll led to depression and anxiety, but for some, post-traumatic stress disorder. PTSD, defined as a "mental disorder that occurs after exposure to a potentially traumatic life event and is characterized by extreme levels of distress," is associated with a 61% increased risk of coronary artery disease, with associations with traditional risk factors. Along with these, anger and hostility, depression and pessimism all have a role in cardiovascular outcomes. With declining mental health, healthy behaviors are less likely to be prevalent, with a reduction in exercise consistency and poor dietary choices [10].

As women have been juggling the traditional roles with increased work stress and decreased income, there is the potential for an increase in heart disease. Perhaps this impact has just begun, and we will start seeing the true burden in years to come. As a cardiologist, I know the toll will roll out increasingly over time and we will continue to see an uptick in heart disease in this same population that, during this intensely stressful time, was more forced to carry the load than ever before.

For women, this mind–body connection is even stronger. Depression and stress may quickly negatively impact physical health with increased weight gain and diminished exercise. The cycle, which has always been a factor in women's heart health is now heightened directly because of the pandemic.

5. The Future Perspective

The long-term impact of the pandemic's attack on women will long be seen in women's hearts.

As we look at the research behind the pandemic, it becomes a concerning issue to conceptualize the toll that this pandemic will take on women's hearts. With the awareness of the psychological and the economic toll, it is essential to discuss the physical toll—no one has spoken of what we are to expect regarding women and heart disease in the future.

As a cardiologist working in prevention for two decades, I am sadly confident that the statistics will soon show the impact that this pandemic has had on women and their hearts.

As the demographic of heart disease changes, it is essential to evaluate and understand this population, the reality behind the increase in risk factors, and the reasons behind the increased risk. This younger group of women is the group of women who are going to be most significantly impacted in terms of their heart health [11]. We are at a critical time in understanding the profound impact of these risks and are lagging behind in fully addressing them.

Much like the past thirty years in general when we slowly evolved from a "man's disease" to the realization that heart disease is the number one killer of women, we are again unprepared for what is to come.

This simple lack of acknowledgement can possibly foreshadow the possibility that women will suffer greatly due to their heart disease. There continues to exist that unconscious, intrinsic, inexplicable bias that is still is pervasive, except when women patients get to see women doctors [12].

6. A Better Way Forward

We can do better, across the board. We need to focus on the needs of women and the true issues at hand. We need to understand the psychosocial impact and the true devastation that COVID-19 has on our population of women, and most importantly, we need to anticipate and address the future.

We have had our wake-up call. We have seen the statistics, and after decades of watching more women die of heart disease than all cancers combined, it is time we pay attention. We need to shift our focus from looking at each patient the same and open our understanding to who women have been during this historical time. They have been carrying the load emotionally, which is taking a toll physically.

The doctors need to be trained and ready to understand the symptoms of heart disease in women, be able to assess the risks, and expediently provide care that could possibly save her life [13].

As a community, we need to get ready for the women whose hearts have suffered and understand that if we do not address their mental well-being and the effects it has on the overall health, we will continue to misdiagnose, undertreat and enable women younger and younger to become ill.

Women have just lived through the ultimate test for their hearts with chronic daily stressors and high levels of stress. It is time we get this issue straight and be prepared. Not only has the essence of women's lives been put on the line, but also their hearts. I hope we are ready for it when the time comes.

Funding: This research received no external funding.

Institutional Review Board Statement: Not applicable.

Conflicts of Interest: The authors declare no conflict of interest.

References

1. Harris, K. The Exodus of Women from the Workforce Is a National Emergency. Available online: https://www.washingtonpost.com/opinions/kamala-harris-women-workforce-pandemic/2021/02/12/b8cd1cb6-6d6f-11eb-9f80-3d7646ce1bc0_story.html (accessed on 12 February 2021).
2. Arnett, D.K.; Blumenthal, R.S.; Albert, M.A.; Buroker, A.B.; Goldberger, Z.D.; Hahn, E.J.; Himmelfarb, C.D.; Khera, A.; Lloyd-Jones, D.; McEvoy, J.W.; et al. 2019 ACC/AHA guideline on the primary prevention of cardiovascular disease: Executive Summary: A Report of the American College of Cardiology/American Heart Association Task Force on Clinical Practice guidelines. *J. Am. Coll. Cardiol.* **2019**, *74*, 1376–1414. [CrossRef] [PubMed]
3. Jin, X.; Chandranouli, C.; Allocco, B.; Gong, E.; Lam, C.; Yan, L.L. Women's Participation in Cardiovascular Clinical Trials from 2010 to 2017. *Circulation* **2020**, *141*, 540–548. [CrossRef] [PubMed]
4. Bairy Merz, C.N.; Anderson, H.; Sprague, E.; Burns, A.; Keida, M.; Walsh, M.N.; Greenberger, P.; Campbell, S.; Pollin, I.; McCullough, C.; et al. Knowledge, Attitudes, and Beliefs Regarding Cardiovascular Disease in Women: The Women's Heart Alliance. *J. Am. Coll. Cardiol.* **2017**, *70*, 123–132. [CrossRef] [PubMed]

5. Pathak, E.B. Is Heart Disease or Cancer the Leading Cause of Death in United States Women? *Women's Health Issues* **2016**, *26*, 589–594. [CrossRef] [PubMed]
6. Van Oosterhout, R.E.; DeBoer, A.R.; Maas, A.H.E.M.; Rutten, F.H.; Bots, M.L.; Peters, S.A.E. Sex Differences in Symptom Presentation in Acute Coronary Syndromes: A Systematic Review and Meta-analysis. *J. Am. Heart Assoc.* **2020**, *9*, e014733. [CrossRef] [PubMed]
7. Sameer, A.; Stouffer, G.A.; Kucharska-Newton, A.M.; Qamar, A.; Vaduganathan, M.; Pandey, A.; Porterfield, D.; Blankstein, R.; Rosamond, W.D.; Bhatt, D.L.; et al. Twenty Year Trends and Sex Differences in Young Adults Hospitalized with Acute Myocardial Infarction: The ARIC Community Surveillance Study. *Circulation* **2019**, *139*, 1047–1056.
8. Brown, M.A.; Magee, L.A.; Kenny, L.C.; Karumanchi, S.A.; McCarthy, F.P.; Saito, S.; Hall, D.R.; Warren, C.E.; Adoyi, G.; Ishaku, S.; et al. Hypertensive Disorders of Pegnancy: ISSHP Classification, Diagnosis and Management Recommendations for International Practice. *Hypertension* **2018**, *72*, 24–43. [CrossRef] [PubMed]
9. Lau, E.S.; Hayes, S.N.; Volgman, A.S.; Lindley, K.; Pepine, C.J.; Wood, M.J.; American College of Cardiology Cardiovascular Disease in Women Section. Does Patient-Physician Gender Concordance Influence Patients Perceptions or Outcomes? *J. Am. Coll. Cardiol.* **2021**, *77*, 1135–1138. [CrossRef] [PubMed]
10. Cho, L.; Davis, M.; Elgendy, I.; Epps, K.; Lindley, K.J.; Mehta, P.K.; Michos, E.D.; Minissian, M.; Pepine, C.; Vaccarino, V.; et al. Summary of Updated Recommendations for Primary Prevention of Cardiovascular Disease in Women: JACC State-of-the-Art Review. *J. Am. Coll. Cardiol.* **2020**, *75*, 2602–2618. [CrossRef] [PubMed]
11. Levine, G.J.; Cohen, B.E.; Commondore-Mensah, Y.; Fleury, J.; Huffman, J.C.; Khalid, U.; Labarthe, D.R.; Lavretsky, H.; Michos, E.D.; Spatz, E.S.; et al. Psychological Health, Well Being, and the Mind-Heart-Body Connection: A Scientific Statement from the American Heart Association. *Circulation* **2021**, *143*, e763–e783. [CrossRef] [PubMed]
12. Lichtman, J.H.; Leifheit, E.C.; Safdar, B. Sex Differences in the Presentation and Perception of Symptoms among Young Patients with Myocardial Infarction: Evidence from the VIRGO Study (Variation in Recovery: Role of Gender on Outcomes of Young AMI Patients). *Circulation* **2018**, *137*, 781–790. [CrossRef] [PubMed]
13. Shah, T.; Haimi, I.; Yang, Y.; Gaston, S.; Taoutel, R.; Mehta, S.; Lee, H.J.; Zambahari, R.; Baumbach, A.; Henry, T.D.; et al. Meta-analysis of gender disparities in in-hospital care and outcomes in patients with ST-segment elevation myocardial infarction. *Am. J. Cardiol.* **2021**, *147*, 23–32. [CrossRef] [PubMed]

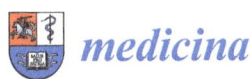

Review

Natural Products and Nutrients against Different Viral Diseases: Prospects in Prevention and Treatment of SARS-CoV-2

Syed Ghazanfar Ali [1,*], Mohammad Azam Ansari [2], Mohammad A. Alzohairy [3], Ahmad Almatroudi [3], Mohammad N. Alomary [4,*], Saad Alghamdi [5], Suriya Rehman [2] and Haris M. Khan [1]

1. Viral Research Diagnostic Laboratory, Department of Microbiology, Jawaharlal Nehru Medical College A.M.U., Aligarh U.P.202002, India; harismk2003@hotmail.com
2. Department of Epidemic Disease Research, Institutes for Research and Medical Consultations (IRMC), Imam Abdulrahman Bin Faisal University, Dammam 31441, Saudi Arabia; maansari@iau.edu.sa (M.A.A.); surrehman@iau.edu.sa (S.R.)
3. Department of Medical Laboratories, College of Applied Medical Sciences, Qassim University, Qassim 51431, Saudi Arabia; dr.alzohairy@gmail.com (M.A.A.); aamtrody@qu.edu.sa (A.A.)
4. National Centre for Biotechnology, King Abdulaziz City for Science and Technology (KACST), P.O. Box 6086, Riyadh 11442, Saudi Arabia
5. Laboratory Medicine Department, Faculty of Applied Medical Sciences, Umm Al-Qura University, Makkah21955, Saudi Arabia; ssalghamdi@uqu.edu.sa
* Correspondence: syedmicro72@gmail.com (S.G.A.); malomary@kacst.edu.sa (M.N.A.)

Abstract: Severe acute respiratory syndrome coronavirus-2 (SARS-CoV-2) has caused a global pandemic and is posing a serious challenge to mankind. As per the current scenario, there is an urgent need for antiviral that could act as a protective and therapeutic against SARS-CoV-2. Previous studies have shown that SARS-CoV-2 is much similar to the SARS-CoV bat that occurred in 2002-03. Since it is a zoonotic virus, the exact source is still unknown, but it is believed bats may be the primary reservoir of SARS-CoV-2 through which it has been transferred to humans. In this review, we have tried to summarize some of the approaches that could be effective against SARS-CoV-2. Firstly, plants or plant-based products have been effective against different viral diseases, and secondly, plants or plant-based natural products have the minimum adverse effect. We have also highlighted a few vitamins and minerals that could be beneficial against SARS-CoV-2.

Keywords: antiviral; medicinal plants; pandemic; SARS-CoV-2; zoonotic virus

1. Introduction

Coronaviruses under the realm of Riboviria belongs to the order Nidovirales, suborder cornidovirinea, family Coronoviridae [1]. Orthocoronavirinae the subfamily of coronoviridae is further divided into four genera alpha (a), beta (b), gamma (c), and delta (d) coronavirus. Further, SARS-CoV belongs to Beta coronavirus and sarbecovirus is the subgenus of SARS-CoV-2 [2]. It shares similar homology with bat coronavirus and it has been estimated that both have 96.2% sequence homology [3].

The two epidemics due to coronavirus have already occurred that were due to SARS-CoV and the Middle East respiratory syndrome (MERS) and both have been the major cause of pneumonia in humans [4]. SARS-CoV emerged in 2002 and remained till 2003 during the period it caused 774 death and more than 800 people were infected. MERS-CoV emerged in Saudi Arabia in 2012, which caused more than 800 deaths, and 2500 people became infected [5].

Coronaviruses have single-stranded RNA as genetic material that can range from 26 kbs to 32 kbs in length. Coronaviruses possess specific genes in Open Reading Frame ORF1 downstream region that are responsible for encoding the proteins responsible for viral replication, nucleocapsid, and spike formation [6]. The structure of SARS-CoV shows the spikes on the outer surface. Furthermore, studies have shown that structural proteins are encoded by the four structural genes, which include spike (S), envelope (E), membrane (M), and nucleocapsid (N) gene. These genes are responsible for viral functionality and structure [7].

SARS-CoV-2 genome is 80% similar to the previous human coronavirus SARS-CoV [8]. For some of the encoded proteins such as coronavirus main proteinase (3CLpro), papain-like protease (PLpro), and RNA-dependent RNA polymerase (RdRp) the sequence similarity is very high (96%) between SARS-CoV, and SARS-CoV-2 [9].

SARS-CoV-2 and SARS-CoV spike protein have 76.5% identical amino acid sequences [10]. The 3D structures of spike proteins of SARS-CoV-2 and SARS-CoV as analyzed by computer imaging revealed that both have identical structures in the receptor-binding domain and maintains the Vander Waals force [10]. The major amino acid residue of SARS-CoV-2 in the receptor-binding domain is Gln-493, which favors the attachment of spike protein S with human cells more specifically with the lungs therefore the attachment results in respiratory infections in humans [11,12]. Zhao et al. [11] have suggested that 83% of the angiotensin-converting enzyme (ACE-2) expressing cells are alveolar epithelial type II, therefore, these cells can be the reservoir for the viral invasion. Some analysts have suggested that SARS-CoV-2 binds to ACE-2 more efficiently as compared with SARS-CoV, therefore, it has a greater ability to transmit from person to person [13].

Initially, for the attachment to the host cells, virus use the spike (S) glycoprotein, which also mediates the host and viral cell membrane fusion during infection [14]. The spike (S) glycoprotein has two regions namely S1 and S2. S1 helps in the binding of host cell receptors, and S2 helps in the fusion with the membrane. The receptor-binding domain (RBD) is located in the S1 region of SARS-CoV and the attachment of the human host cell with the virus is mediated by the RBD protein of the RBD domain with the angiotensin-converting enzyme (ACE-2) as a receptor similar to the one required by SARS-CoV [15,16]. Since SARS-CoV and SARS-CoV-2 are much similar, it is believed that SARS-CoV-2 uses a similar receptor (ACE-2) for entering into human host cells [10,13].

The initial clinical symptoms that appear after SARS-CoV-2 infection are pneumonia, fever, dry cough, headache dyspnea, and in acute cases leads to respiratory failure and eventually, death occurs [17–19]. Although the healing depends upon immunity, pre-existing conditions such as hypertension, diabetes, cardiovascular diseases, or kidney diseases further enhances the severity of the pathogenesis of SARS-CoV-2 [17,19]. Different drugs are available in the market against SARS-CoV-2 but none has shown accurate results. None of the drugs has been approved by FDA against SARS-CoV-2.

Plants have been used as a medicine in the traditional Chinese and Ayurvedic systems [20]. Some of the herbal medicines have safety margins above those of reference drugs, which shows that they can be used against mild SARS-CoV-2 infection [21]. Plants in the form of herbal medicine or dietary components act as immunomodulators and can be a potent antiviral against SARS-CoV-2 infection [22].

Medicinal plants contain diverse secondary metabolites, therefore, they have been the source of drugs against viral, bacterial, and protozoal infection, including cancer [23,24]. The secondary metabolites present in the medicinal plants can interrupt viral proteins and enzymes by binding with them and preventing viral penetration and replication [25–28]. When consumed without knowing the appropriate dosage, herbal medicines may be toxic [29]. The genetically modified (GM) plants also pose serious health issues because the unnatural change in naturally occurring protein or the metabolic pathways results in toxins or allergens [30]. Therefore, the selection of medicinal plants is also an important aspect.

Vitamins play a major role in preventing established respiratory infection and intensive care settings. Vitamins enhance natural barriers because of their antioxidant and immunomodulatory effect and this could be beneficial against SARS-CoV-2 [31]. Mineral elements such as selenium and zinc have shown antiviral effects by enhancing the immune responses [32,33].

In this review article, we have tried to highlight the use of medicinal plants against different viral diseases including SARS-CoV-2, and also the possible factors (vitamins and minerals) that could be helpful against SARS-CoV-2.

2. Plants as a Source of Medicine against SARS-CoV-2

2.1. Glycyrrhiza Glabra

Glycyrrhiza glabra belongs to the family Fabaceae and is commonly known as licorice. Dried roots from the plant have a characteristic odor and sweet taste. Glycyrrhizin is the main component isolated from the roots. Glycyrrhizin inhibited 50% hepatitis C virus (HCV) in a dose-dependent manner at a concentration of 14 ± 2 µg [34].

Glycyrrhizin also protects from the influenza A virus and caused a reduction in influenza-infected lung cells [35]. In addition to being effective against hepatitis and influenza virus, it has also shown its effect on SARS CoV [31]. Cinatal et al. [36] showed that glycyrrhizin effectively inhibited the SARS-CoV virus replication at an early stage. They were also of opinion that glycyrrhizin affected cellular signaling pathways such as protein kinase C, casein kinase II, and transcription factors such as protein 1 and nuclear factor B. Furthermore, they also concluded the upregulation of nitrous oxide that inhibits the virus.

Sinha et al. [37] through in silico approach showed that the replication process of SARS-CoV-2 was affected by the two components of licorice (glyasperin A and glycyrrhizic acid) They concluded that the ACE-2 receptor of the virus was disturbed by glycyrrhizic acid and the replication process was inhibited by glyasperin A (Table 1).

2.2. Alnus Japonica

Alnus japonica, also known as the East Asian alder tree, grows approximately up to 22 m. It is deciduous with a very fast growth rate. It belongs to the family Betulaceae, also known as the birch family, which includes six genera having nut-bearing deciduous trees and shrubs. The extract of leaves and bark of *Alnus japonica* have been used as food that boosts immunity against influenza [38]. Studies have shown that methanolic extract of *Alnus japonica* bark possesses strong antiviral activity against the H9N2 subtype avian influenza virus [39]. Further, the chromatographic separation revealed the presence of four lupine type triterpenes and one steroid [39].

Diarylheptanoids isolated from *Alnus japonica* showed inhibitory activity against papain-like protease (required for replication of SARS-CoV) [40]. Nine diarylheptanoids were isolated, namely, platyphyllenone, hirsutenone, hirsutanonol, oregonin, rubranol, rubranoside B, and rubranoside A. Furthermore, hirsutenone, hirsutanonol, oregonin, rubranol, rubranoside B, and rubranoside A showed dose-dependent inhibitory activity against the papain-like protease. They also showed that hirsutenone possessed the most potent inhibitory activity against papain-like protease. Furthermore, the analysis of Park et al. [40] showed that catechol and α,β-unsaturated carbonyl moiety were present in the molecule, which are the key requirements for SARS-CoV cysteine protease inhibition.

Furthermore, Kwon et al. [41] described that *Alnus japonica* extract is useful for prevention from viral diseases, such as influenza of humans and of other mammalian and avian species. They also said that the extract exhibits very low toxicity in normal cell conditions but has high antiviral activity. Lastly, the extract from *Alnus japonica* could be effectively used in foods and pharmaceutical industries against the influenza virus.

2.3. Allium Sativum(Garlic)

Allium sativum belongs to the Amaryllidaceae family. It is a perennial flowering plant that grows from a bulb and comprises a tall flowering stem that attains a height of upto 1 m. *Allium sativum* is commonly called garlic, which is also an ingredient in Indian food. A peculiar smell can be noticed from the bulb of garlic, which is due to the presence of sulfur compounds. In addition to possessing antibacterial activity, *Allium sativum* (garlic) also has antiviral properties. *Allium sativum* extract hasan inhibitory effect on avian infectious bronchitis virus, which is a single-stranded RNA and belongs to coronaviruses. It has also shown its effect on other viruses including influenza A and B [42], cytomegalovirus [43], herpes simplex virus 1 [44], and herpes simplex virus-2 [45].

Molecular docking studies have revealed that garlic can inhibit SARS-CoV-2 [46]. Molecular docking has shown that 17 organosulfur compounds from garlic essential oil can effectively interact with the amino acid of angiotensin-converting enzyme (ACE-2), a receptor in the human body and main protease (PDB6LU7) of SARS-CoV-2. The highest efficacy was observed by allyl disulfide and allyl trisulfide. Furthermore, it was predicted that garlic essential oil or extract can be used as a source of antiviral against SARS-CoV-2 [46].

2.4. Houttuynia Cordata

Houttuynia cordata belongs to the family Saururaceae and is mostly confined to the moist habitat. It is an aromatic medicinal plant that has a creeping rootstock. Ethyl acetate extract of *Houttuynia cordata* is effective in inhibiting the infectivity of the dengue virus (DENV). Some workers have shown the inhibition of DENV-2 by ethyl acetate extract of *Houttuynia cordata* [47,48]. *Houttuynia cordata* extract also inhibited the avian infectious bronchitis virus [49]. Quercetin 3-rhamnoside from *Houttuynia cordata* showed anti-influenza (inf-A) activity and inhibited virus replication in the initial stages of infection [50]. Stem distillate from the *Houttuynia cordata* has shown inhibitory activity against herpes simplex virus-1, influenza virus, and human immunodeficiency virus-1 without any cytotoxicity [51]. The three major components from the distillate were methyl *n*–nonyl ketone, lauryl aldehyde, and capryl aldehyde.

Houttuynia cordata showed significant inhibition on SARS-CoV. The *Houttuynia cordata* (HC) extract successfully inhibited the SARS-CoV3C such as protease (3CLpro) and RNA-dependent RNA polymerase (RdRp) [52]. Furthermore, it was also observed that *Houttuynia cordata* extract was non-toxic to animal models at an oral administration dose of 16 g/kg. Through flow cytometric analysis, Lau et al. [52] showed that *Houttuynia cordata* extract in mice model significantly increases the CD4+ and CD8+ T cells with a significant increase in the secretion of IL-2 and IL-10 cytokine in mouse splenic lymphocytes.

2.5. Lycoris Radiata

Lycoris radiata, which is commonly known as red spider lily, hell flower, red magic lily, or sometimes called equinox flower, belongs to the family Amaryllidaceae. *Lycoris radiata* has shown its effect against H5N1 [53]. Lycorine the active component of *Lycoris radiata* successfully inhibited the influenza virus, which is responsible for avian influenza infection [54]. Proteomic analysis revealed that lycorine alters protein expression in avian influenza virus-infected cells and the treatment with lycorine also decreased the levels of nuclear pore complex protein 93(Nup93, E2RSV7), which is a part of nuclear-cytoplasmic transport [54]. Lycoricidine derivatives obtained from the bulb of *Lycoris radiata* have also shown the anti-hepatitis C virus activity [55]. Furthermore, it has also been observed that Lycorocidine derivates possess inhibitory activity against the tobacco mosaic virus [56].

Ethanolic extract of the stem cortex of the plant successfully inhibited the SARS-CoV. [57]. The active component that probably inhibited the SARS-CoV was lycorine (C16H17NO4), which was analyzed by high-performance liquid chromatography (HPLC). Although the mechanism of action of lycorine on the SARS-CoV is still unclear, it has shown promising results as an antiviral. Li et al. [57] also showed that commercially available lycorine inhibited the SARS-CoV.

2.6. Tinospora Cordifolia

Tinospora cordifolia, commonly called Guduchi or Giloy, belongs to the family Menispermaceae. The plant is an herbaceous vine that bears heart-shaped leaves. *Tinospora cordifolia* extract has shown an increase in IFN-α, IL-1, IL-2,and IL-4 levels in the peripheral blood mononuclear cells in the chickens infected with infectious bursal disease virus, which causes infectious bursal disease [58]. Further, the reduction in the mortality rate of chickens treated with *Tinospora cordifolia* extract was also observed when compared with uninfected chickens [58].

The stem extract of *Tinospora cordifolia* has antibacterial, antifungal, and antiviral properties. The stem extract of *Tinospora cordifolia* successfully inhibited the herpes simplex virus by 61.43% in the Vero cell line [59]. Kalikar et al. [60] showed that 60% of the patients who received *Tinospora cordifolia* extract and 20% on placebo showed a decrease in the incidence of various symptoms associated with HIV. However, they did not study all the parameters but hypothesized that *Tinospora cordifolia* extract could be used as an adjunct to HIV management. The in silico approach against SARS-CoV-2 was tested by Sagar and Kumar [61]. The key targets they considered for the docking were surface glycoprotein, receptor-binding domain, RNA-dependent RNA polymerase, and protease. The natural compounds from *Tinospora cordifolia* such as berberine, isocolumbin, magnoflorine, and tinocordiside showed high binding efficacy against all four key targets [61].

2.7. *Vitex Trifolia*

Vitex trifolia belongs to the family Verbenaceae. The leaves of the plants are compound and oppositely arranged with three linear leaflets ranges between1–12 cm in length. The upper surface of the leaf is mostly green, whereas the lower surface is grayish.

Fruits of the plants contain essential oils, monoterpenes, diterpenes, beta-sitosterol [62–68]. The leaves and bark of the plant contain essential oils, flavones, and artemetin [65]. Furthermore, the essential oil of *Vitex trifolia* is used as an anti-inflammatory and against headache, cold, cough, liver disorders, and HIV [66,67]. Extract from the leaves of *vitex trifolia* inhibited TNF-α and IL-1 β production in human U937 macrophages [68]. The components that were isolated from leaf extract were artemetin, casticin, vitexilactone, and maslinic acid. Wee et al. [68] also suggested that artemetin could be the active compound that suppressed TNF-α and IL-1β production.

Due to the high contents of the phenolic compounds such as phenolic acid, flavones, and flavonols, it was analyzed that methanolic extract contains antioxidant and anticancer properties [69]. *Vitex trifolia* has also been found to block the NK-kB pathways that reduce inflammatory cytokines; this is a similar pathway that is being used in respiratory distress in SARS-CoV [70,71].

Table 1. Plants and their activity against different viral diseases.

Plants	Family	Plant Part	References
Glycyrrhiza glabra	Fabaceae	Roots	Hepatitis C [34] Influenza-A [35] SARS-CoV [36] SARS-CoV-2 [37]
Alnus japonica	Betulaceae	Leaves and bark	Influenza [38] H9N2 Avian influenza virus [39] SARS CoV [40]
Allium sativum	Amaryllidaceae	Bulb	Influenza A and B [42] Cytomegalovirus [43] Herpes simplex virus 1 [44] Herpes simplex virus 2 [45] SARS CoV [46]
Houttuynia cordata	Saururaceae	Leaves, roots	DEN V-2 [47,48] Avian infection bronchitis virus [49] Influenza-A [50] Herpes simplex virus-1 [51] SARS CoV [52]

Table 1. Cont.

Plants	Family	Plant Part	References
Lycoris radiata	Amaryllidaceae	Bulb, stem cortex	H5N1 [53] Hepatitis C [55] Tobacco mosaic virus [56] SARS CoV [57]
Tinospora cordifolia	Menispermaceae	Stem	HSV-1 [59] HIV [60] SARS-CoV [61]
Vitex trifolia	Verbenaceae	Leaves	HIV [66,67] SARS-CoV [70,71]

3. Vitamins and Minerals

Vitamins and minerals are an essential requirement of our body since they help in wound healing, enhancing the immune system, etc. They are also required for converting food into energy and play a major role in cellular damage. There are two types of vitamins, fat-soluble and water-soluble, and here we have discussed only those vitamins and minerals that could have a probable role against SARS-CoV (Table 2).

Vitamin A also called retinol is the fat-soluble vitamin that has β-carotene as its plant-derived precursor. Vitamin A is also called as an anti-infective vitamin since many of the defensive mechanism of the body depends upon the supply of this vitamin. It has already been reported that calves having low vitamin A content are more susceptible to the infection since they lose the effectiveness of the bovine coronavirus vaccine [72]. Bronchitis virus, which is a kind of coronavirus, was more prominent in the chickens that were fed with vitamin A deficient diet [73].

Vitamin B is a complex of different vitamins together designated as vitamin B complex because it comprises of different vitamins (B1 and B2 up to B-12). Each vitamin has its specific requirement, and its deficiency is related to different diseases. Elderly people are more prone to vitamin B2 deficiency [74]. Vitamin B2, along with UV light, effectively reduced the titer of MERS-CoV in human plasma products [75]. Vitamin B3 inhibited neutrophil infiltration into the lungs causing a strong anti-inflammatory response during the ventilator-associated lung injury but also led to hypoxemia [76]. Vitamin B-12 improves sustained viral response in patients with hepatitis C [77]. Narayan and Nair [78], through computational analysis using different software, also predicted that Vitamin B12 inhibited RNA-dependent RNA polymerase activity of an nsp-12 protein in SARS-CoV-2. nsp-12protein is associated with RNA-dependent RNA polymerase activity and is responsible for viral replication.

Vitamin C has shown a significant lowering of pneumonia in lower respiratory tract infections during clinical trials [79]. Therefore, it is suggested that vitamin C might work against SARS-CoV-2. There are reports that suggest that vitamin C had increased the resistance of chicken embryo organ culture against avian coronavirus infection [80].

Vitamin D is a prohormone vitamin and is produced during exposure to sunlight, although smaller amounts are obtained from the food as well. It has many roles, including the enhancement of cellular immunity through the induction of antimicrobial peptides [81,82]. SARS-CoV-2 infection can be lowered by targeting an unbalanced Renin-angiotensin system (RAS) with Vitamin D supplements [83]. The current pandemic of SARS-CoV-2 has led to a call for the widespread use of vitamin D supplements [83–86]. Some reviews have suggested vitamin D loading doses of 200,000–300,000 IU in 50,000 IU capsules reduce the severity of COVID-19 [87].

Table 2. Vitamins and their role.

Vitamins	Role
Vitamin-A	Deficiency of Vit-A leads to enhancement of Bronchitis virus in chicken [73]
Vitamin B2	Effectively reduced titer of MERS-CoV in human plasma products [75]
Vitamin B3	Strong anti-inflammatory response during the ventilator-associated lung injury [76]
Vitamin B-12	Improves sustained viral response in patients with hepatitis C [77] Inhibits RNA Dependent RNA polymerase activity of an nsp-12 protein in SARS-CoV-2 [78]
Vitamin C	Lowering of pneumonia in lower respiratory tract infection [79]. Increase the resistance of chicken embryo organ culture against avian coronavirus infection [80]
Vitamin D	Enhancement of cellular immunity through induction of antimicrobial peptides [81,82]. Lowering of SARS-CoV-2 infection by targeting unbalanced RAS [83].
Vitamin E	Deficiency of Vit-E along with Vit-D caused the bovine coronavirus in calves [88]

Vitamin E, along with Vitamin D, deficiency has caused the bovine coronavirus in calves [88].

Zinc is required for the functioning and maintenance of immune cells. Zinc also increases interferon α (IFNα) production by leukocytes [89] and mediates its antiviral activity in cells infected with the rhinovirus [90]. In combination with pyrithione, zinc inhibits the RNA transcription in SARS-CoV and SARS-CoV RNA polymerase activity in RNA-dependent RNA polymerase. Selenium could also be another alternative to treat against SARS-CoV. The synergistic effect of selenium with ginseng stem-leaf saponins could induce an immune response to a bronchitis coronavirus vaccine in chicken [91].

4. Conclusions

From this review, we attempted to highlight natural medicines that could be used against SARS-CoV-2. Different companies and institutes have launched vaccines after getting approval from World Health Organization (WHO), whereas some vaccines are still under clinical trials. Different antivirals that have been previously used against SARS, MERS, and influenza have been evaluated alone or in combination, but still, no fruitful response has been achieved. Furthermore, it has been reported that the virus has a high rate of mutation, which is again a hurdle in the development of a vaccine [92].

This review is based on the treatments given in the case of SARS-CoV and MERS, which could also be effective against SARS-CoV-2 since SARS-CoV-2 is closely related to SARS-CoV and have 80% sequence identical [8]. Plants are a good source of natural medication and an alternative to antibiotic treatment because the excessive use of antibiotics is responsible for drug resistance. Secondly, the main advantage of using plants is that they are economically efficient, have high scalability and safety because the plants can be cultivated in a very low amount, and they also do not support the growth of human pathogens [93]. Plants have produced a large range of antivirals lectins, including griffithsin [94,95], cyanovirin [96–99] and cyanovirin-N-fusion proteins [100], and also the transgenic rice lines that express griffithsin and cyanovirin-N in the seeds, with or without antibody 2G12 [101]. Medicinal plants may be a good source of antivirals, but the accurate dosage and plant parts that have medicinal properties, such as root, shoot, etc., should be known prior to the consumption; otherwise, the adverse effect could also exist. Although the exact mechanism of action of plants on to the virus is still unknown, we are of opinion that healthy food helps in boosting the immune system, which further prevents disease including SARS-CoV-2. Therefore, a nutritious diet that includes different vitamins, minerals should be consumed regularly.

5. Future Perspectives

Plants could be a better alternative to modern medicines in the future. To validate the hypothesis of plants as a medicine further, extensive research should be carried out on different medicinal plants so that correct dosage and toxicity levels may be known prior to application.

Author Contributions: Conceptualization, S.G.A., M.A.A. (Mohammad Azam Ansari) and H.M.K.; methodology, S.G.A. and M.A.A. (Mohammad Azam Ansari).; validation, M.A.A. (Mohammad A. Alzohairy), A.A., M.N.A., S.A. and S.R.; investigation, S.G.A., M.A.A. (Mohammad Azam Ansari), A.A. and S.A.; resources, writing—original draft preparation, S.G.A. and M.A.A. (Mohammad Azam Ansari); writing—review and editing, M.A.A. (Mohammad A. Alzohairy), A.A., M.N.A., S.A., S.R. and H.M.K.; All authors have read and agreed to the published version of the manuscript.

Funding: Deanship of Scientific Research, Imam Abdulrahman Bin Faisal University, Dammam, Saudi Arabia, Grant number-Covid19-2020-002-IRMC.

Institutional Review Board Statement: Not Applicable.

Informed Consent Statement: Not Applicable.

Data Availability Statement: Not Applicable.

Acknowledgments: Syed Ghazanfar Ali would like to acknowledge Viral Research Diagnostic Laboratory (funded by DHR-ICMR-New Delhi) in Aligarh U.P India for giving an opportunity to work as a Research Scientist (Non-medical).

Conflicts of Interest: The authors declare no conflict of interest.

References

1. Gorbalenya, A.E.; Baker, S.C.; Baric, R.S.; de Groot, R.J.; Drosten, C.; Gulyaeva, A.A.; Haagmans, B.L.; Lauber, C.; Leontovich, A.M.; Neuman, B.W.; et al. The species severe acute respiratory syndrome-related coronavirus: Classifying 2019-nCoV and naming it SARS-CoV-2. *Nat. Microbiol.* **2020**, *5*, 536–544. [CrossRef]
2. Ansari, M.A.; Almatroudi, A.; Alzohairy, M.A.; AlYahya, S.; Alomary, M.N.; Al-Dossary, H.A.; Alghamdi, S. Lipid-based nano delivery of Tat-peptide conjugated drug or vaccine–promising therapeutic strategy for SARS-CoV-2 treatment. *Expert Opin. Drug Deliv.* **2020**, *17*, 1671–1674. [CrossRef]
3. Chan, J.F.W.; Kok, K.H.; Zhu, Z.; Chu, H.; To, K.K.W.; Yuan, S.; Yuen, K.Y. Genomic characterization of the 2019 novel human-pathogenic coronavirus isolated from a patient with atypical pneumonia after visiting Wuhan. *Emerg. Microbes Infect.* **2020**, *9*, 221–236. [CrossRef]
4. Song, Z.; Xu, Y.; Bao, L.; Zhang, L.; Yu, P.; Qu, Y.; Zhu, H.; Zhao, W.; Han, Y.; Qin, C. From SARS to MERS, thrusting coronaviruses into the spotlight. *Viruses* **2019**, *11*, 59. [CrossRef] [PubMed]
5. Zaki, A.M.; Van Boheemen, S.; Bestebroer, T.M.; Osterhaus, A.D.; Fouchier, R.A. Isolation of a novel coronavirus from a man with pneumonia in Saudi Arabia. *N. Engl. J. Med.* **2012**, *367*, 1814–1820. [CrossRef]
6. van Boheemen, S.; de Graaf, M.; Lauber, C.; Bestebroer, T.M.; Raj, V.S.; Zaki, A.M.; Osterhaus, A.D.M.E.; Haggmans, B.L.; Gorbalenya, A.E.; Snijder, E.J.; et al. Genomic characterization of a newly discovered coronavirus associated with acute respiratory distress syndrome in humans. *MBio* **2012**, *3*, e00473-12. [CrossRef]
7. Schoeman, D.; Fielding, B.C. Coronavirus envelope protein: Current knowledge. *Virology* **2019**, *16*, 69. [CrossRef]
8. Ansari, M.A.; Jamal, Q.M.S.; Rehman, S.; Almatroudi, A.; Alzohairy, M.A.; Alomary, M.N.; Tripathi, T.; Alharbi, A.H.; Adil, S.F.; Khan, M.; et al. TAT-peptide conjugated repurposing drug against SARS-CoV-2 main protease (3CLpro): Potential therapeutic intervention to combat COVID-19. *Arab. J. Chem.* **2020**, *13*, 8069–8079. [CrossRef]
9. Chan, J.F.-W.; Yuan, S.; Kok, K.-H.; To, K.K.-W.; Chu, H.; Yang, J.; Xing, F.; BNurs, J.L.; Yip, C.C.-Y.; Poon, R.W.-S.; et al. A familial cluster of pneumonia associated with the 2019 novel coronavirus indicating person-to person transmission: A study of a family cluster. *Lancet* **2020**, *395*, 514–523. [CrossRef]
10. Xu, X.; Chen, P.; Wang, J.; Feng, J.; Zhou, H.; Li, X.; Zhong, W.; Hao, P. Evolution of the novel coronavirus from the ongoing Wuhan outbreak and modeling of its spike protein for risk of human transmission. *Sci. China Life Sci.* **2020**, *63*, 457–460. [CrossRef]

11. Zhao, Y.; Zhao, Z.; Wang, Y.; Zhou, Y.; Ma, Y.; Zuo, W. Single-cell RNA expression profiling of ACE2, the putative receptor of Wuhan 2019-nCov. *Am. J. Respir. Crit. Care Med.* **2020**, *202*, 756–759. [CrossRef]
12. Yin, Y.; Wunderink, R.G. MERS, SARS and other coronaviruses as causes of pneumonia. *Respirology* **2018**, *23*, 130–137. [CrossRef] [PubMed]
13. Wan, Y.; Shang, J.; Graham, R.; Baric, R.S.; Li, F. Receptor recognition by novel coronavirus from Wuhan: An analysis based on decade-long structural studies of SARS. *J. Virol.* **2020**, *94*, e00127-20. [CrossRef]
14. Li, F. Structure, Function, and Evolution of Coronavirus Spike Proteins. *Annu. Rev. Virol.* **2016**, *3*, 237–261. [CrossRef]
15. Song, W.; Gui, M.; Wang, X.; Xiang, Y. Cryo-EM structure of the SARS coronavirus spike glycoprotein in complex with its host cell receptor ACE2. *PLoS Pathog.* **2018**, *14*, e1007236. [CrossRef] [PubMed]
16. Li, W.; Moore, M.J.; Vasilieva, N.; Sui, J.; Wong, S.K.; Berne, M.A.; Somasundaran, M.; Sullivan, J.L.; Luzuriaga, K.; Greenough, T.C.; et al. Angiotensin-converting enzyme 2 is a functional receptor for the SARS coronavirus. *Nature* **2003**, *426*, 450–454. [CrossRef] [PubMed]
17. Gralinski, L.E.; Menachery, V.D. Return of the coronavirus: 2019-nCoV. *Viruses* **2020**, *12*, 135. [CrossRef]
18. Zhou, P.; Yang, X.L.; Wang, X.G.; Hu, B.; Zhang, L.; Zhang, W.; Si, H.-R.; Zhu, Y.; Li, B.; Huang, C.-L.; et al. A pneumonia outbreak associated with a new coronavirus of probable bat origin. *Nature* **2020**, *579*, 270–273. [CrossRef] [PubMed]
19. Huang, C.; Wang, Y.; Li, X.; Ren, L.; Zhao, J.; Hu, Y. Clinical features of patients infected with 2019 novel coronavirus in Wuhan, China. *Lancet* **2020**, *395*, 497–506. [CrossRef]
20. Jaiswal, Y.; Liang, Z.; Zhao, Z. Botanical drugs in Ayurveda and traditional Chinese medicine. *J. Ethnopharmacol.* **2016**, *194*, 245–259. [CrossRef]
21. Silveira, D.; Prieto-Garcia, J.M.; Boylan, F.; Estrada, O.; Fonseca-Bazzo, Y.M.; Jamal, C.M.; Magalhães, P.O.; Pereira, E.O.; Tomczyk, M.; Heinrich, M. COVID-19: Is There Evidence for the Use of Herbal Medicines as Adjuvant Symptomatic Therapy? *Front. Pharmacol.* **2020**, *11*, 581840. [CrossRef]
22. Panyod, S.; Ho, C.-T.; Sheen, L.-Y. Dietary therapy and herbal medicine for COVID-19 prevention: A review and perspective. *J. Trad. Complement. Med.* **2020**, *10*, 420–427. [CrossRef]
23. Gurib-Fakim, A. Medicinal plants: Traditions of yesterday and drugs of tomorrow. *Mol. Asp. Med.* **2006**, *27*, 1–93. [CrossRef]
24. Harvey, A.L. Natural products as a screening resource. *Curr. Opin. Chem. Biol.* **2007**, *11*, 480–484. [CrossRef]
25. Li, T.; Peng, T. Traditional Chinese herbal medicine as a source of molecules with antiviral activity. *Antivir. Res.* **2013**, *97*, 1–9. [CrossRef]
26. Arbab, A.H.; Parvez, M.K.; Al-Dosari, M.S.; Al-Rehaily, A.J. In vitro evaluation of novel antiviral activities of 60 medicinal plants extracts against hepatitis B virus. *Exp. Ther. Med.* **2017**, *14*, 626–634. [CrossRef] [PubMed]
27. Akram, M.; Tahir, I.M.; Shah, S.M.A.; Mahmood, Z.; Altaf, A.; Ahmad, K.; Munir, N.; Daniyal, M.; Nasir, S.; Mehboob, H. Antiviral potential of medicinal plants against HIV, HSV, influenza, hepatitis, and coxsackievirus: A systematic review. *Phytother. Res.* **2018**, *32*, 811–822. [CrossRef]
28. Dhama, K.; Karthik, K.; Khandia, R.; Munjal, A.; Tiwari, R.; Rana, R.; Khurana, S.K.; Ullah, S.; Khan, R.U.; Alagawany, M. Medicinal and therapeutic potential of herbs and plant metabolites/extracts countering viral pathogens-current knowledge and future prospects. *Curr. Drug Metab.* **2018**, *19*, 236–263. [CrossRef] [PubMed]
29. Fatima, N.; Nayeem, N. Toxic effects as a result of herbal medicine intake. In *Toxicology—New Aspects to This Scientific Conundrum*; Intech Open: London, UK, 2016; pp. 193–204.
30. Fagan, J.; Antoniou, M.; Robinson, C. *GMO Myths and Truths*; Earth Open Source: London, UK, 2014.
31. Jovic, T.H.; Ali, S.R.; Ibrahim, N.; Jessop, Z.M.; Tarassoli, S.P.; Dobbs, T.D.; Holford, P.; Thornton, C.A.; Whitaker, I.S. Could Vitamins Help in the Fight Against COVID-19? *Nutrients* **2020**, *12*, 2550. [CrossRef]
32. Acevedo-Murillo, J.A.; Leon, M.L.G.; Firo-Reyes, V.; Santiago-Cordova, J.L.; Gonzalez-Rodrigues, A.P.; Wong-Chew, R.M. Zinc supplementation promotes a Th1 response and improves clinical symptoms in fewer hours in children with pneumonia younger than 5 Years old. A randomized controlled clinical trial. *Front. Pediatrics* **2019**, *7*, 431. [CrossRef] [PubMed]
33. Rayman, M.P. Selenium and human health. *Lancet* **2012**, *379*, 1256–1268. [CrossRef]
34. Ashfaq, U.A.; Masoud, M.S.; Nawaz, Z.; Riazuddin, S. Glycyrrhizin as antiviral agent against Hepatitis C Virus. *J. Transl. Med.* **2011**, *9*, 112. [CrossRef]
35. Wolkerstorfer, A.; Kurz, H.; Bachhofner, N.; Szolar, O.H. Glycyrrhizin inhibits influenza A virus uptake into the cell. *Antivir. Res.* **2009**, *83*, 171–178. [CrossRef]
36. Cinatl, J.; Morgenstern, B.; Bauer, G.; Chandra, P.; Rabenau, H.; Doerr, H.W. Glycyrrhizin, an active component of liquorice roots, and replication of SARS-associated coronavirus. *Lancet* **2003**, *361*, 2045–2046. [CrossRef]
37. Sinha, S.K.; Prasad, S.K.; Islam, M.A.; Gaurav, S.S.; Patil, R.B.; Al-Faris, N.A.; Aldayel, T.S.; AlKehayez, N.M.; Wabaidur, S.M.; Shakya, A. Identification of bioactive compounds from *Glycyrrhiza glabra* as possible inhibitor of SARS-CoV-2 spike glycoprotein and non-structural protein-15: A pharmacoinformatics study. *J. Biomol. Struct. Dyn.* **2020**, 1–15. [CrossRef] [PubMed]
38. Ra, J.C.; Kwon, H.J.; Kim, B.G.; You, S.H. Anti-Influenza Viral Composition Containing Bark or Stem Extract of *Alnus japonica*. US Patent US 2010/0285160 A1, 11 November 2010.
39. Tung, N.H.; Kwon, H.J.; Kim, J.H.; Ra, J.C.; Kim, J.A.; Kim, Y.H. An anti-influenza component of the bark of *Alnus japonica*. *Arch. Pharm. Res.* **2010**, *33*, 363–367. [CrossRef] [PubMed]

40. Park, J.Y.; Jeong, H.J.; Kim, J.H.; Kim, Y.M.; Park, S.J.; Kim, D.; Park, K.H.; Lee, W.S.; Ryu, Y.B. Diarylheptanoids from Alnus japonica inhibit papain-like protease of severe acute respiratory syndrome coronavirus. *Biol. Pharm. Bull.* **2012**, *35*, 2036–2042. [CrossRef] [PubMed]
41. Kwon, J.H.; Cho, S.H.; Kim, S.J.; Ahn, Y.J.; Ra, J.C. Antiviral Composition Comprising Alnus Japonica Extracts. US Patent US 2010/0189827 A1, 29 July 2010.
42. Fenwick, G.R.; Hanley, A.B. Allium species poisoning. *Vet. Rec.* **1985**, *116*, 28. [CrossRef] [PubMed]
43. Meng, Y.; Lu, D.; Guo, N.; Zhang, L.; Zhou, G. Anti-HCMV effect of garlic components. *Virol. Sin.* **1993**, *8*, 147–150.
44. Tsai, Y.; Cole, L.L.; Davis, L.E.; Lockwood, S.J.; Simmons, V.; Wild, G.C. Antiviral properties of garlic: In vitro effects on influenza B, herpes simplex and coxsackie viruses. *Planta Med.* **1985**, *5*, 460–461. [CrossRef] [PubMed]
45. Weber, N.D.; Andersen, D.O.; North, J.A.; Murray, B.K.; Lawson, L.D.; Hughes, B.G. In vitro virucidal effects of Allium sativum (garlic) extract and compounds. *Planta Med.* **1992**, *58*, 417–423. [CrossRef]
46. Thuy, B.T.P.; My, T.T.A.; Hai, N.T.T.; Hieu, L.T.; Hoa, T.T.; Loan, H.T.T.P.; Triet, N.T.; Anh, T.T.V.; Quy, P.T.; Tat, P.V.; et al. Investigation into SARS-CoV-2 Resistance of Compounds in Garlic Essential Oil. *ACS Omega* **2020**, *5*, 8312–8320. [CrossRef] [PubMed]
47. Chiow, K.H.; Phoon, M.C.; Putti, T.; Tan, B.K.; Chow, V.T. Evaluation of Antiviral Activities of Houttuynia CordataThunb. Extract, Quercetin, Quercetrin and Cinanserin on Murine Coronavirus and Dengue Virus Infection. *Asian Pac. J. Trop. Med.* **2016**, *9*, 1–7. [CrossRef]
48. Xie, M.L.; Phoon, M.C.; Dong, S.X.; Tan, B.K.H.; Chow, V.T. Houttuynia cordata extracts and constituents inhibit the infectivity of dengue virus type 2 in vitro. *Int. J. Integr. Biol.* **2013**, *14*, 78–85.
49. Yin, J.; Li, G.; Li, J.; Yang, Q.; Ren, X. In vitro and in vivo effects of Houttuynia cordata on infectious bronchitis virus. *Avian Pathol.* **2011**, *40*, 491–498. [CrossRef]
50. Choi, H.J.; Song, J.H.; Park, K.S.; Kwon, D.H. Inhibitory effects of quercetin 3-rhamnoside on influenza A virus replication. *Eur. J. Pharm. Sci.* **2009**, *37*, 329–333.
51. Hayashi, K.; Kamiya, M.; Hayashi, T. Virucidal effects of the steam distillate from Houttuynia cordata and its components on Hsv-1, Influenza-Virus, and HIV. *Planta Med.* **1995**, *61*, 237–241. [CrossRef] [PubMed]
52. Lau, K.M.; Lee, K.M.; Koon, C.M.; Cheung, C.S.; Lau, C.P.; Ho, H.M.; Lee, M.Y.-H.; Au, S.W.-N.; Cheng, C.H.-K.; Lau, C.B.-S.; et al. Immunomodulatory and anti-SARS activities of Houttuynia cordata. *J. Ethnopharmacol.* **2008**, *118*, 79–85. [CrossRef]
53. He, J.; Qi, W.B.; Wang, L.; Tian, J.; Jiao, P.R.; Liu, G.Q.; Ye, W.-C.; Liao, M. Amaryllidaceae alkaloids inhibit nuclear-to-cytoplasmic export of ribonucleoprotein (RNP) complex of highly pathogenic avian influenza virus H5N1. *Influenza Other Respir. Viruses* **2012**, *7*, 922–931. [CrossRef]
54. Yang, L.; Zhang, J.H.; Zhang, X.L.; Lao, G.J.; Su, G.M.; Wang, L.; Li, Y.L.; Ye, W.C.; He, J. Tandem mass tag-based quantitative proteomic analysis of lycorine treatment in highly pathogenic avian influenza H5N1 virus infection. *Peer J.* **2019**, *7*, e7697. [CrossRef] [PubMed]
55. Chen, D.Z.; Jiang, J.D.; Zhang, K.Q.; He, H.P.; Di, Y.T.; Zhang, Y.; Cai, J.-Y.; Wang, L.; Li, S.-L.; Yi, P.; et al. Evaluation of anti-HCV activity and SAR study of (+)-lycoricidine through targeting of host heat-stress cognate 70 (Hsc70). *Bioorg. Med. Chem. Lett.* **2013**, *23*, 2679–2682. [CrossRef] [PubMed]
56. Yang, D.Q.; Chen, Z.R.; Chen, D.Z.; Hao, X.J.; Li, S.L. Anti-TMV Effects of Amaryllidaceae Alkaloids Isolated from the Bulbs of *Lycoris radiata* and Lycoricidine Derivatives. *Nat. Prod. Bioprospect.* **2018**, *8*, 189–197. [CrossRef] [PubMed]
57. Li, S.Y.; Chen, C.; Zhang, H.Q.; Guo, H.Y.; Wang, H.; Wang, L. Identification of natural compounds with antiviral activities against SARS-associated coronavirus. *Antivir. Res.* **2005**, *67*, 18–23. [CrossRef]
58. Sachan, S.; Dhama, K.; Latheef, S.K.; Samad, H.A.; Mariappan, A.K.; Munuswamy, P.; Singh, R.; Singh, K.P.; Malik, Y.S.; Singh, R.K. Immunomodulatory Potential of Tinosporacordifolia and CpG ODN (TLR21 Agonist) against the Very Virulent, Infectious Bursal Disease Virus in SPF Chicks. *Vaccines (Basel)* **2019**, *7*, 106. [CrossRef]
59. Pruthvish, R.; Gopinatha, S.M. Antiviral prospective of Tinospora cordifolia on HSV-1. *Int. J. Curr. Microbiol. Appl. Sci.* **2018**, *7*, 3617–3624.
60. Kalikar, M.V.; Thawani, V.R.; Varadpande, U.K.; Sontakke, S.D.; Singh, R.P.; Khiyani, R.K. Immunomodulatory effect of Tinospora cordifolia extract in human immuno-deficiency virus positive patients. *Indian J. Pharmacol.* **2008**, *40*, 107–110.
61. Sagar, V.; Kumar, A.H.S. Efficacy of natural compounds from Tinospora cordifolia against SARS-CoV-2 protease, surface glycoprotein and RNA polymerase. *BEMS Rep.* **2020**, *6*, 6–8. [CrossRef]
62. Cousins, M.M.; Briggs, J.; Gresham, C.; Whetstone, J. Beach Vitex (*Vitex rotundifolia*) an invasive coastal species. *Invasive Plant Sci. Manag. (Weed Sci. Soc. Am.)* **1991**, *6*, 101–103. [CrossRef]
63. Zeng, X.; Fang, Z.; Wu, Y.; Zhang, H. Chemical constituents of the fruits of Vitex trifolia L. *Zhongguo Zhong Yao Za Zhi* **1996**, *21*, 167–168. [PubMed]
64. Ono, M.; Sawamura, H.; Ito, Y.; Mizuki, K.; Nohara, T. Diterpenoids from the fruits of Vitex trifolia. *Phytochemistry* **2000**, *55*, 873–877. [CrossRef]
65. Chan, E.W.C.; Baba, S.; Chan, H.T.; Kainumaz, M.; Tangah, J. Medicinal plants of sandy shores a short review on *V trifolia* L. and Iomoea pes caprae. *Indian J. Nat. Prod. Resour.* **2016**, *7*, 107–115.
66. Devi, W.R.; Singh, C.B. Chemical composition, anti-dermatophytic activity, antioxidant and total phenolic content within the leaves essential oil of *Vitex trifolia*. *Int. J. Phytocosmetics Nat. Ingred.* **2014**, *1*, 5–10. [CrossRef]

67. Suksamrarn, A.; Werawattanametin, K.; Brophy, J.J. Variation of essential oil constituents in *Vitex trifolia* species. *FlavourFragr. J.* **1991**, *6*, 97–99.
68. Wee, H.N.; Neo, S.Y.; Singh, D.; Yew, H.C.; Qiu, Z.Y.; Tsai, X.R.C.; How, S.Y.; Yip, K.-Y.C.; Tan, C.-H.; Koh, H.-L. Effects of *Vitex trifolia* L. Leaf Extracts and Phytoconstituents on Cytokine Production in Human U937 Macrophages. *BMC Complement. Med. Ther.* **2020**, *20*, 91. [CrossRef] [PubMed]
69. Yao, J.L.; Fang, S.M.; Liu, R.; Oppong, M.B.; Liu, E.W.; Fan, G.W.; Zhang, H. A Review on the Terpenes from Genus Vitex. *Molecules* **2016**, *21*, 1179. [CrossRef]
70. Alam, G.; Wahyuono, S.; Ganjar, I.G.; Hakim, L.; Timmerman, H.; Verpoorte, R. Tracheospasmolytic activity of viteosin-A and vitexicarpin isolated from *Vitex trifolia*. *Planta Med.* **2002**, *68*, 1047–1049. [CrossRef]
71. Srivastava, R.A.K.; Mistry, S.; Sharma, S. A novel anti-inflammatory natural product from *Sphaeranthus indicus* inhibits expression of VCAM1 and ICAM1, and slows atherosclerosis progression independent of lipid changes. *Nutr. Metab.* **2015**, *12*, 20. [CrossRef] [PubMed]
72. Jee, J.; Hoet, A.E.; Azevedo, M.P.; Vlasova, A.N.; Loerch, S.C.; Pickworth, C.L.; Hanson, J.; Saif, L.J. Effects of dietary vitamin A content on antibody responses of feedlot calves inoculated intramuscularly with an inactivated bovine coronavirus vaccine. *Am. J. Vet. Res.* **2013**, *74*, 1353–1362. [CrossRef]
73. West, C.E.; Sijtsma, S.R.; Kouwenhoven, B.; Rombout, J.H.; van der Zijpp, A.J. Epithelia-damaging virus infections affect vitamin A status in chickens. *J. Nutr.* **1992**, *122*, 333–339. [CrossRef] [PubMed]
74. Powers, H.J. Riboflavin (vitamin B-2) and health. *Am. J. Clin. Nutr.* **2003**, *77*, 1352–1360. [CrossRef]
75. Keil, S.D.; Bowen, R.; Marschner, S. Inactivation of Middle East respiratory syndrome coronavirus (MERS-CoV) in plasma products using a riboflavin-based and ultraviolet light-based photochemical treatment. *Transfusion* **2016**, *56*, 2948–2952. [CrossRef]
76. Jones, H.D.; Yoo, J.; Crother, T.R.; Kyme, P.; Shlomo, A.B.; Khalafi, R.; Tseng, C.W.; Parks, W.C.; Arditi, M.; Liu, G.Y.; et al. Nicotinamide exacerbates hypoxemia in ventilator-induced lung injury independent of neutrophil infiltration. *PLoS ONE* **2015**, *10*, e0123460. [CrossRef]
77. Rocco, A.; Compare, D.; Coccoli, P.; Esposito, C.; Spirito, A.D.; Barbato, A.; Strazzullo, P.; Nardone, G. Vitamin B12 Supplementation Improves Rates of Sustained Viral Response in Patients Chronically Infected With Hepatitis C Virus. *Hepatology* **2013**, *62*, 766–773.
78. Narayanan, N.; Nair, D.T. Vitamin B12 May Inhibit RNA-Dependent-RNA Polymerase Activity of nsp12 from the SARS-CoV-2 Virus. *IUBMB Life* **2020**, *72*, 2112–2120. [CrossRef] [PubMed]
79. Hemila, H. Vitamin C intake and susceptibility to pneumonia. *Pediatr. Infect. Dis.J.* **1997**, *16*, 836–837. [CrossRef]
80. Atherton, J.G.; Kratzing, C.C.; Fisher, A. The effect of ascorbic acid on infection chick-embryo ciliated tracheal organ cultures by coronavirus. *Arch. Virol.* **1978**, *56*, 195–199. [CrossRef]
81. Liu, P.T.; Stenger, S.; Li, H.; Wenzel, L.; Tan, B.H.; Krutzik, S.R.; Ochoa, M.T.; Schauber, J.; Wu, K.; Meinken, C.; et al. Toll-like receptor triggering of a vitamin D-mediated human antimicrobial response. *Science* **2006**, *311*, 1770–1773. [CrossRef] [PubMed]
82. Adams, J.S.; Ren, S.; Liu, P.T.; Chun, R.F.; Lagishetty, V.; Gombart, A.F.; Borregaard, N.; Modlin, R.L.; Hewison, M. Vitamin d-directed rheostatic regulation of monocyte antibacterial responses. *J. Immunol.* **2009**, *182*, 4289–4295. [CrossRef]
83. Garami, A.R. Preventing a covid-19 pandemic—Is there a magic bullet to save COVID-19 patients? We can give it a try! *BMJ* **2020**, *368*, m810.
84. Grant, W.B.; Lahore, H.; McDonnell, S.L.; Baggerly, C.A.; French, C.B.; Aliano, J.L.; Bhattoa, H.P. Evidence that vitamin D supplementation could reduce risk of influenza and COVID-19 infections and deaths. *Nutrients* **2020**, *12*, 988. [CrossRef]
85. McCartney, D.M.; Byrne, D.G. Optimisation of vitamin D status for enhanced Immuno-protection against Covid-19. *Ir. Med. J.* **2020**, *113*, 58.
86. Schwalfenberg, G.K. Preventing a COVID-19 pandemic. Covid 19, Vitamin D deficiency, Smoking, Age and Lack of Masks Equals the Perfect Storm: Rapid response. *BMJ* **2020**, *368*, m810.
87. Wimalawansa, S.J. Global epidemic of coronavirus–COVID-19: What we can do to minimzeriskl. *Eur. J. Biomed. Pharm. Sci.* **2020**, *7*, 432–438.
88. Nonnecke, B.J.; McGill, J.L.; Ridpath, J.F.; Sacco, R.E.; Lippolis, J.D.; Reinhardt, T.A. Acute phase response elicited by experimental bovine diarrhea virus (BVDV) infection is associated with decreased vitamin D and E status of vitamin-replete preruminant calves. *J. Dairy Sci.* **2014**, *97*, 5566–5579. [CrossRef]
89. Cakman, I.; Kirchner, H.; Rink, L. Zinc supplementation reconstitutes the production of interferon-α by leukocytes from elderly persons. *J. Interferon Cytokine Res.* **1997**, *17*, 469–472. [CrossRef]
90. Berg, K.; Bolt, G.; Andersen, H.; Owen, T.C. Zinc potentiates the antiviral action of human IFN-α tenfold. *J. Interferon CytokineRes.* **2001**, *21*, 471–474. [CrossRef]
91. Ma, X.; Bi, S.; Wang, Y.; Chi, X.; Hu, S. Combined adjuvant effect of ginseng stem-leaf saponins and selenium on immune responses to a live bivalent vaccine of Newcastle disease virus and infectious bronchitis virus in chickens. *Poult. Sci.* **2019**, *98*, 3548–3556. [CrossRef]
92. Vellingiri, B.; Jayaramayya, K.; Iyer, M.; Narayasamy, A.; Govindasamy, V.; Giridharan, B.; Ganesan, S.; Venugopal, A.; Venkatesan, D.; Ganesan, H. Covid-19: A promising cure for the global panic. *Sci. Total Environ.* **2020**, *725*, 138277. [CrossRef] [PubMed]
93. Ma, J.K.; Drake, P.M.; Chritou, P. The production of recombinant pharmaceutical proteins in plants. *Nat. Rev. Genet.* **2003**, *4*, 794–805. [CrossRef] [PubMed]

94. Keefe, B.R.O.; Vojdani, F.; Buffa, V.; Shattock, R.J.; Montefiori, D.C.; Bakke, J.; Mirsalis, J.; d'Andrea, A.-L.; Hume, S.D.; Bratcher, B.; et al. Scaleable manufacture of HIV-1 entry inhibitor griffithsin and validation of its safety and efficacy as a topical microbicide component. *Proc. Natl. Acad. Sci. USA* **2009**, *106*, 6099–6104. [CrossRef]
95. Vamvaka, E.; Arcalis, E.; Ramessar, K.; Evans, A.; Keefe, B.R.O.; Shattock, R.J.; Medina, V.; Stoger, E.; Christou, P.; Capell, T. Rice endosperm is cost-effective for the production of recombinant griffithsin with potent activity against HIV. *Plant Biotechnol. J.* **2016**, *14*, 1427–1437. [CrossRef] [PubMed]
96. Sexton, A.; Drake, P.M.; Mahmood, N.; Harman, S.J.; Shatoock, R.; Ma, J.K.C. Transgenic plant production of cyanovirin-N, an HIV microbicide. *FASEB J.* **2006**, *20*, 356–358. [CrossRef]
97. Drake, P.M.W.; Madeira, L.D.M.; Szeto, T.H.; Ma, J.K.C. Transformation of *Althaea officinalis* L. by Agrobacterium rhizogenes for the production of transgenic roots expressing the anti-HIV microbicide cyanovirin-N. *Transgenic Res.* **2013**, *22*, 1225–1229. [CrossRef] [PubMed]
98. Keefe, B.R.O.; Murad, A.M.; Vianna, G.R.; Ramessar, K.; Saucedo, C.J.; Wilson, J.; Buckheit, K.W.; da-Cunha, N.B.; Araujo, A.C.G.; Lacorte, C.C.; et al. Engineering soya bean seeds as a scalable platform to produce cyanovirin-N, a non-ARV microbicide against HIV. *Plant Biotechnol. J.* **2015**, *13*, 884–892. [CrossRef] [PubMed]
99. Vamvaka, E.; Evans, A.; Ramessar, K.; Krumpe, L.R.H.; Shattock, R.J.; Keefe, B.R.O.; Christou, P.; Capell, T. Cyanovirin-N produced in rice endosperm offers effective pre-exposure prophylaxis against HIV-1BaL infection in vitro. *Plant Cell Rep.* **2016**, *35*, 1309–1319. [CrossRef]
100. Sexton, A.; Harman, S.; Shattock, R.J.; Ma, J.K.C. Design, expression, and characterization of a multivalent, combination HIV microbicide. *FASEB J.* **2009**, *23*, 3590–3600. [CrossRef]
101. Vamvaka, E.; Farre, G.; Molinos-Albert, L.M.; Evans, A.; Canela-Xandri, A.; Twyman, R.M.; Carrillo, J.; Ordonez, R.A.; Shattock, R.J.; O'Keefe, B.R.; et al. Unexpected synergistic HIV neutralization by a triple microbicide produced in rice endosperm. *Proc. Natl. Acad. Sci. USA* **2018**, *115*, E7854–E7862. [CrossRef] [PubMed]

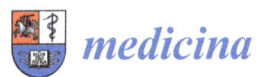

Review

Antiviral and Immunomodulation Effects of Artemisia

Suhas G. Kshirsagar [1],* and Rammohan V. Rao [2],*

[1] College of Ayurveda, Mount Madonna Institute, 445 Summit Road, Watsonville, CA 95076, USA
[2] California College of Ayurveda, 700 Zion Street, Nevada City, CA 95959, USA
* Correspondence: drsuhashi@yahoo.com (S.G.K.); rrao2006@gmail.com (R.V.R.)

Abstract: *Background and Objectives:* Artemisia is one of the most widely distributed genera of the family Astraceae with more than 500 diverse species growing mainly in the temperate zones of Europe, Asia and North America. The plant is used in Chinese and Ayurvedic systems of medicine for its antiviral, antifungal, antimicrobial, insecticidal, hepatoprotective and neuroprotective properties. Research based studies point to Artemisia's role in addressing an entire gamut of physiological imbalances through a unique combination of pharmacological actions. Terpenoids, flavonoids, coumarins, caffeoylquinic acids, sterols and acetylenes are some of the major phytochemicals of the genus. Notable among the phytochemicals is artemisinin and its derivatives (ARTs) that represent a new class of recommended drugs due to the emergence of bacteria and parasites that are resistant to quinoline drugs. This manuscript aims to systematically review recent studies that have investigated artemisinin and its derivatives not only for their potent antiviral actions but also their utility against the severe acute respiratory syndrome coronavirus 2 (SARS-CoV-2). *Materials and Methods*: PubMed Central, Scopus and Google scholar databases of published articles were collected and abstracts were reviewed for relevance to the subject matter. *Conclusions:* The unprecedented impact that artemisinin had on public health and drug discovery research led the Nobel Committee to award the Nobel Prize in Physiology or Medicine in 2015 to the discoverers of artemisinin. Thus, it is clear that Artemisia's importance in indigenous medicinal systems and drug discovery systems holds great potential for further investigation into its biological activities, especially its role in viral infection and inflammation.

Keywords: Artemisia; Artemisinin; ARTs; phytochemicals; SARS-CoV-2

1. Introduction

Medicinal plants, which are undervalued, have an important place in modern medicine owing to the multitude of active principles that nature provided through millions of years of evolution. These numerous plant chemicals or phytochemicals possess far reaching, biologically active, beneficial effects and provide protection to the plants from insects, bacteria, virus and other predators. These phytochemicals either alone or in combination affect multiple pathways simultaneously to produce the desired pharmacological effect. Many medicinal plants or herbs are revered by the ancient medical traditions (Chinese medicine, Ayurveda, Native Americans, etc.) due to their healing benefits and about 40% of modern medicines are derived from plants [1–3]. The development of antibacterial and anti-infectious agents is a major focus in modern medical research. Plant-based antiviral formulations have been studied for their therapeutic potential in the management of various viral diseases including influenza, human immunodeficiency virus (HIV), herpes simplex virus (HSV), hepatitis, and coxsackievirus infections [4–7].

One particular plant that has garnered a lot of attention in lieu of the COVID-19 epidemic is Artemisia which is one of the largest and most widely distributed genera of the family Astraceae (Compositae) [6,8]. Artemisia is a varied genus consisting of more than 500 diverse species and is found in the temperate zones of Europe, Asia and North America [9–11]. Evidence-based in vitro and in vivo studies on several species of

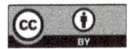

Artemisia resulted in the identification of numerous phytochemicals with varied pharmacological activities, including terpenoids, flavonoids, coumarins, caffeoylquinic acids and sterols [12,13]. The first clinical trial of Artemisia extract in human patients with malaria was conducted in August 1972. Following that trial, the active compound in the Artemisia extract was isolated and identified as artemisinin. Several derivatives or synthetic compounds with key structures similar to artemisinin have now been developed including artesunate and piperaquine from *A. annua* and piperitone and trans-ethyl cinnamate from *A. judaica* that have potent antiviral and anti-inflammatory activities [9,14–16]. A combination of artemisinin and its derivatives (ARTs) is now recommended by the World Health Organization (WHO) for the treatment of malaria.

2. Methods

For the review, we conducted a search of PubMed Central, Scopus and Google scholar databases of articles published from 2000 to 2020 to include the most recent literature. The search was limited to articles in English and abstracts were reviewed for relevance to the subject matter of pharmacological perspective on Artemisia. Articles containing combinations of MeSH terms 'Artemisia' 'artemisinin', 'artesunate', 'phytochemistry', 'diseases or conditions', 'in vitro or in vivo experiments', 'COVID-19', 'SARS-CoV-2' and 'mechanistic actions' were collected. Boolean terms (AND/OR/NOT) were added to combine or exclude keywords in the search resulting in more focused literature.

3. Ethnopharmacology

The isolation and identification of potent compounds from the genus Artemisia, particularly artemisinin and its derivatives using novel drug discovery methods, prompted the Nobel Committee to award the Nobel Prize in Physiology or Medicine in 2015 for its impact on public health [17,18]. This spurred the interest of several researchers to study the phytochemical and pharmacological properties of other species of the genus Artemisia.

Nearly 45 different species of Artemisia grow in India and in the Indian subcontinent and is mainly used as a medicinal plant [8,19]. Ayurveda describes two species *A. absinthium* and *A. maritima*, popularly known as Mugwort that vary slightly in their qualities and actions as shown in Table 1.

Table 1. Ayurveda describes two species *A. absinthium* and *A. maritima* that vary slightly in their qualities and actions. Both plants popularly known as Mugwort are revered in Ayurveda for their anti-infectious and insecticidal (*krimighna*) properties [20].

	A. absinthium	*A. maritima*
Names	Mugwort, Indian wormseed, Damanaka, Davana, Dona, Douna, Davanamu	Old woman, Mugwort, worm seed, Kirmani, Chuhara, Dirmana
Qualities (*guna*)	Light (laghu), Dry (ruksha), Hot (teekshana)	Light (laghu), Dry (ruksha), Hot (teekshana)
Taste (*rasa*)	Asringent (kashaya), Bitter (tikta)	Pungent (katu), Bitter (tikta)
Potency (*veerya*)	Hot (Ushna)	Hot (Ushna)
Post-digestive effect (*vipaka*)	Pungent (katu)	Pungent (katu)
Special Intrinsic Action (*prabhava*)	Insecticidal (*krimighna*), anti-pyretic (*jwaraghna*)	Insecticidal (*krimighna*), anti-pyretic (*jwaraghna*)
Uses	Optimizes kapha, pitta and vata (tridosha shamaka), anti-infectious, improves digestion, wound healing, respiratory and liver tonic	Optimizes kapha and vata (Kaphavata shamaka), anti-infectious, improves digestion, wound healing
Parts of plant used	Root, leaves, bark	Root, leaves, bark

In the Ayurvedic system of medicine, the term *'prabhava'* refers to the 'instinct intelligence' of a plant in eliciting a wide range of medicinal effects [21,22]. *A. absinthium* and *A. maritima* are revered, owing to their *prabhava* and are recommended in Ayurveda for infections, inflammation, skin and liver diseases, respiratory conditions, neurological conditions and as an insecticidal (*krimighna*) [6,8].

The pharmacological actions and properties of the various Artemisia species from several geographic locations are listed in Table 2. Basically, the plant has been used as an anti-malarial, anti-spasmodic, anti-inflammatory, febrifuge, cardiac stimulant, anthelmintic, headaches, dyspepsia, liver and kidney tonic, to improve memory, for digestive and respiratory issues and as a hypertensive and anticoagulant.

Table 2. The pharmacological actions and properties of a subset of Artemisia species.

Species	Uses	Phytochemicals Isolated
A. absinthium	cardiac stimulant, anthelmintic, liver function, memory booster	Sesquiterpene lactones, polyphenolic compounds, flavonoids, tannins, lignins [23,24].
A. abrotanum	Insecticide, liver conditions	Flavonols, tannins, coumarins [6,8,25].
A. afra	coughs, colds, malaria, diabetes, bladder and kidney disorders	monoterpenoids, sesquiterpenes, glaucolides, guaianolides; flavonoids [23,26].
A. annua	Fever, malaria, fibrosis	Volatile oils, sesquiterpene lactones, phenolic compounds, flavones [23,27–29].
A. asiatica	cancer, inflammation, infections and ulcers	Volatile oils, flavones, alkaloids [6,30].
A. arborescens	Anti-inflammatory, Antihistaminic, Blood decongestant	Terpenes, flavone, fatty acids [6,31].
A. douglasiana	premenstrual syndrome and dysmenorrhea	Monoterpenes, sesquiterpene lactones [23,32]
A. dracunculus	antidiabetic and anticoagulant	Volatile oils, coumarins, polyphenolic compounds, glucoside [33,34].
A. judaica	Gastrointestinal disorders	Volatile components, phenolic compounds [6,35]
A. maritima	anthelmintic, liver function, GI issues	Volatile oils, fatty acids, polyphenolic compounds, sesquiterpene lactones [6,23]
A. scoparia	antibacterial, antiseptic, antipyretic	Volatile oils, fatty acids, coumarins, pyrogallol tannins, cholagogic components, flavonoids, flavones [6,36,37].
A. t ripartite	cold, sore throats, tonsillitis, headaches and wounds	Guaianolides, polysaccharides [6,38]
A. verlotorum	hypertension	Volatile oils, fatty acids [6,39,40].
A. vestita	inflammatory diseases	Volatile oils, flavonoids [41,42].
A. vulgaris	analgesic, anti-inflammatory, antispasmodic and liver disease	Terpenes, coumarins [6,43].

The wide variety of actions stems from the fact that these various species of Artemisia possess high content of alkaloids, lactones, flavonoids, phenols, quinines, tannins and terpenoids all of which play a role in the growth of the plant or provide protection from pathogens or predators [6,9,44,45].

4. In Vitro and In Vivo Studies

We review some of the recent in vivo and in vitro studies of various extracts and formulations of Artemisia. The research studies utilized aqueous, methanol, chloroform or acetone extracts, essential oils or oil based extracts or dried powders of various species of Artemisia. The studies were performed on bacterial, viral or fungal cultures, cultured cells or animal models with limited studies on humans.

In the light of the COVID-19 pandemic, some species of Artemisia including but not limited to *A. annua, A. absinthium, A. vulgaris, A. maritima* and *A. indhana* are receiving greater attention from researchers as they hold great potential for their powerful anti-infectious, antiviral and anti-inflammatory activities [6,12,46–48]. Recent studies are now pointing to the exciting roles of artemisinin and its derivatives (ARTs) as potential drug candidates against SARS-CoV-2 owing to their potent antiviral and anti-inflammatory properties.

4.1. Anti-Carcinogenic Activity

Various species of the Artemisia plant have been shown to suppress the growth of numerous cancer cell lines including leukemia, colon cancer, renal cell carcinoma and breast cancer cells [28,49,50]. Phytochemical analysis of the various extracts revealed the presence of coumarins, flavonoids, anthocyanins, cardiac glycosides and tannins. These phytochemicals and their derivatives exhibit growth inhibitory properties through multiple actions including blocking angiogenesis, triggering apoptosis or cell cycle arrest and disrupting cell migration [51–53]. Researchers are now focusing their efforts on ARTs that appear to be broad-spectrum antitumor agents based on their efficacy and safety [54,55].

In a randomized, double-blind, placebo-controlled pilot trial involving 23 subjects, the anticancer effect and tolerability of oral artesunate in colorectal cancer (CRC) was determined. The primary outcome measure was the proportion of tumor cells undergoing apoptosis. Despite the fact that it was a small study size with variability in quantitating immunohistochemical markers, the results clearly indicated selective cytotoxicity of oral artesunate.

In addition to the above mentioned study, other clinical trials involving patients with solid tumors including colorectal carcinoma, breast cancer, hepatocellular carcinoma and lung cancer have been completed with encouraging results. In all these studies, ARTs inhibited growth of solid tumors with no evident toxicity and with a low incidence of adverse effects thus highlighting their role as promising anti-cancer agents [54,56,57].

4.2. Anti-Oxidant Activity

The phytochemicals and their derivatives, extracts and essential oils derived from the Artemisia plant have a unique property of being reactive oxygen species (ROS) modulators. In some cases they exhibit strong antioxidant and radical scavenging activity against hydroxyl ion and hydrogen peroxide and display excellent protective effect by strengthening the antioxidant defense system and lowering the generation of ROS [6,58].

In other situations, especially involving cancer cells, ARTs triggered ROS production leading to mitochondrial dysfunction and autophagy of leukemia cell lines. ARTs-induced ROS production triggered apoptosis in various tumor cell lines studies, including neuroblastoma, glioblastoma, T-cell lymphoma and breast cancer cells [54]. In studies using mouse models of cancer, ARTs induced ROS production leading to the inhibition of growth of ovarian cancer [54].

The mechanism of action of ARTs involves binding to ferrous iron (e.g., heme) and triggering the generation of ROS, which results in cytostatic or cytotoxic effects. The production of ROS can also trigger cellular damage through the peroxidation of membrane lipids, activation of pro-apoptotic pathways or creating genomic and mitochondrial DNA instability [59]. Thus, the ROS modulating properties exhibited by the various phytochemicals isolated from different species of Artemisia highlight the importance of exploring the therapeutic uses of these compounds in pathological conditions that feature oxidative stress.

4.3. Anti-Bacterial and Anti-Parasitic Activity

The plant extracts and compounds obtained from Artemisia species have been shown to be powerful inhibitors of bacteria and parasites [9]. Mechanistic studies demonstrate the bactericidal properties of some of these phytochemicals against Gram-negative or Gram-positive bacteria involving the destruction of the bacterial membrane [6,28,60,61]. Notable among the phytochemicals is ARTs that represent a new class of antibacterial drugs [9,14,15].

ARTs also possess potent antimalarial properties and are effective against both asexual and sexual parasite stages. In several clinical trials involving both ARTs and quinine, ARTs outperformed quinine in terms of mean parasite clearance time, fever clearance time, coma resolution times and incidence of adverse effects [14–16,62]. Artemisinin-based therapies are now recommended due to the resistance displayed by bacteria and parasites to quinoline drugs.

4.4. Anti-Fibrotic Effects

In addition to the above mentioned pharmacological properties, ARTs are also known for their anti-fibrotic effects [29,63,64]. The role of ARTs in blocking the development or progression of fibrotic phenotypes has been studied in animal models of pulmonary fibrosis, renal fibrosis, hepatic fibrosis, and other types of tissue fibrosis suggesting the potential utility of these compounds as anti-fibrotic agents. The effects of ARTs against profibrotic processes include induction of apoptosis, inhibition of proliferation, blocking differentiation of tissue-specific myofibroblast precursors or preventing the accumulation of tissue myofibroblasts that provoke tissue fibrosis [6,63]. In addition, ARTs block the expression of extracellular matrix (ECM) genes and pro-fibrotic genes in myofibroblasts thereby antagonizing cellular processes that promote accumulation of fibrotic tissue. ARTs also inhibit angiogenesis either through direct effects on endothelial cells or indirectly by down-regulating pro-angiogenic gene expression in angiogenesis-supporting non-endothelial cells. With its anti-fibrotic role in disease models across several species and multiple tissues involving diverse mechanisms, artemisinin-based therapeutics for treatment of fibrotic diseases may prove efficacious in humans [64].

4.5. Role in Neurodegeneration

Extracts of several Artemisia species exhibit neuroprotective effects against focal ischemia-reperfusion-induced cerebral injury, microglial cytotoxicity and glutamate excitotoxicity [65]. Furthermore, Artemisia protects neurons against mitochondrial potential loss, attenuates reactive oxygen species and protects neurons against H_2O_2-induced death by upregulating the Nrf2 pathway [66]. ARTs improve learning and memory in mouse models of Alzheimer's disease mice by blocking Aβ25-35-induced increase in the levels of inflammatory cytokines IL-1β, IL-6 and TNF-α and by restoring the autophagic flux and promoting the clearance of Aβ fibrils [67,68].

Recently, three different subtypes of Alzheimer's disease (AD) have been described [69]. The type-3 AD classified as infectious or Krimi (ayurveda classification of AD) is the result of exposure to virus or biotoxins, such as mycotoxins, and features chronic inflammation [69,70]. Owing to their powerful antiviral and anti-inflammatory properties, ARTs may serve as excellent drug candidates for type-3 AD.

4.6. Anti-Inflammatory Activity

Artemisia species exhibit powerful anti-inflammatory effects. Several sesquiterpenes derived from Artemisia and their derivatives including artemisinin, artesunate, dihydroarteannuin, artemisolide, eupatilin, scoparone, capillarisin and scopoletin have received special attention due to their role in blocking inflammation. Using animal models, ARTs were found to be effective in treating inflammatory conditions including rheumatoid arthritis, systemic lupus erythematosus, multiple sclerosis and allergic disorders [71].

Some of the anti-inflammatory mechanisms include: (1) inhibition of the iNOS and COX-2 pathways; (2) suppression of ERK and NF-κB signaling; (3) inhibition of pathogenic T cell activation; (4) suppressing B cells activation and antibody production; and (5) inhibition of Akt phosphorylation and IκB degradation through the PI3K/Akt signaling pathway downstream of TNF-α [72–75]. Thus, the varied mechanisms through which these phytochemicals derived from Artemisia exhibit their anti-inflammatory effects warrant investigation into their role as therapeutic candidates for inflammatory conditions and autoimmune disorders.

4.7. Anti-Viral

Several phytochemicals isolated from various Artemisia species exhibit significant antiviral activity [76]. ARTs have turned out to be the most promising antiviral drug candidates with activities against hepatitis B and C viruses, human herpes viruses HSV-1 and HSV-2, HIV-1 and influenza virus A in the low micromolar range [77–82]. In most cases, ARTs inhibited the central regulatory processes of viral-infected cells (NF-κB or Sp1-dependent pathways), thus blocking the host-cell–type and metabolic requirements for viral replication [80].

Owing to their potent anti-inflammatory, immunoregulatory and antiviral properties, ARTs are being pursued for their activity against SARS-CoV-2 infection. Researchers used in silico approaches to investigate if artemisinin or its derivatives could physically bind any of the COVID-19 target proteins including SARS-CoV-2 spike glycoprotein, spike ectodomain structural protein, the main protease of the virus (M^{Pro}) or spike receptor-binding domain, thereby preventing SARS-CoV-2 from binding to the host receptor ACE2 [83–89]. AD-MET (absorption, distribution, metabolism, excretion and toxicity) analysis of artemisinin showed that it was non-cytotoxic, had good aqueous solubility and a good permeability through the blood–brain barrier with a promising therapeutic potential. Furthermore, molecular docking studies revealed that artemisinin bound to all four proteins and in some cases displayed better binding modes than hydroxychloroquine [85–89]. Thus, ARTs could serve as best leads for further drug development process for SARS-CoV-2 infection.

Several investigators have now shown that extracts from different species of Artemisia are active against SARS-CoV-2 [79,86,90,91]. Results from recent studies indicate that ARTs impair SARS-CoV-2 viral infection by modulating several host cell metabolic pathways thus making them attractive candidates for COVID-19 [85,86,92]. The mechanism of antiviral activity may be through the induction of cellular ROS, blunting the PI3K/Akt/p70S6K signaling pathway, binding to NF-κB/Sp1 or inducing a endocytosis inhibition mechanism, all of which lead to inhibition of viral replication and growth [85,93,94]. The above mentioned results have spurred the interest of few groups to embark on clinical trials to evaluate the safety and efficacy of ARTs in the treatment of subjects with SARS-CoV-2 viral infection.

In a recently published controlled clinical trial, 41 patients with confirmed COVID-19 were divided into two groups. While 18 subjects served as the control group, the experimental group (n = 23) received a combination of artemisinin-piperaquine (AP). AP was orally administered with a loading dose of two tablets (artemisinin 125 mg and piperaquine 750 mg) on the first day, followed by a low dose of one tablet/day (artemisinin 62.5 mg and piperaquine 375 mg) for six days [95]. The primary outcome was the percentage of participants with undetectable SARS-CoV-2 on days 7, 10, 14, and 28 following the treatment. The results indicated that: (1) the average time to achieve undetectable SARS-CoV-2 RNA in the AP group was significantly less than that in the control group; (2) the elimination rate of SARS-CoV-2 RNA in the AP group was significantly higher than that in the control group; and (3) the length of hospital stay for the AP group was significantly lower than that in the control group. Although the study had insufficient sample size and trial design, nevertheless, the safe toxicity profile and immunoregulatory activities makes AP an excellent drug candidate against SARS-CoV-2 infection [95].

Transforming Growth Factor-beta (TGF-β) plays an important role in modulating the immune system and displays different activities on different types of immune cells. SARS-

CoV-2 infection is accompanied by a cytokine storm together with edema and pulmonary fibrosis at the end stage of the infection. SARS-CoV-2 also up-regulates TGF-β expression which may partly explain the cytokine storm and fibrosis in the lung [94,96,97]. Efforts are underway to discover novel and specific small molecules that can potently block TGF-β expression with negligible side-effects. Artemisinin and its derivatives have been shown to be suppressors of TGF-β in several models of inflammatory diseases [64,98–100]. A randomized, open-label Phase IV study is underway to evaluate the safety and efficacy of a proprietary formulation of ARTs in adult COVID-19 patients with symptomatic mild-moderate COVID-19 [101]. In addition to its potent antiviral activity, the drug is expected to mitigate the TGF-β mediated inflammatory injury associated with the cytokine storm and viral sepsis in these patients. Initial results show that the ARTs-based drug has a very favorable safety profile and significantly accelerated the recovery of patients with mild-moderate COVID-19 infection [101]. Thus inhibition of TGF-β signaling by ARTs may be an attractive therapeutic strategy making them excellent drug candidates against SARS-CoV-2 infection.

5. Conclusions and Future Direction

Several phytochemical derivatives and lead molecules have been developed from medicinal plants for various significant therapeutic activities [4,5,94,102,103]. Scientists routinely investigate medicinal plants just for that one single and potent compound responsible for the therapeutic effect [104]. Studies comparing the action of whole plant extracts to the action of purified preparation show that, in many cases, the potency of the purified preparation declines at each step of fractionation [105]. Since the therapeutic effect may be the result of the combination of several compounds present in the medicinal plant, a complex mixture of compounds has a greater effect than isolated compounds [106]. The advantages of a combinatorial approach may be the synergy exhibited by the various components, enhanced bioavailability, cumulative effects and affecting an entire network of pathways in tandem [107].

Artemisia has prominence in Chinese and Ayurvedic medicinal systems for its numerous therapeutic properties. Among the phytochemicals present in the plant, the lactone derivative artemisinin and its derivatives—termed ARTs—are very promising owing to their multiple pharmacological actions [4,7,85,93,94]. Recent studies point to ARTs as attractive candidates for SARS-CoV-2 and they are a major focus in medical research [4,85,92,103]. SARS-CoV-2 infection manifests as a mild respiratory tract infection and influenza-like illness to a severe disease with accompanying lung injury (in severe cases lung fibrosis), oxidative stress, multisystem inflammatory conditions, multi-organ failure and neurological issues [108–111]. The role of ARTs as an antioxidant and anti-inflammatory and to be able to block tissues fibrosis together with its safety and low toxicity profile makes it an excellent drug candidate against SARS-CoV-2 infection [85,94].

Author Contributions: Conceptualization, S.G.K. and R.V.R.; Methodology, S.G.K. and R.V.R.; Data curation, S.G.K. and R.V.R.; Original draft preparation and Writing, R.V.R.; Reviewing and Editing, S.G.K. and R.V.R. Both authors have read and agreed to the published version of the manuscript.

Funding: The research study did not receive any specific grant from funding agencies in the public, commercial, or not-for-profit sectors.

Institutional Review Board Statement: Not Applicable.

Informed Consent Statement: Not Applicable.

Data Availability Statement: Not Applicable.

Conflicts of Interest: This manuscript is not under consideration by another journal, nor has it been published. SGK is a paid consultant-at-large with Oncotelic, Inc., a wholly-owned subsidiary of Mateon Therapeutics, the sponsor for the clinical development of the proprietary formulation of ARTs for SARS-CoV-2 infection. RVR declares no competing financial interests.

References

1. Rao, R.V.; Descamps, O.; John, V.; Bredesen, D.E. Ayurvedic medicinal plants for Alzheimer's disease: A review. *Alzheimers Res. Ther.* **2012**, *4*, 22. [CrossRef] [PubMed]
2. Parasuraman, S.; Thing, G.S.; Dhanaraj, S.A. Polyherbal formulation: Concept of ayurveda. *Pharmacogn. Rev.* **2014**, *8*, 73–80. [CrossRef]
3. Barkat, M.A.; Goyal, A.; Barkat, H.A.; Salauddin, M.; Pottoo, F.H.; Anwer, E.T. Herbal medicine: Clinical perspective & regulatory status. *Comb. Chem. High Throughput Screen.* **2020**. [CrossRef]
4. Vellingiri, B.; Jayaramayya, K.; Iyer, M.; Narayanasamy, A.; Govindasamy, V.; Giridharan, B.; Ganesan, S.; Venugopal, A.; Venkatesan, D.; Ganesan, H.; et al. COVID-19: A promising cure for the global panic. *Sci. Total Environ.* **2020**, *725*, 138277. [CrossRef]
5. Akram, M.; Tahir, I.M.; Shah, S.M.A.; Mahmood, Z.; Altaf, A.; Ahmad, K.; Munir, N.; Daniyal, M.; Nasir, S.; Mehboob, H. Antiviral potential of medicinal plants against HIV, HSV, influenza, hepatitis, and coxsackievirus: A systematic review. *Phytother. Res.* **2018**, *32*, 811–822. [CrossRef] [PubMed]
6. Bora, K.S.; Sharma, A. The genus *Artemisia*: A comprehensive review. *Pharm. Biol.* **2011**, *49*, 101–109. [CrossRef] [PubMed]
7. Mishra, K.P.; Sharma, N.; Diwaker, D.; Ganju, L.; Singh, S.B. Plant derived antivirals: A potential source of drug development. *J. Virol. Antivir. Res.* **2013**, *2*. [CrossRef]
8. Koul, B.; Taak, P.; Kumar, A.; Khatri, T.; Sanyal, I. The *Artemisia* genus: A review on traditional uses, phytochemical constituents, pharmacological properties and germplasm conservation. *J. Glycom. Lipidom.* **2018**, *7*, 1–7. [CrossRef]
9. Pandey, A.K.; Singh, P. The Genus *Artemisia*: A 2012–2017 literature review on chemical composition, antimicrobial, insecticidal and antioxidant activities of essential oils. *Medicines* **2017**, *4*, 68. [CrossRef]
10. Poiata, A.; Tuchilus, C.; Ivanescu, B.; Ionescu, A.; Lazar, M.I. Antibacterial activity of some *Artemisia* species extract. *Revista Medico Chirurgicala a Societatii de Medici si Naturalisti din Iasi* **2009**, *113*, 911–914.
11. Tan, R.X.; Zheng, W.F.; Tang, H.Q. Biologically active substances from the genus *Artemisia*. *Planta Medica* **1998**, *64*, 295–302. [CrossRef]
12. Obistioiu, D.; Cristina, R.T.; Schmerold, I.; Chizzola, R.; Stolze, K.; Nichita, I.; Chiurciu, V. Chemical characterization by GC-MS and in vitro activity against *Candida albicans* of volatile fractions prepared from *Artemisia dracunculus*, *Artemisia abrotanum*, *Artemisia absinthium* and *Artemisia vulgaris*. *Chem. Cent. J.* **2014**, *8*, 6. [CrossRef] [PubMed]
13. Semwal, B.R.; Semwal, D.K.; Mishra, S.P.; Semwal, R. Chemical composition and antibacterial potential of essential oils from *Artemisia capillaris*, *Artemisia nilagirica*, *Citrus limon*, *Cymbopogon flexuosus*, *Hedychium spicatum* and *Ocimum tenuiflorum*. *Nat. Prod. J.* **2015**, *5*, 199–205. [CrossRef]
14. Antoine, T.; Fisher, N.; Amewu, R.; O'Neill, P.M.; Ward, S.A.; Biagini, G.A. Rapid kill of malaria parasites by artemisinin and semi-synthetic endoperoxides involves ROS-dependent depolarization of the membrane potential. *J. Antimicrob. Chemother.* **2014**, *69*, 1005–1016. [CrossRef]
15. Shah, N.K.; Tyagi, P.; Sharma, S.K. The impact of artemisinin combination therapy and long-lasting insecticidal nets on forest malaria incidence in tribal villages of India, 2006–2011. *PLoS ONE* **2013**, *8*, e56740. [CrossRef]
16. WWARN Artemisinin Based Combination Therapy (ACT) Africa Baseline Study Group. Clinical determinants of early parasitological response to ACTs in African patients with uncomplicated falciparum malaria: A literature review and meta-analysis of individual patient data. *BMC Med.* **2015**, *13*, 212.
17. Tambo, E.; Khater, E.I.; Chen, J.H.; Bergquist, R.; Zhou, X.N. Nobel prize for the artemisinin and ivermectin discoveries: A great boost towards elimination of the global infectious diseases of poverty. *Infect. Dis. Poverty* **2015**, *4*, 58. [CrossRef]
18. Su, X.Z.; Miller, L.H. The discovery of artemisinin and the Nobel prize in physiology or medicine. *Sci. China Life Sci.* **2015**, *58*, 1175–1179. [CrossRef]
19. Joshi, R.K.; Satyal, P.; Setzer, W.N. Himalayan aromatic medicinal plants: A review of their ethnopharmacology, volatile phytochemistry, and biological activities. *Medicines* **2016**, *3*, 6. [CrossRef]
20. Joshi, V.K.; Joshi, A.; Dhiman, K.S. The ayurvedic pharmacopoeia of India, development and perspectives. *J. Ethnopharmacol.* **2017**, *197*, 32–38. [CrossRef]
21. Kumar, D.; Arya, V.; Kaur, R.; Bhat, Z.A.; Gupta, V.K.; Kumar, V. A review of immunomodulators in the Indian traditional health care system. *J. Microbiol. Immunol. Infect.* **2012**, *45*, 165–184. [CrossRef] [PubMed]
22. Katiyar, C.K. Ayurpathy: A modern perspective of Ayurveda. *Ayu* **2011**, *32*, 304–305. [CrossRef]
23. Ivanescu, B.; Miron, A.; Corciova, A. Sesquiterpene lactones from *Artemisia* genus: Biological activities and methods of analysis. *J. Anal. Methods Chem.* **2015**, *2015*. [CrossRef]
24. Batiha, G.E.; Olatunde, A.; El-Mleeh, A.; Hetta, H.F.; Al-Rejaie, S.; Alghamdi, S.; Zahoor, M.; Magdy Beshbishy, A.; Murata, T.; Zaragoza-Bastida, A.; et al. Bioactive compounds, pharmacological actions, and pharmacokinetics of wormwood (*Artemisia absinthium*). *Antibiotics* **2020**, *9*, 353. [CrossRef]
25. Kumar, S.; Kumari, R. *Artemisia*: A medicinally important genus. *J. Complement. Med. Alt. Healthcare* **2018**, *7*. [CrossRef]
26. Liu, N.Q.; Van der Kooy, F.; Verpoorte, R. *Artemisia afra*: A potential flagship for African medicinal plants? *South Afr. J. Bot.* **2009**, *75*, 185–195. [CrossRef]

27. Fu, C.; Yu, P.; Wang, M.; Qiu, F. Phytochemical analysis and geographic assessment of flavonoids, coumarins and sesquiterpenes in *Artemisia annua* L. based on HPLC-DAD quantification and LC-ESI-QTOF-MS/MS confirmation. *Food Chem.* **2020**, *312*, 126070. [CrossRef] [PubMed]
28. Feng, X.; Cao, S.; Qiu, F.; Zhang, B. Traditional application and modern pharmacological research of *Artemisia annua* L. *Pharmacol. Ther.* **2020**, *216*, 107650. [CrossRef] [PubMed]
29. Septembre-Malaterre, A.; Lalarizo Rakoto, M.; Marodon, C.; Bedoui, Y.; Nakab, J.; Simon, E.; Hoarau, L.; Savriama, S.; Strasberg, D.; Guiraud, P.; et al. *Artemisia annua*, a traditional plant brought to light. *Int. J. Mol. Sci.* **2020**, *21*, 4986. [CrossRef] [PubMed]
30. Ahuja, A.; Yi, Y.S.; Kim, M.Y.; Cho, J.Y. Ethnopharmacological properties of *Artemisia asiatica*: A comprehensive review. *J. Ethnopharmacol.* **2018**, *220*, 117–128. [CrossRef]
31. Costa, R.; Ragusa, S.; Russo, M.; Certo, G.; Franchina, F.A.; Zanotto, A.; Grasso, E.; Mondello, L.; Germano, M.P. Phytochemical screening of *Artemisia arborescens* L. by means of advanced chromatographic techniques for identification of health-promoting compounds. *J. Pharm. Biomed. Anal.* **2016**, *117*, 499–509. [CrossRef]
32. Adams, J.D.; Garcia, C.; Garg, G. Mugwort (*Artemisia vulgaris*, *Artemisia douglasiana*, *Artemisia argyi*) in the treatment of menopause, premenstrual syndrome, dysmenorrhea and Attention Deficit Hyperactivity Disorder. *Chin. Med.* **2012**, *3*, 116–123. [CrossRef]
33. Allerton, T.D.; Kowalski, G.M.; Stampley, J.; Irving, B.A.; Lighton, J.R.B.; Floyd, Z.E.; Stephens, J.M. An ethanolic extract of *Artemisia dracunculus* L. enhances the metabolic benefits of exercise in diet-induced obese mice. *Med. Sci. Sports Exerc.* **2020**. [CrossRef] [PubMed]
34. Majdan, M.; Kiss, A.K.; Halasa, R.; Granica, S.; Osinska, E.; Czerwinska, M.E. Inhibition of neutrophil functions and antibacterial effects of tarragon (*Artemisia dracunculus* L.) infusion-phytochemical characterization. *Front. Pharmacol.* **2020**, *11*. [CrossRef]
35. Mokhtar, A.B.; Ahmed, S.A.; Eltamany, E.E.; Karanis, P. Anti-blastocystis activity in vitro of Egyptian herbal extracts (family: Asteraceae) with emphasis on *Artemisia judaica*. *Int. J. Environ. Res. Public Health* **2019**, *16*, 1555. [CrossRef]
36. Cho, J.Y.; Park, K.H.; Hwang, D.Y.; Lee, S.Y.; Moon, J.H.; Ju Lee, Y.; Park, K.D.; Ham, K.S. Three new decenynol glucosides from *Artemisia scoparia* (Asteraceae). *J. Asian Nat. Prod. Res.* **2020**, *22*, 795–802. [CrossRef] [PubMed]
37. Boudreau, A.; Poulev, A.; Ribnicky, D.M.; Raskin, I.; Rathinasabapathy, T.; Richard, A.J.; Stephens, J.M. Distinct fractions of an *Artemisia scoparia* extract contain compounds with novel adipogenic bioactivity. *Front. Nutr.* **2019**, *6*. [CrossRef]
38. Xie, G.; Schepetkin, I.A.; Siemsen, D.W.; Kirpotina, L.N.; Wiley, J.A.; Quinn, M.T. Fractionation and characterization of biologically-active polysaccharides from *Artemisia tripartita*. *Phytochemistry* **2008**, *69*, 1359–1371. [CrossRef] [PubMed]
39. Calderone, V.; Martinotti, E.; Baragatti, B.; Breschi, M.C.; Morelli, I. Vascular effects of aqueous crude extracts of *Artemisia verlotorum* Lamotte (Compositae): In vivo and in vitro pharmacological studies in rats. *Phytother. Res.* **1999**, *13*, 645–648. [CrossRef]
40. De Lima, T.C.; Morato, G.S.; Takahashi, R.N. Evaluation of the central properties of *Artemisia verlotorum*. *Planta Medica* **1993**, *59*, 326–329. [CrossRef]
41. Ding, Y.H.; Wang, H.T.; Shi, S.; Meng, Y.; Feng, J.C.; Wu, H.B. Sesquiterpenoids from *Artemisia vestita* and their antifeedant and antifungal activities. *Molecules* **2019**, *24*, 3671. [CrossRef]
42. Tian, S.H.; Zhang, C.; Zeng, K.W.; Zhao, M.B.; Jiang, Y.; Tu, P.F. Sesquiterpenoids from *Artemisia vestita*. *Phytochmistry* **2018**, *147*, 194–202. [CrossRef] [PubMed]
43. Ragasa, C.Y.; de Jesus, J.P.; Apuada, M.J.; Rideout, J.A. A new sesquiterpene from *Artemisia vulgaris*. *J. Nat. Med.* **2008**, *62*, 461–463. [CrossRef]
44. Willcox, M. *Artemisia* species: From traditional medicines to modern antimalarials—And back again. *J. Altern. Complement. Med.* **2009**, *15*, 101–109. [CrossRef] [PubMed]
45. Nigam, M.; Atanassova, M.; Mishra, A.P.; Pezzani, R.; Devkota, H.P.; Plygun, S.; Salehi, B.; Setzer, W.N.; Sharifi-Rad, J. Bioactive compounds and health benefits of *Artemisia* species. *Nat. Prod. Commun.* **2019**. [CrossRef]
46. Ekiert, H.; Pajor, J.; Klin, P.; Rzepiela, A.; Slesak, H.; Szopa, A. Significance of *Artemisia vulgaris*, L. (common mugwort) in the history of medicine and its possible contemporary applications substantiated by phytochemical and pharmacological studies. *Molecules* **2020**, *25*, 4415. [CrossRef]
47. Abad, M.J.; Bedoya, L.M.; Apaza, L.; Bermejo, P. The *Artemisia* L. genus: A review of bioactive essential oils. *Molecules* **2012**, *17*, 2542–2566. [CrossRef] [PubMed]
48. Lee, Y.J.; Thiruvengadam, M.; Ching, I.M.; Nagella, P. Polyphenol composition and antioxidant activity from the vegetable plant *Artemisia absinthium* L. *Aust. J. Crop Sci.* **2013**, *7*, 1921–1926.
49. Kiani, B.H.; Kayani, W.K.; Khayam, A.U.; Dilshad, E.; Ismail, H.; Mirza, B. Artemisinin and its derivatives: A promising cancer therapy. *Mol. Biol. Rep.* **2020**, *47*, 6321–6336. [CrossRef]
50. Firestone, G.L.; Sundar, S.N. Anticancer activities of artemisinin and its bioactive derivatives. *Expert Rev. Mol. Med.* **2009**, *11*. [CrossRef]
51. Ly, B.T.K.; Ly, D.M.; Linh, P.H.; Son, H.K.; Ha, N.L.; Chi, H.T. Screening of medicinal herbs for cytotoxic activity to leukemia cells. *J. BUON* **2020**, *25*, 1989–1996.
52. Kumar, M.S.; Yadav, T.T.; Khair, R.R.; Peters, G.J.; Yergeri, M.C. Combination therapies of artemisinin and its derivatives as a viable approach for future cancer treatment. *Curr. Pharm. Des.* **2019**, *25*, 3323–3338. [CrossRef] [PubMed]

53. Jia, L.; Song, Q.; Zhou, C.; Li, X.; Pi, L.; Ma, X.; Li, H.; Lu, X.; Shen, Y. Dihydroartemisinin as a putative STAT3 inhibitor, suppresses the growth of head and neck squamous cell carcinoma by targeting Jak2/STAT3 signaling. *PLoS ONE* **2016**, *11*, e0147157. [CrossRef] [PubMed]
54. Slezakova, S.; Ruda-Kucerova, J. Anticancer activity of artemisinin and its derivatives. *Anticancer Res.* **2017**, *37*, 5995–6003.
55. Pulito, C.; Strano, S.; Blandino, G. Dihydroartemisinin: From malaria to the treatment of relapsing head and neck cancers. *Ann. Transl. Med.* **2020**, *8*, 612. [CrossRef] [PubMed]
56. Krishna, S.; Ganapathi, S.; Ster, I.C.; Saeed, M.E.; Cowan, M.; Finlayson, C.; Kovacsevics, H.; Jansen, H.; Kremsner, P.G.; Efferth, T.; et al. A randomised, double blind, placebo-controlled pilot study of oral artesunate therapy for colorectal cancer. *EBioMedicine* **2015**, *2*, 82–90. [CrossRef] [PubMed]
57. Berger, T.G.; Dieckmann, D.; Efferth, T.; Schultz, E.S.; Funk, J.O.; Baur, A.; Schuler, G. Artesunate in the treatment of metastatic uveal melanoma—First experiences. *Oncol. Rep.* **2005**, *14*, 1599–1603. [CrossRef] [PubMed]
58. Du, L.; Chen, J.; Xing, Y.Q. Eupatilin prevents H_2O_2-induced oxidative stress and apoptosis in human retinal pigment epithelial cells. *Biomed. Pharmacother.* **2017**, *85*, 136–140. [CrossRef]
59. Krishna, S.; Uhlemann, A.C.; Haynes, R.K. Artemisinins: Mechanisms of action and potential for resistance. *Drug Resist. Updates* **2004**, *7*, 233–244. [CrossRef]
60. Yang, M.T.; Kuo, T.F.; Chung, K.F.; Liang, Y.C.; Yang, C.W.; Lin, C.Y.; Feng, C.S.; Chen, Z.W.; Lee, T.H.; Hsiao, C.L.; et al. Authentication, phytochemical characterization and anti-bacterial activity of two *Artemisia* species. *Food Chem.* **2020**, *333*, 127458. [CrossRef] [PubMed]
61. Huang, J.; Qian, C.; Xu, H.; Huang, Y. Antibacterial activity of *Artemisia asiatica* essential oil against some common respiratory infection causing bacterial strains and its mechanism of action in *Haemophilus influenzae*. *Microb. Pathog.* **2018**, *114*, 470–475. [CrossRef]
62. Cui, L.; Su, X.Z. Discovery, mechanisms of action and combination therapy of artemisinin. *Expert Rev. Anti Infect. Ther.* **2009**, *7*, 999–1013. [CrossRef]
63. Dolivo, D.; Weathers, P.; Dominko, T. Artemisinin and artemisinin derivatives as anti-fibrotic therapeutics. *Acta Pharmaceutica Sinica B* **2021**, *11*, 322–339. [CrossRef]
64. Wang, Y.; Wang, Y.; You, F.; Xue, J. Novel use for old drugs: The emerging role of artemisinin and its derivatives in fibrosis. *Pharmacol. Res.* **2020**, *157*, 104829. [CrossRef] [PubMed]
65. Lu, B.W.; Baum, L.; So, K.F.; Chiu, K.; Xie, L.K. More than anti-malarial agents: Therapeutic potential of artemisinins in neurodegeneration. *Neural Regen. Res.* **2019**, *14*, 1494–1498.
66. Sajjad, N.; Wani, A.; Sharma, A.; Ali, R.; Hassan, S.; Hamid, R.; Habib, H.; Ganai, B.A. *Artemisia amygdalina* upregulates Nrf2 and protects neurons against oxidative stress in Alzheimer disease. *Cell Mol. Neurobiol.* **2019**, *39*, 387–399. [CrossRef]
67. Qiang, W.; Cai, W.; Yang, Q.; Yang, L.; Dai, Y.; Zhao, Z.; Yin, J.; Li, Y.; Li, Q.; Wang, Y.; et al. Artemisinin B improves learning and memory impairment in AD dementia mice by suppressing neuroinflammation. *Neuroscience* **2018**, *395*, 1–12. [CrossRef]
68. Zhao, Y.; Long, Z.; Ding, Y.; Jiang, T.; Liu, J.; Li, Y.; Liu, Y.; Peng, X.; Wang, K.; Feng, M.; et al. Dihydroartemisinin ameliorates learning and memory in Alzheimer's disease through promoting autophagosome-lysosome fusion and autolysosomal degradation for abeta clearance. *Front. Aging Neurosci.* **2020**, *12*. [CrossRef] [PubMed]
69. Bredesen, D.E. Inhalational Alzheimer's disease: An unrecognized—And treatable—Epidemic. *Aging* **2016**, *8*, 304–313. [CrossRef] [PubMed]
70. Bredesen, D.E.; Rao, R.V. Ayurvedic profiling of Alzheimer's disease. *Altern. Ther. Health Med.* **2017**, *23*, 46–50. [PubMed]
71. Shi, C.; Li, H.; Yang, Y.; Hou, L. Anti-inflammatory and immunoregulatory functions of artemisinin and its derivatives. *Mediators Inflamm.* **2015**, *2015*. [CrossRef] [PubMed]
72. Qin, D.P.; Li, H.B.; Pang, Q.Q.; Huang, Y.X.; Pan, D.B.; Su, Z.Z.; Yao, X.J.; Yao, X.S.; Xiao, W.; Yu, Y. Structurally diverse sesquiterpenoids from the aerial parts of *Artemisia annua* (Qinghao) and their striking systemically anti-inflammatory activities. *Bioorg. Chem.* **2020**, *103*, 104221. [CrossRef]
73. Boudreau, A.; Burke, S.J.; Collier, J.J.; Richard, A.J.; Ribnicky, D.M.; Stephens, J.M. Mechanisms of *Artemisia scoparia*'s anti-inflammatory activity in cultured adipocytes, macrophages, and pancreatic β-cells. *Obesity* **2020**, *28*, 1726–1735. [CrossRef]
74. Zamani, S.; Emami, S.A.; Iranshahi, M.; Zamani Taghizadeh Rabe, S.; Mahmoudi, M. Sesquiterpene fractions of *Artemisia* plants as potent inhibitors of inducible nitric oxide synthase and cyclooxygenase-2 expression. *Iran. J. Basic Med. Sci.* **2019**, *22*, 774–780. [PubMed]
75. Cheng, C.; Ho, W.E.; Goh, F.Y.; Guan, S.P.; Kong, L.R.; Lai, W.Q.; Leung, B.P.; Wong, W.S. Anti-malarial drug artesunate attenuates experimental allergic asthma via inhibition of the phosphoinositide 3-kinase/Akt pathway. *PLoS ONE* **2011**, *6*, e20932. [CrossRef] [PubMed]
76. Efferth, T. Beyond malaria: The inhibition of viruses by artemisinin-type compounds. *Biotechnol. Adv.* **2018**, *36*, 1730–1737. [CrossRef]
77. Obeid, S.; Alen, J.; Nguyen, V.H.; Pham, V.C.; Meuleman, P.; Pannecouque, C.; Le, T.N.; Neyts, J.; Dehaen, W.; Paeshuyse, J. Artemisinin analogues as potent inhibitors of in vitro hepatitis C virus replication. *PLoS ONE* **2013**, *8*, e81783. [CrossRef] [PubMed]
78. Romero, M.R.; Efferth, T.; Serrano, M.A.; Castano, B.; Macias, R.I.; Briz, O.; Marin, J.J. Effect of artemisinin/artesunate as inhibitors of hepatitis B virus production in an "in vitro" replicative system. *Antiviral Res.* **2005**, *68*, 75–83. [CrossRef] [PubMed]

79. Uzun, T.; Toptas, O. Artesunate: Could be an alternative drug to chloroquine in COVID-19 treatment? *Chin. Med.* **2020**, *15*, 54. [CrossRef]
80. Efferth, T.; Romero, M.R.; Wolf, D.G.; Stamminger, T.; Marin, J.J.; Marschall, M. The antiviral activities of artemisinin and artesunate. *Clin. Infect. Dis.* **2008**, *47*, 804–811. [CrossRef]
81. D'Alessandro, S.; Scaccabarozzi, D.; Signorini, L.; Perego, F.; Ilboudo, D.P.; Ferrante, P.; Delbue, S. The use of antimalarial drugs against viral infection. *Microorganisms* **2020**, *8*, 85. [CrossRef] [PubMed]
82. Jang, E.; Kim, B.J.; Lee, K.T.; Inn, K.S.; Lee, J.H. A survey of therapeutic effects of *Artemisia capillaris* in liver diseases. *Evid. Based Complement. Alternat. Med.* **2015**, *2015*. [CrossRef] [PubMed]
83. Rolta, R.; Salaria, D.; Kumar, V.; Sourirajan, A.; Dev, K. Phytocompounds of *Rheum emodi, Thymus serpyllum* and *Artemisia annua* inhibit COVID-19 binding to ACE2 receptor: In silico approach. *Res. Square* **2020**. [CrossRef]
84. Sharma, S.; Deep, S. In-silico drug repurposing for targeting SARS-CoV-2 Mpro. *J. Biomol. Struct. Dyn.* **2020**. [CrossRef]
85. Cao, R.; Hu, H.; Li, Y.; Wang, X.; Xu, M.; Liu, J.; Zhang, H.; Yan, Y.; Zhao, L.; Li, W.; et al. Anti-SARS-CoV-2 potential of artemisinins in vitro. *ACS Infect. Dis.* **2020**, *6*, 2524–2531. [CrossRef]
86. Sehailia, M.; Chemat, S. Antimalarial-agent artemisinin and derivatives portray more potent binding to Lys353 and Lys31-binding hotspots of SARS-CoV-2 spike protein than hydroxychloroquine: Potential repurposing of artenimol for COVID-19. *J. Biomol. Struct. Dyn.* **2020**. [CrossRef]
87. Rai, K.K.; Sharma, L.; Pandey, N.; Meena, R.P.; Rai, S.P. Repurposing *Artemisia annua* L. flavonoids, artemisinin and its derivatives as potential drugs against novel coronavirus (SARS-nCoV) as revealed by in-silico studies. *Int. J. Appl. Sci. Biotechnol.* **2020**, *84*, 374–393. [CrossRef]
88. Tomic, N.; Pojskic, L.; Kalajdzic, A.; Ramic, J.; Kadric, N.L.; Ikanovic, T. Screening of preferential binding affinity of selected natural compounds to SARS-CoV-2 proteins using in silico methods. *EJMO* **2020**, *4*, 319–323.
89. Alazmi, M.; Motwalli, O. Molecular basis for drug repurposing to study the interface of the S protein in SARS-CoV-2 and human ACE2 through docking, characterization, and molecular dynamics for natural drug candidates. *J. Mol. Model.* **2020**, *26*, 338. [CrossRef]
90. Gilmore, K.; Zhou, Y.; Ramirez, S.; Pham, L.V.; Fahnøe, U.; Feng, S.; Offersgaard, A.; Trimpert, J.; Bukh, J.; Osterrieder, K.; et al. In vitro efficacy of artemisinin-based treatments against SARS-CoV-2. *BioRxiV* **2020**. [CrossRef]
91. Nair, M.S.; Huang, Y.; Fidock, D.A.; Polyak, S.J.; Wagoner, J.; Towler, M.J.; Weathers, P.J. *Artemisia annua* L. extracts prevent in vitro replication of SARS-CoV-2. *BioRxiV* **2020**. [CrossRef]
92. Gendrot, M.; Duflot, I.; Boxberger, M.; Delandre, O.; Jardot, P.; Le Bideau, M.; Andreani, J.; Fonta, I.; Mosnier, J.; Rolland, C.; et al. Antimalarial artemisinin-based combination therapies (ACT) and COVID-19 in Africa: In vitro inhibition of SARS-CoV-2 replication by mefloquine-artesunate. *Int J. Infect. Dis.* **2020**, *99*, 437–440. [CrossRef] [PubMed]
93. Krishna, S.; Bustamante, L.; Haynes, R.K.; Staines, H.M. Artemisinins: Their growing importance in medicine. *Trends Pharmacol. Sci.* **2008**, *29*, 520–527. [CrossRef] [PubMed]
94. Chen, W. A potential treatment of COVID-19 with TGF-beta blockade. *Int J. Biol. Sci.* **2020**, *16*, 1954–1955. [CrossRef]
95. Li, G.; Yuan, M.; Li, H.; Deng, C.; Wang, Q.; Tang, Y.; Zhang, H.; Yu, W.; Xu, Q.; Zou, Y.; et al. Safety and efficacy of artemisinin-piperaquine for treatment of COVID-19: An open-label, non-randomized, and controlled trial. *Int J. Antimicrob. Agents* **2020**, *18*, 106216. [CrossRef] [PubMed]
96. Evans, R.M.; Lippman, S.M. Shining light on the COVID-19 pandemic: A vitamin D receptor checkpoint in defense of unregulated wound healing. *Cell Metab.* **2020**, *32*, 704–709. [CrossRef] [PubMed]
97. Uckun, F.M.; Hwang, L.; Trieu, V. Selectively targeting TGF-β with trabedersen/OT-101 in treatment of evolving and mild ARDS in COVID-19. *Clin. Investig.* **2020**, *10*, 167–176.
98. Yao, Y.; Guo, Q.; Cao, Y.; Qiu, Y.; Tan, R.; Yu, Z.; Zhou, Y.; Lu, N. Artemisinin derivatives inactivate cancer-associated fibroblasts through suppressing TGF-beta signaling in breast cancer. *J. Exp. Clin. Cancer Res.* **2018**, *37*, 282. [CrossRef]
99. Wu, X.; Zhang, W.; Shi, X.; An, P.; Sun, W.; Wang, Z. Therapeutic effect of artemisinin on lupus nephritis mice and its mechanisms. *Acta Biochimica et Biophysica Sinica* **2010**, *42*, 916–923. [CrossRef] [PubMed]
100. Cao, Y.; Feng, Y.H.; Gao, L.W.; Li, X.Y.; Jin, Q.X.; Wang, Y.Y.; Xu, Y.Y.; Jin, F.; Lu, S.L.; Wei, M.J. Artemisinin enhances the anti-tumor immune response in 4T1 breast cancer cells in vitro and in vivo. *Int. Immunopharmacol.* **2019**, *70*, 110–116. [CrossRef] [PubMed]
101. Trieu, V.; Saund, S.; Rahate, P.S.; Barge, V.B.; Nalk, K.S.; Windlass, H.; Uckun, F.M. Targeting TGF-β pathway with COVID-19 drug candidate ARTIVeda/PulmoHeal accelerates recovery from mild-moderate COVID-19. *MedRxiv* **2020**. [CrossRef]
102. Cragg, G.M.; Newman, D.J.; Snader, K.M. Natural products in drug discovery and development. *J. Nat. Prod.* **1997**, *60*, 52–60. [CrossRef] [PubMed]
103. Haq, F.U.; Roman, M.; Ahmad, K.; Rahman, S.U.; Shah, S.M.A.; Suleman, N.; Ullah, S.; Ahmad, I.; Ullah, W. *Artemisia annua*: Trials are needed for COVID-19. *Phytother. Res.* **2020**, *34*, 2423–2424. [CrossRef]
104. Williamson, E.M. Synergy and other interactions in phytomedicines. *Phytomedicine* **2001**, *8*, 401–409. [CrossRef]
105. Rasoanaivo, P.; Wright, C.W.; Willcox, M.L.; Gilbert, B. Whole plant extracts versus single compounds for the treatment of malaria: Synergy and positive interactions. *Malar. J.* **2011**, *10*, S4. [CrossRef] [PubMed]
106. Raskin, I.; Ripoll, C. Can an apple a day keep the doctor away? *Curr. Pharm. Des.* **2004**, *10*, 3419–3429. [CrossRef] [PubMed]
107. Wagner, H.; Ulrich-Merzenich, G. Synergy research: Approaching a new generation of phytopharmaceuticals. *Phytomedicine* **2009**, *16*, 97–110. [CrossRef] [PubMed]

108. Thevarajan, I.; Buising, K.L.; Cowie, B.C. Clinical presentation and management of COVID-19. *Med. J. Aust.* **2020**, *213*, 134–139. [CrossRef]
109. Lipman, M.; Chambers, R.C.; Singer, M.; Brown, J.S. SARS-CoV-2 pandemic: Clinical picture of COVID-19 and implications for research. *Thorax* **2020**, *75*, 614–616. [CrossRef]
110. Cecchini, R.; Cecchini, A.L. SARS-CoV-2 infection pathogenesis is related to oxidative stress as a response to aggression. *Med. Hypotheses* **2020**, *143*, 110102. [CrossRef] [PubMed]
111. Ritchie, K.; Chan, D.; Watermeyer, T. The cognitive consequences of the COVID-19 epidemic: Collateral damage? *Brain Commun.* **2020**, *2*, fcaa069. [CrossRef] [PubMed]

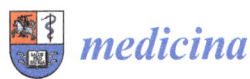

Hypothesis

Integrative Medicine and Plastic Surgery: A Synergy—Not an Antonym

Ioannis-Fivos Megas [1], Dascha Sophie Tolzmann [1], Jacqueline Bastiaanse [1], Paul Christian Fuchs [2], Bong-Sung Kim [3], Matthias Kröz [4,5,6], Friedemann Schad [6], Harald Matthes [6,7] and Gerrit Grieb [1,8,*]

1. Department of Plastic Surgery and Hand Surgery, Gemeinschaftskrankenhaus Havelhoehe, Kladower Damm 221, 14089 Berlin, Germany; fivos.megas@gmail.com (I.-F.M.); d.tolzmann@live.de (D.S.T.); jacqueline.bastiaanse@havelhoehe.de (J.B.)
2. Department of Plastic Surgery and Hand Surgery, Burn Center, University of Witten/Herdecke, Kliniken der Stadt Köln, Ostmerheimer Str. 200, 51109 Köln, Germany; FuchsP@kliniken-koeln.de
3. Department of Plastic Surgery and Hand Surgery, University Hospital Zurich, Rämistrasse 100, 8091 Zurich, Switzerland; bong-sung.kim@usz.ch
4. Institute of Integrative Medicine, University of Witten/Herdecke, Alfred-Herrhausen-Straße 50, 58448 Witten, Germany; matthias.kroez@klinik-arlesheim.ch
5. Research Department Klinik Arlesheim, Pfeffingerweg 1, 4144 Arlesheim, Switzerland
6. Research Institute Havelhoehe, Kladower Damm 221, 14089 Berlin, Germany; friedemann.schad@havelhoehe.de (F.S.); harald.matthes@havelhoehe.de (H.M.)
7. Institute of Social Medicine, Epidemiology and Health Economics CCM, Charité University Medicine, Charitéplatz 1, 10117 Berlin, Germany
8. Department of Plastic Surgery and Hand Surgery, Burn Center, Medical Faculty, RWTH Aachen University, Pauwelsstrasse 30, 52074 Aachen, Germany
* Correspondence: gerritgrieb@gmx.de

Abstract: Background: Integrative medicine focuses on the human being as a whole—on the body, mind, and spirit—to achieve optimal health and healing. As a synthesis of conventional and complementary treatment options, integrative medicine combines the pathological with the salutogenetic approach of therapy. The aim is to create a holistic system of medicine for the individual. So far, little is known about its role in plastic surgery. Hypothesis: We hypothesize that integrative medicine based on a conventional therapy with additional anthroposophic therapies is very potent and beneficial for plastic surgery patients. Evaluation and consequence of the hypothesis: Additional anthroposophic pharmacological and non-pharmacological treatments are promising for all areas of plastic surgery. We are convinced that our specific approach will induce further clinical trials to underline its therapeutic potential.

Keywords: integrative medicine; complementary medicine; plastic surgery; anthroposophic medicine

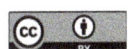

1. Introduction

The concept of integrative medicine (IM) combines conventional and complementary medicine and has become an increasingly emerging area of interest for patients and professionals alike. The regulations of complementary medicine are constantly developing, and the professional licensing and health insurance programmes are multiplying rapidly [1–5]. While the conventional understanding of medical treatment was predominantly in reacting to pathologic values, modern integrative medicine rather aims at promoting salutogenetic and hygiogenetic health as sources in a proactive manner [6].

IM in the context of anthroposophic medicine focuses on the human being as a whole—on the body, vitality, mind, and spirit—to achieve optimal health and healing [6]. The most widely used approach to complementary medicine can be divided into two subcategories: natural products, as well as mind and body practices and acupuncture [7]. This includes appropriate therapeutic and lifestyle approaches as well as healthcare professionals and most modern disciplines.

As a synthesis of conventional and complementary treatment options, IM combines the pathogenetic with the salutogenetic or hygiogenetic approach of therapy [6]. The aim is to create a holistic system of medicine for the individual. Precisely this concept addresses the patient's needs and requirements of the present; a period of time in which self-determination and personal responsibility have become more and more important [8].

For example, in anthroposophic integrative oncology, it is an established concept to propose mistletoe therapy (*Viscum album* L., VA) concomitant to antineoplastic treatment in cancer patients in order to improve the tolerability of oncology-induced toxicity [9]. In anthroposophic cardiology, for example, the influence of rhythmic massage on heart rate variability has been studied [10].

The field of complementary medicine, as far as natural products are involved, is already present in plastic surgery [11]. For example, *Arnica montana*, onion extract, Vitamin E products, and *Melitolus* are considered beneficial [11]. Mind and body practices, such as hypnosis and meditation, are also known to have a positive effect on the postoperative course of plastic surgery patients [11]. It should also be mentioned that therapeutic concepts of integrative medicine can be applied in all four pillars of plastic surgery (aesthetic surgery, reconstructive surgery, burns, and hand surgery) [2,11–14]. However, little is known about the impact of a broader integrative concept that is based on anthroposophic medicine and combines these individual offerings and procedures, as the utilisation of IM in plastic surgery departments seems to be under-frequented [2]. We aim to share our encouraging first experiences of anthroposophic medicine integrated into standard plastic surgery treatments.

2. Hypothesis

We hypothesize, that integrative medicine based on a conventional therapy with additional anthroposophic therapies is potent and beneficial for healing and post-operative recovery of plastic surgery patients.

As a general hospital, the "Gemeinschaftskrankenhaus Havelhoehe (GKH)" provides a broad spectrum of surgery with an integrative approach [15]. The demand of complementary therapy concepts next to conventional medicine leads to a very attractive and healthy environment at the GKH, even for patients with an international background.

The newly established department of plastic surgery (2016) offers a broad spectrum of treatments, which ranges from reconstructive surgery, breast surgery, hand surgery, and burn surgery to aesthetic surgery. Our department pays special attention to continuing the extraordinary offer of integrative medicine, which was introduced in our breast cancer center (BCC) by the gynaecological and oncological departments [15].

During in-patient stay, complementary treatment options are offered, such as anthroposophical massage (rhythmical massage and streaming massage), breathing therapy, ergotherapy, eurythmy therapy, hyperthermia, painting therapy, clay modelling therapy, music therapy, physiotherapy, and psychotherapy. Therefore, not only functional and physical approaches are stressed, but also the mental state, creativity, and self-determination are focused on and promoted. Next to these mind body practices, anthroposophical care therapy and natural products are provided, such as *Arnica montana* salve for haematoma, *Bryophyllum pinnatum* for calming, aroma oils for wellbeing, and *aurum/lavendulan/rosae* unguents against agitation with tachycardia and (cardiac) restlessness.

The described IM concept is regularly integrated into the daily clinical routine and individually adapted to the wishes of the patients, as every patient has their individual requirements and expects individual support: for example, patients with chronic wounds walk through an exhaustingly long hospital stay and additionally expect variety and social assistance. Hand-surgery patients with functional impairments also need physical and interactive challenges and oncological patients with a life-shortening prognosis certainly require mental encouragement.

In this article, we hypothesize that integrative medicine based on a conventional therapy with additional anthroposophic therapies is potent and beneficial for plastic surgery patients, leading to faster wound healing, less complications, and a more effective treatment for the body as a whole, also including the mind and spiritual dimensions.

Over a period of three years (2018–2020), about 150 patients have received the anthroposophic program and complementary therapies in our plastic surgery department at Havelhoehe. These patients have accepted and fully completed the offered program for at least six days. Specifically, the program included as standard: eurythmy therapy, music therapy, painting therapy, rhythmic massage, physiotherapy, psychoeducation, a biographical interview, and the application of aromatic wet packs and embrocations (with, e.g., *thyme* or *aurum/lavendulan/rosae*). The heterogeneous patient population included cases with chronic wounds, extensive skin soft tissue defects, hand surgical clinical pictures, acute burns, as well as burn complications, but also aesthetic operations. Based on the feedback from these patients, we have developed our hypothesis.

3. Evaluation of the Hypotheses

Broadly speaking, despite the experienced demand for complementary therapy methods in plastic surgery [2,13]. The first publications mentioning plastic surgery in combination with complementary medicine was published in the 1970s [16]. However, as already reported, the current published data on these aspects are sparse. Still, the positive effects on the emotional state of the patients and the perception and processing of a perioperative and postoperative course are indisputable [17–19]. Surveys have even shown that patients expect plastic surgeons to be familiar with integrative medicine [13,20]. One of these surveys, by Patel et al., described that 80% of plastic surgery patients received integrative medicine services, such as natural products and mind–body practices. The majority of the questioned patients (71%) strongly believe in self-healing [13]. This elective surgery population seeks and examines the possibility of complementary treatments [21]. Patients undergoing aesthetic surgery are reported to have a high incidence of psychosocial issues [22,23]. A department offering a surgical therapy in combination with a holistic approach that stresses the importance of mental wellness is promising. However, so far, no studies have been performed with respect to treatment based on anthroposophic medicine.

If applied, the effects of natural products and of course potential complications have to be monitored in a standardized way. Possible complications of natural products are, for example, postoperative bleeding, hypertension, and dry eyes [24–26]. The use of herbals like *Gingko* caused bleeding in a blepharoplasty patient and a perioperative therapy with acupuncture was associated with a risk of wound-site infections in a lipoplasty patient [27,28]. Taking into account this important information, we believe that all integrative approaches, which have been described so far mainly in aesthetic-surgical patients, can be applied to all areas of plastic surgery [11,27].

In the US, nearly two thirds of medical schools have incorporated courses and/or clerkships in complementary and alternative medicine and the National Center for Complementary and Integrative Health states that 40% of the American population utilizes IM concepts [1,29]. In Germany, a cross-sectional survey of a nationally representative sample of women and men aged 18–69 years was conducted, which showed that overall the effectiveness and usefulness of natural therapies was positively evaluated by the majority of the study population and 58% of those surveyed would like to see such therapies prescribed more often [30].

In daily clinical practice, IM is used to relieve symptoms associated with chronic or terminal illnesses or side effects of conventional treatments [31]. In pain therapy, complementary, non-pharmacologic approaches show a positive effect and have already begun to replace some of the conventional medication in times of opioid epidemics [31].

Therapies such as acupuncture, massage, biofeedback, and natural remedies help to manage pain and limit reliance on opioids. Although the literature so far indicates that modern integrative in-patient treatment is mostly cost-equivalent to conventional treatment therapies, there could also be a favourable economic aspect here, saving costs for opioids by weaning patients off them early [32–35].

In oncology, the concept is not only based on curing, prolongation of life, or symptom relief, but also on the enhancement of physical, emotional, and or spiritual well-being, as well as maintenance of control over cancer and its treatment [15]. In this context, the addition of mistletoe (*Viscum album*) to targeted therapy significantly reduced the probability of adverse-event-induced oncological treatment discontinuation by 70% [9]. In addition, transcendental meditation can lead to a higher quality of life in older breast cancer patients [36].

As the meta-analysis by Hole et al., shows, music, which we regularly offer in our clinic, is extremely helpful perioperatively. In the 73 randomised controlled trials included in the study, the choice of music, timing, and duration varied. However, it was found that postoperative pain and analgesic consumption were lower and patient satisfaction was higher than in the control group without perioperative music [37].

It is further reported that there is a beneficial use of *Arnica montana* to decrease postoperative oedema and ecchymosis after rhinoplasty, as well as a positive impact of onion extract on improving scar pigmentation, hypnosis approaches to alleviate perioperative anxiety, as well as acupuncture as a methodology to improve perioperative nausea [14,34,38–42].

While IM centres are becoming more established, the referrals to these centres in the US (02/2017) were analysed by Ruan et al. In total, 73.8% of the patients were primarily referred from departments of medicine; only 13.1% were from the departments of surgery. From this 13.1%, merely 0.77% (0.077% of all referrals) were primarily referred from the department of plastic and reconstructive surgery [2]. These facts also suggest the assumption that even in hospitals where IM is offered, it is rarely applied by plastic surgery departments. Because of this, we would like to emphasise our hypothesis that plastic surgery in combination with IM based on anthroposophic medicine is a promising treatment.

A large part of the daily work of our department concerns chronic wounds. The risk factors for such wounds are manifold. Systemic risk factors, such as malnutrition, obesity, vascular disease, diabetes mellitus, cancer, immunosuppression, and personal habits (e.g., smoking), favour the detrimental conditions as much as local risk factors such as neuropathy, local pressure, repetitive trauma, or radiation [43]. Optimised health behaviours would have a positive effect on many of these points, as some studies have already shown [44,45]. Therefore, in our hospital we try to support patients in this respect, to give them an impulse or to reinforce them with our holistic offer.

Even though the demand for IM and the utilisation in plastic surgery is obviously high, to the best of our knowledge, there are no other hospitals in Germany that provide IM in their departments of plastic surgery and offer complementary therapy options aiming at a holistic approach.

The Gemeinschaftskrankenhaus Havelhoehe found a way to include anthroposophic medicine in plastic surgery during in-patient time. This synergistic concept meets the requirements of the present and empowers the patient's sanitary self-determination and holistic concept.

Nevertheless, the limitations of a complementary approach should be mentioned. In many cases, for example, the dosages of the prescribed medications are an empirical value of the physician and are not suggested in a guideline. Further, there is a huge lack in terms of randomized trials, especially in the field of general or plastic surgery. To date, there is no randomized study dealing with plastic surgery and complementary medicine or anthroposophic medicine. However, some studies concerning chronic pain or diabetic polyneuropathy have surgical aspects [46–48]. Expanding the included literature reveals a variety of negative and positive studies related to integrative therapy approaches and the corresponding issues investigated [46,49–53].

4. Consequence of the Hypothesis

Our patients report that they have perceived our integrative therapies very positively. In addition, plastic surgery departments can increase their attractiveness and patient satisfaction in general by offering IM. Finally, an economic factor not to be neglected could be present, for example, through earlier weaning off pain medication. Thus, we are convinced that our approach will provide a strong impulse for further randomized controlled trials, which are definitely necessary in this area.

Author Contributions: Conceptualization: I.-F.M., H.M. and G.G.; methodology: I.-F.M., M.K. and G.G.; validation: I.-F.M., J.B., P.C.F., B.-S.K., M.K., and G.G.; formal analysis I.-F.M., P.C.F., F.S. and G.G.; investigation, I.-F.M., D.S.T., B.-S.K. and G.G.; resources, I.-F.M., J.B., F.S. and G.G.; writing—original draft preparation: I.-F.M. and D.S.T.; writing—reviewing and editing: I.-F.M., J.B., P.C.F., B.-S.K., D.S.T., M.K., F.S., H.M. and G.G.; supervision: H.M. and G.G.; project administration: G.G. All authors have read and agreed to the published version of the manuscript.

Funding: This research received no external funding.

Institutional Review Board Statement: Not applicable.

Informed Consent Statement: Not applicable.

Data Availability Statement: Not applicable.

Conflicts of Interest: M.K. received a grant from Weleda, A.G. Otherwise; all other authors declare that there is no conflict of interest.

References

1. Complementary, Alternative, or Integrative Health: What's in a Name? NCCIH. 2011. Available online: https://nccih.nih.gov/health/integrative-health (accessed on 15 September 2019).
2. Ruan, Q.Z.; Chen, A.D.; Tobias, A.M.; Fukudome, E.Y.; Lin, S.J.; Lee, B.T.; Singhal, D. Referrals of Plastic Surgery Patients to Integrative Medicine Centers: A Review of Resource Utility. *Ann. Plast. Surg.* **2019**, *83*, 3–6. [CrossRef] [PubMed]
3. Maizes, V.; Schneider, C.; Bell, I.; Weil, A. Integrative medical education: Development and implementation of a comprehensive curriculum at the University of Arizona. *Acad. Med.* **2002**, *77*, 851–860. [CrossRef] [PubMed]
4. WHO global strategy on traditional and alternative medicine. *Public Health Rep.* **2002**, *117*, 300–301.
5. Yun, H.; Sun, L.; Mao, J.J. Growth of Integrative Medicine at Leading Cancer Centers between 2009 and 2016: A Systematic Analysis of NCI-Designated Comprehensive Cancer Center Websites. *J. Natl. Cancer Inst. Monographs* **2017**, *2017*, lgx004. [CrossRef]
6. Fan, D. Holistic integrative medicine: Toward a new era of medical advancement. *Front. Med.* **2017**, *11*, 152–159. [CrossRef] [PubMed]
7. Powell, S.K. Integrative Medicine and Case Management. *Prof. Case Manag.* **2016**, *21*, 111–113. [CrossRef]
8. Adams, J. Complementary and Integrative Medicine and Patient Self-Management of Health. *Complement. Med. Res.* **2017**, *4*, 205–206. [CrossRef]
9. Thronicke, A.; Oei, S.L.; Merkle, A.; Matthes, H.; Schad, F. Clinical Safety of Combined Targeted and *Viscum album* L. Therapy in Oncological Patients. *Medicines* **2018**, *5*, 100. [CrossRef]
10. Seifert, G.; Kanitz, J.-L.; Rihs, C.; Krause, I.; Witt, K.; Voss, A. Rhythmical massage improves autonomic nervous system function: A single-blind randomised controlled trial. *J. Integr. Med.* **2018**, *16*, 172–177. [CrossRef]
11. Ruan, Q.Z.; Chen, A.D.; Tran, B.N.N.; Epstein, S.; Fukudome, E.Y.; Tobias, A.M.; Lin, S.J.; Lee, B.T.; Yeh, G.Y.; Singhal, D. Integrative Medicine in Plastic Surgery: A Systematic Review of Our Literature. *Ann. Plast. Surg.* **2019**, *82*, 459–468. [CrossRef]
12. Fan, D.M. Holistic integrative medicine: The road to the future of the development of burn medicine. *Zhonghua Shao Shang Za Zhi* **2017**, *33*, 1–3.
13. Patel, N.; Pierson, J.; Lee, T.; Mast, B.; Lee, B.T.; Estores, I.; Singhal, D. Utilization and Perception of Integrative Medicine Among Plastic Surgery Patients. *Ann. Plast. Surg.* **2017**, *78*, 557–561. [CrossRef] [PubMed]
14. Karagoz, H.; Yuksel, F.; Ulkur, E.; Evinc, R. Comparison of efficacy of silicone gel, silicone gel sheeting, and topical onion extract including heparin and allantoin for the treatment of postburn hypertrophic scars. *Burns* **2009**, *35*, 1097–1103. [CrossRef]
15. Schad, F.; Thronicke, A.; Merkle, A.; Steele, M.L.; Kröz, M.; Herbstreit, C.; Matthes, H. Implementation of an Integrative Oncological Concept in the Daily Care of a German Certified Breast Cancer Center. *Complement. Med. Res.* **2018**, *25*, 85–91. [CrossRef]
16. Franklyn, R.A. Experience with acupuncture anesthesia in cosmetic plastic surgery. *Am. J. Chin. Med.* **1974**, *2*, 345. [CrossRef]
17. Matheson, G.; Drever, J.M. Psychological preparation of the patient for breast reconstruction. *Ann. Plast. Surg.* **1990**, *24*, 238–247. [CrossRef]
18. Ginandes, C.; Brooks, P.; Sando, W.; Jones, C.; Aker, J. Can medical hypnosis accelerate post-surgical wound healing? Results of a clinical trial. *Am. J. Clin. Hypn.* **2003**, *45*, 333–351. [CrossRef]
19. Zysman, S.A.; Zysman, S.H. Hypnosis as a primary anesthetic in reconstructive and cosmetic facial surgery. *J. Am. Soc. Psychosom. Dent. Med.* **1983**, *30*, 102–106.

20. Harnett, J.E.; McIntyre, E.; Steel, A.; Foley, H.; Sibbritt, D.; Adams, J. Use of complementary medicine products: A nationally representative cross-sectional survey of 2019 Australian adults. *BMJ Open* **2019**, *9*, e024198. [CrossRef]
21. Ring, M.; Mahadevan, R. Introduction to Integrative Medicine in the Primary Care Setting. *Prim. Care* **2017**, *44*, 203–215. [CrossRef]
22. Sansone, R.A.; Sansone, L.A. Cosmetic surgery and psychological issues. *Psychiatry (Edgmont)* **2007**, *4*, 65–68.
23. Constantian, M.B. The new criteria for body dysmorphic disorder: Who makes the diagnosis? *Plast. Reconstr. Surg.* **2013**, *132*, 1759–1762. [CrossRef]
24. Mohan, A.; Lahiri, A. Herbal medications and plastic surgery: A hidden danger. *Aesthetic Plast. Surg.* **2014**, *38*, 479–481. [CrossRef]
25. Broughton, G.; Crosby, M.A.; Coleman, J.; Rohrich, R.J. Use of herbal supplements and vitamins in plastic surgery: A practical review. *Plast. Reconstr. Surg.* **2007**, *119*, 48e–66e. [CrossRef]
26. Chin, S.H.; Cristofaro, J.; Aston, S.J. Perioperative management of antidepressants and herbal medications in elective plastic surgery. *Plast. Reconstr. Surg.* **2009**, *123*, 377–386. [CrossRef]
27. Mesquita, C.J. About "top-10 list of herbal and supplemental medicines used by cosmetic patients: What the plastic surgeon needs to know". *Plast. Reconstr. Surg.* **2006**, *118*, 821. [CrossRef]
28. Choi, H.J. Cervical necrotizing fasciitis resulting in acupuncture and herbal injection for submental lipoplasty. *J. Craniofacial Surg.* **2014**, *25*, e507–e509. [CrossRef] [PubMed]
29. Wetzel, M.S.; Eisenberg, D.M.; Kaptchuk, T.J. Courses involving complementary and alternative medicine at US medical schools. *JAMA* **1998**, *280*, 784–787. [CrossRef] [PubMed]
30. Härtel, U.; Volger, E. Use and acceptance of classical natural and alternative medicine in Germany—Findings of a representative population-based survey. *Forsch. Komplement. Klass. Naturheilkd.* **2004**, *11*, 327–334.
31. Hillinger, M.G.; Wolever, R.Q.; McKernan, L.C.; Elam, R. Integrative Medicine for the Treatment of Persistent Pain. *Prim. Care* **2017**, *44*, 247–264. [CrossRef] [PubMed]
32. Ostermann, T.; Lauche, R.; Cramer, H.; Dobos, G. Comparative cost analysis of inpatient integrative medicine—Results of a pilot study. *Complement. Ther. Med.* **2017**, *32*, 129–133. [CrossRef]
33. Taw, M.B. Integrative medicine, or not integrative medicine: That is the question. *J. Integr. Med.* **2015**, *13*, 350–352. [CrossRef]
34. Larson, J.D.; Gutowski, K.A.; Marcus, B.C.; Rao, V.K.; Avery, P.G.; Stacey, D.H.; Yang, R.Z. The effect of electroacustimulation on postoperative nausea, vomiting, and pain in outpatient plastic surgery patients: A prospective, randomized, blinded, clinical trial. *Plast. Reconstr. Surg.* **2010**, *125*, 989–994. [CrossRef]
35. Scott, D.L. Hypnosis in plastic surgery. *Am. J. Clin. Hypn.* **1975**, *18*, 98–104. [CrossRef]
36. Nidich, S.I.; Fields, J.Z.; Rainforth, M.V.; Pomerantz, R.; Cella, D.; Kristeller, J.; Salerno, J.W.; Schneider, R.H. A randomized controlled trial of the effects of transcendental meditation on quality of life in older breast cancer patients. *Integr. Cancer Ther.* **2009**, *8*, 228–234. [CrossRef]
37. Hole, J.; Hirsch, M.; Ball, E.; Meads, C. Music as an aid for postoperative recovery in adults: A systematic review and meta-analysis. *Lancet* **2015**, *386*, 1659–1671. [CrossRef]
38. Totonchi, A.; Guyuron, B. A randomized, controlled comparison between arnica and steroids in the management of postrhinoplasty ecchymosis and edema. *Plast. Reconstr. Surg.* **2007**, *120*, 271–274. [CrossRef]
39. Simsek, G.; Sari, E.; Kilic, R.; Bayar Muluk, N. Topical Application of Arnica and Mucopolysaccharide Polysulfate Attenuates Periorbital Edema and Ecchymosis in Open Rhinoplasty: A Randomized Controlled Clinical Study. *Plast. Reconstr. Surg.* **2016**, *137*, 530e–535e. [CrossRef]
40. Hosnuter, M.; Payasli, C.; Isikdemir, A.; Tekerekoglu, B. The effects of onion extract on hypertrophic and keloid scars. *J. Wound Care* **2007**, *16*, 251–254. [CrossRef] [PubMed]
41. Jenwitheesuk, K.; Surakunprapha, P.; Jenwitheesuk, K.; Kuptarnond, C.; Prathanee, S.; Intanoo, W. Role of silicone derivative plus onion extract gel in presternal hypertrophic scar protection: A prospective randomized, double blinded, controlled trial. *Int. Wound J.* **2012**, *9*, 397–402. [CrossRef] [PubMed]
42. Chuangsuwanich, A.; Arunakul, S.; Kamnerdnakta, S. The efficacy of combined herbal extracts gel in reducing scar development at a split-thickness skin graft donor site. *Aesthetic Plast. Surg.* **2013**, *37*, 770–777. [CrossRef]
43. Morton, L.M.; Phillips, T.J. Wound healing and treating wounds: Differential diagnosis and evaluation of chronic wounds. *J. Am. Acad. Dermatol.* **2016**, *74*, 589–605. [CrossRef]
44. Wolever, R.Q.; Caldwell, K.L.; McKernan, L.C.; Hillinger, M.G. Integrative Medicine Strategies for Changing Health Behaviors: Support for Primary Care. *Prim. Care* **2017**, *44*, 229–245. [CrossRef]
45. Wolever, R.Q.; Abrams, D.I.; Kligler, B.; Dusek, J.A.; Roberts, R.; Frye, J.; Edman, J.S.; Amoils, S.; Pradhan, E.; Spar, M.; et al. Patients Seek Integrative Medicine for Preventive Approach to Optimize Health. *Explore* **2012**, *8*, 348–352. [CrossRef]
46. Lederer, A.-K.; Schmucker, C.; Kousoulas, L.; Fichtner-Feigl, S.; Huber, R. Naturopathic Treatment and Complementary Medicine in Surgical Practice. *Dtsch. Ärzteblatt Int.* **2018**, *115*, 815–821. [CrossRef]
47. Gardiner, P.; Luo, M.; D'Amico, S.; Gergen-Barnett, K.; White, L.F.; Saper, R.; Mitchell, S.; Liebschutz, J.M. Effectiveness of integrative medicine group visits in chronic pain and depressive symptoms: A randomized controlled trial. *PLoS ONE* **2019**, *14*, e0225540. [CrossRef]
48. Chao, M.T.; Schillinger, D.; Nguyen, U.; Santana, T.; Liu, R.; Gregorich, S.; Hecht, F.M. A Randomized Clinical Trial of Group Acupuncture for Painful Diabetic Neuropathy among Diverse Safety Net Patients. *Pain Med.* **2019**, *20*, 2292–2302. [CrossRef]

49. Hashemi, S.A.; Madani, S.A.; Abediankenari, S. The Review on Properties of Aloe Vera in Healing of Cutaneous Wounds. *Biomed Res. Int.* **2015**, *2015*, 714216. [CrossRef]
50. Fazlollahpour-Rokni, F.; Shorofi, S.A.; Mousavinasab, N.; Ghafari, R.; Esmaeili, R. The effect of inhalation aromatherapy with rose essential oil on the anxiety of patients undergoing coronary artery bypass graft surgery. *Complement. Ther. Clin. Pract.* **2019**, *34*, 201–207. [CrossRef]
51. Bahrami-Taghanaki, H.; Azizi, H.; Hasanabadi, H.; Jokar, M.H.; Iranmanesh, A.; Khorsand-Vakilzadeh, A.; Badiee-Aval, S. Acupuncture for Carpal Tunnel Syndrome: A Randomized Controlled Trial Studying Changes in Clinical Symptoms and Electrodiagnostic Tests. *Altern. Ther. Health Med.* **2020**, *26*, 10–16.
52. Attias, S.; Keinan Boker, L.; Arnon, Z.; Ben-Arye, E.; Bar'am, A.; Sroka, G.; Matter, I.; Somri, M.; Schiff, E. Effectiveness of integrating individualized and generic complementary medicine treatments with standard care versus standard care alone for reducing preoperative anxiety. *J. Clin. Anesth.* **2016**, *29*, 54–64. [CrossRef] [PubMed]
53. Liu, E.H.; Turner, L.M.; Lin, S.X.; Klaus, L.; Choi, L.Y.; Whitworth, J.; Ting, W.; Oz, M.C. Use of alternative medicine by patients undergoing cardiac surgery. *J. Thorac. Cardiovasc. Surg.* **2000**, *120*, 335–341. [CrossRef] [PubMed]

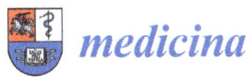

Review

Asthma: New Integrative Treatment Strategies for the Next Decades

Diego A. Arteaga-Badillo [1], Jacqueline Portillo-Reyes [1], Nancy Vargas-Mendoza [2], José A. Morales-González [2], Jeannett A. Izquierdo-Vega [1], Manuel Sánchez-Gutiérrez [1], Isela Álvarez-González [3], Ángel Morales-González [4], Eduardo Madrigal-Bujaidar [3] and Eduardo Madrigal-Santillán [2],*

[1] Instituto de Ciencias de la Salud, Universidad Autónoma del Estado de Hidalgo, Ex-Hacienda de la Concepción, Tilcuautla, Pachuca de Soto 42080, Mexico; diego060195@hotmail.com (D.A.A.-B.); jacke_star230990@hotmail.com (J.P.-R.); jizquierdovega@gmail.com (J.A.I.-V.); spmtz68@yahoo.com.mx (M.S.-G.)

[2] Escuela Superior de Medicina, Instituto Politécnico Nacional, "Unidad Casco de Santo Tomas", Ciudad de México 11340, Mexico; nvargas_mendoza@hotmail.com (N.V.-M.); jmorales101@yahoo.com.mx (J.A.M.-G.)

[3] Escuela Nacional de Ciencias Biológicas, Instituto Politécnico Nacional, "Unidad Profesional A. López Mateos", Ciudad de México 07738, Mexico; isela.alvarez@gmail.com (I.Á.-G.); eduardo.madrigal@lycos.com (E.M.-B.)

[4] Escuela Superior de Cómputo, Instituto Politécnico Nacional, "Unidad Profesional A. López Mateos", Ciudad de México 07738, Mexico; anmorales@ipn.mx

* Correspondence: eomsmx@yahoo.com.mx; Tel.: +52-555-729-6300 (ext. 62753)

Received: 18 June 2020; Accepted: 24 August 2020; Published: 28 August 2020

Abstract: Asthma is a chronic disease whose main anatomical–functional alterations are grouped into obstruction, nonspecific bronchial hyperreactivity, inflammation and airway remodeling. Currently, the Global Initiative of Asthma 2020 (GINA 2020) suggests classifying it into intermittent cases, slightly persistent, moderately persistent and severely persistent, thus determining the correct guidelines for its therapy. In general, the drugs used for its management are divided into two groups, those with a potential bronchodilator and the controlling agents of inflammation. However, asthmatic treatments continue to evolve, and notable advances have been made possible in biological therapy with monoclonal antibodies and in the relationship between this disease and oxidative stress. This opens a new path to dietary and herbal strategies and the use of antioxidants as a possible therapy that supports conventional pharmacological treatments and reduces their doses and/or adverse effects. This review compiles information from different published research on risk factors, pathophysiology, classification, diagnosis and the main treatments; likewise, it synthesizes the current evidence of herbal medicine for its control. Studies on integrative medicine (IM) therapies for asthmatic control are critically reviewed. An integrative approach to the prevention and management of asthma warrants consideration in clinical practice. The intention is to encourage health professionals and scientists to expand the horizons of basic and clinical research (preclinical, clinical and integrative medicine) on asthma control.

Keywords: asthma; diagnosis; treatment strategies; oxidative stress; antioxidants

1. Introduction

Asthma is a syndrome that can present different superimposed phenotypes with defined clinical and physiological characteristics, and with sub-adjacent inflammatory processes with identifiable biomarkers whose risk factors can be genetic, environmental, and/or represent the interaction of both of these [1]. Due to its alterations in respiratory function, its different clinical expressions (which can vary with age at presentation), and its presenting a multifactorial etiology, it is complicated to find an exact definition that fully describes this entity. The Global Initiative for Asthma 2006 (GINA 2006) considers the functional as well as the cellular aspect, and proposed its definition as a chronic inflammatory disease of the airways in which diverse cells and cellular products play an important role [2].

In general, asthma is characterized by a chronic inflammation of the airways, which is distinguished by classic respiratory symptomology that encompasses wheezing, respiratory difficulty (principally at night or during the early morning hours) thoracic oppression, and a cough. In this entity, there is the participation of the cells as well as of inflammatory mediators that together develop its pathology and cause the hyperreactivity of the smooth muscles of the airway, culminating in its obstruction and the restriction of airflow, avoiding the achievement of adequate hematosis (that is, a correct gaseous exchange of O_2 and CO_2 in the blood) [3]. According to the latest GINA 2020 update, the data suggest that asthma affects approximately 300 million persons worldwide. Therefore, it is considered a public health problem that generates high management costs for the health systems of different governments [4]. In Mexico, it is estimated that 7.0% of the population suffers from asthma, that is, 8.5 million inhabitants, according to the World Health Organization (WHO) database. With respect to mortality, in 2011, the Mexican National Institute of Geography and Statistics (INEGI) showed a statistical datum of 291 deaths per 100,000 inhabitants [5,6]. It was confirmed that this entity similarly affects the different socioeconomic strata, being distributed worldwide in all geographic regions. In the last 30 years, its prevalence and incidence have increased in highly industrialized countries, a situation probably related to the factor of environmental contamination. Asthma can appear at any age, and its prevalence is observed in the masculine gender in boys aged less than 10 years. Later, during puberty, its prevalence levels off in both sexes, while at adult age, its incidence focuses preferentially on the feminine gender [7]. It has been suggested that this prevalence in the female gender is associated with hormonal fluctuations during menstruation, pregnancy and menopause. Animal studies using genetic deletions of estrogen receptors have shown that estrogen signaling promotes allergen-mediated type 2 airway inflammation. In addition, ovarian hormones have been shown to be important for interleukin 17 A-mediated airway inflammation [8].

2. Overview of Asthmatic Pathophysiology

Diverse studies and/or publications have fully described the physiology of asthma. In general, it is considered a chronic disease of the airways whose main anatomical–functional alterations comprise the following:

(a) Airflow obstruction: In the airway of a patient with asthma, we find the generation of hypertrophy and cellular hyperplasia, giving rise to an increase in the bronchial smooth muscle mass. Generally, this increase is induced by the fibroblasts and pericytes (also denominated Rouget cells) present in the vascular endothelium, which possess the capacity to convert into muscle cells through a process of differentiation. A bronchospasm (the sudden response of an individual with asthma) generates the contraction of the bronchial smooth muscle on being confronted with diverse stimuli, causing the narrowing of the airway with the diminution of the flow. It is known that different factors can regulate bronchial smooth muscle tone, highlighting the epithelial and endothelial cells, mastocytes, and macrophages, as well as inflammatory cells (eosinophils, lymphocytes, neutrocytes, and basophils), which release proinflammatory substances (such as histamine, eicosanoids, and platelet activating factor (PAF)). In addition, direct stimuli release acetylcholine, which induces the bronchospasm to a greater degree [2,9].

(b) Nonspecific bronchial hyperreactivity (NBH): NBH in an asthmatic is an exaggerated response to a stimulus (contaminant, allergen, exercise) that induces a more intense bronchospasm than that of a normal individual [3,9].

(c) Inflammation and remodeling of the airway: Inflammation, the principal contributor to the expression of asthma, generates an increase in the reactivity of the airway and recurrent episodes of wheezing, respiratory difficulty, cough, and thoracic oppression. Generally, this inflammation produces edema, angiogenesis with dilation and congestion, and smooth muscle hypertrophy and hyperplasia. Thus, the increase and size of the vessels contributes to the thickening of the bronchial wall, favoring the limitation of the airflow and generating bronchoconstriction. There is evidence that the inflammatory process produces an alteration in the respiratory epithelium. The extension of this alteration or damage may be attributed to a dysfunction in the epidermal growth factor receptors (EGFR), which regulate the epidermal growth factor (EGF), which are indispensable for normal and adequate re-epithelization. The EGF stimulates epithelial proliferation and the production of matrix metalloproteases (MMP), which degrade the extracellular matrix (ECM) and maintain an equilibrium with transforming growth factor beta (TGF-β), which increases the synthesis of the ECM components and inhibits the production of MMP [3,9–13].

Airway remodeling is characterized by the thickening of the reticular lamina (generally with deposits of subepithelial and perivascular fibrin, hyperplasia, the mucosal glands, and vascular and smooth muscle). The fibroblast possesses a relevant function during this process, due to the fact that it produces a large number of cytokines, of growth factors, and that it induces the synthesis of hyaluronic acid and other ECM proteoglycans. In addition, fibroblasts activate compensatory mechanisms of bronchial inflammatory damage (epithelial regeneration and the deposit of collagen between the muscle layers) induction of angiogenesis, vascular infiltration, and vasodilation. Taken together, all of these changes tend to be the result of direct damage to the epithelium to produce remodeling [3,9–13].

It is noteworthy that atopia, also called allergy (current concept), is the most identifiable factor of asthmatic crises, due to the fact that it is genetically predisposed to producing Immunoglobin E (IgE) as an antigen-specific response to allergens (such as dust, animal epithelia, pollen, or synthetic fibers), which are commonly innocuous for the majority of non-asthmatic individuals. In general, the production of IgE depends on the B lymphocytes, and it is regulated by Interleukin 4 (IL-4) and interferon gamma (IFN-γ), synthetized by the TH2 lymphocytes (type 2 cooperator T lymphocytes) and the TH1 lymphocytes (type 1 cooperator T lymphocytes), respectively. Thus, when an individual is sensitive to an allergen, the latter adheres to their IgE and in turn, this interleukin binds to the mastocyte's cellular membrane to release inflammatory mediators that favor the clinical manifestations of asthma. The synthesis of IgE initiates, after repeated exposure to an allergen, for it to be carried to the lymph nodes, which is where the immunologic memory is imprinted [3,14,15].

3. Risk Factors for Asthma

It has been established that, in order for diseases to occur, it is necessary for them to coincide with different elements. Asthma, as a multifactorial disease, conforms to the incidence of different factors of the patient's macro- and microenvironment. The risk factors and triggers of this disease are multiple, the most relevant of these being genetic, infectious (viral, bacterial, fungal, and parasitic), occupational and environmental (aeroallergens, dust, pollen, suspended particles, chemical irritants, tobacco), related to climate changes, dietetic, and obesity-related. In addition, it is thought that the severity of this entity is influenced by age, sex, pregnancy, immaturity of the immunological system, and the atopic march. Likewise, the interaction of the previously mentioned phenomena (obstruction, NBH, inflammation, and airway remodeling) determines its clinical responses and treatment responses [3,16].

The association of asthma with the atopic march or allergies: At present, this is considered to be factor number one for developing asthma. The respiratory system, the skin, the mucosa and the digestive tract participate in this association, as a consequence of a complex immunological disorder. The factors that exert an influence on the atopic course are hereditary in type, related to intrauterine sensitivity and/or maternal immunity, as well as environmental and infectious factors related to habits and/or lifestyle. It tends to be characterized by a course denominated the "clinical triad", in which atopical dermatitis, allergic rhinitis, and/or the induction of asthma are present. In general, it is observed that atopical dermatitis presents between birth and 6 months of age. Later, gastrointestinal disorders appear, mainly during the second year of life. Between 3 and 7 years of age, there can be the initiation of disorders in the upper respiratory tract, culminating in the establishment of asthmatic crises between the ages of 7 and 15 years. To speak of the "atopic march" is to refer to the allergic progression mediated by IgE, which begins with atopic dermatitis and a food allergy in infancy, followed by aeroallergen sensitization at preschool age [8,16,17].

Infectious antecedents: The respiratory epithelium separates the external environment of the internal pulmonary medium, controlling the inter- and transcellular permeability of the passage of pathogens and access to the antigen-presenting cells involved in the immune inflammatory response. Infections produced by bacteria, viruses, fungi, or parasites activate different cellular responses and/or signaling pathways that generate changes on the cellular surface and modify the response to stimuli and/or the previously mentioned infections. Diverse receptors can act during the induction of asthma, the most representative being pattern recognition receptors (PRRs), protease-activated receptors (PARs), and those denominated Toll-like receptors (TLRs), which together favor the identification of microbe-specific molecules and pathogen-associated molecular patterns (PAMPs) [16,18].

Viral infections are an important cause of asthmatic exacerbation and tend to be a causal factor for the development of childhood asthma. It is considered that the first white cells that can be infected by rhinoviruses (RV) are the epithelial cells (between approximately 45 and 50% of cases), while the syncytial respiratory virus (SRV) can initiate an infection in 21% of cases. Both viruses are significantly associated with a high probability of inducing asthma and producing early exacerbations, especially in individuals younger than 2 years of age [16,19,20].

In the case of fungal infections, the fungus-synthesized proteases that tend to grow in humid places can comprise an important factor in producing and increasing the incidence of rhinitis, asthma, and other respiratory diseases. In general, these proteases are related to an increase in the granulomatous response and/or in the production of immunoglobins (principally E and G) [16,21].

With respect to microbial infections, it is convenient to consider the so-called "hygiene theory", which suggests that the lack of exposure to bacteria and/or endotoxins favors the persistence of the TH2 response, increasing the possibility of presenting an atopic disease. Contrariwise, it is suggested that exposure at a young age to bacterial products can prevent subsequent allergic sensitization; therefore, the asthma being directed toward the TH1 pathway; that is, its differentiation is directed toward Interleukin 12 (IL-12) and IFN-γ. Such is the case of the use of lactobacilli in allergic and non-allergic children, where these lactobacilli have been proposed to possess a potential benefit, especially in the treatment of atopic dermatitis. In this context, it is known that probiotics are potent inducers of IL-12, stimulating TH1 immunity and, together the natural maturation process of the digestive immunological barrier, has allowed the digestive tract to be more resistant to the distinct bacterial aggressions, reducing the presence and/or the incidence of asthma [16,22,23].

Dietetic factors and obesity: Epidemiologic data suggest that a poor diet, together with obesity (individuals with a body mass index (BMI) above 30 kg/m^2) can increase the risk of suffering from asthma. In the specific case of a diet high in saturated fats and deficient in polyunsaturated omega-3 fats, fiber, vitamins (especially A, C, and D), magnesium, and selenium, this has been related to the inflammatory induction of the respiratory tract and a direct association with the presence and/or incidence of asthma [17,24,25]. A study conducted by Maciag and Phipatanakul (2019) indicated that pregnant women treated with high doses of 25-hydroxyvitamin D (Calcidiol (2400 and 4000 IU daily)) can reduce by 25% the risk of their offspring having asthma. The latter suggests a balanced diet, one with adequate concentrations of Calcidiol, induces beneficial effects in the uterus and diminishes the possibility of developing asthma [17]. Arias-López et al. (2018) consider that, over the past 30 years, vitamin D levels have diminished in the population in general (particularly in pediatric individuals). Such a reduction suggests that it is related to an increase in some diseases, such as asthma [25].

On the other hand, it has been observed that obesity can exert different negative effects on the lungs, highlighting a reduction in pulmonary function (maximal expiratory volume at the end of the first second (FEV1)/forced vital capacity (FVC)), as well as an increase in the appearance of dyspnea and wheezing. Thus, it has been suggested that obese non-asthmatic patients manifest cardiorespiratory symptoms similar to those of individuals with asthma, principally brought about by a narrowing of the airway due to the accumulation of fat in the thorax. Additionally, obesity can generate a state of systemic inflammation (due to the high concentration of adipocytokines, such as leptin, resistin, an inhibitor of the activation of the plasminogen, tumor necrosis factor alpha (TNF-α), IL-6, and angiotensinogen), which, to a certain degree, acts on the lungs, precipitating the initiation of asthma. Likewise, epidemiologic evidence indicates that patients with asthma who are obese or overweight experience a higher number of emergency room hospitalizations in comparison with asthmatic non-obese individuals. Asthmatic persons with obesity are also considered to have a reduced response to glucocorticoids. Thus, they need higher doses of the latter to improve the control of their asthmatic condition, a situation that, in the long term, can give rise to more significant secondary effects [16,26,27].

Genetic factors: The majority of scientific evidence indicates that the genes play a determining role in asthma. Its heritability ranges from 36–79%, without the existence of a well-defined pattern. Studies have been conducted in various chromosomal regions that contribute to the susceptibility of inducing asthma, although these principally address chromosome 5q31–33,35, which maintains a relation with TH2 and Interleukins 4, 5, 9, and 13. However, despite the presence of these polymorphisms, the participation of other triggers is necessary to determine the type, severity, prognosis, and treatment of this pathology. To date, there are more than 100 genes reported in association with asthma or related to their phenotypes. Table 1 shows the main chromosomes related to this entity [9,16].

Table 1. Main chromosomes involved in the development and expression of asthma.

Chromosome and Region	Genes, Function and/or Association
1q21.3, 1p31, 1q21 and 1q41	Related to asthma and atopic march. Possible association with filaggrin, PTGR3, FLG, LELP, and TGFβ2
2q32q33	(CTLA-4) associated with cytotoxic T lymphocytes and IgE regulation (ICOS) related to TH2 lymphocytes and cytokine activation (IL-4, IL-5, IL-13)
3q21, 3p25, 3p21.3	(CD80/86, PPARG CX3CR1) associated with asthma and exacerbations. Activation and regulation of leukotrienes and cytokines from TH1/TH2 lymphocytes
4q11–q13, 4q21–23	(CXCL9, CXCL10, CXCL11 SPP1, GSNOR) associated with asthma and rhinitis.
5q31–33,35	Increases production of IgE, eosinophils, cytokines, and interleukins (IL-4, IL-5, IL-9, and IL-13). Relationship with CD14, GRL, GM-FSC and β2AA and/or steroidal receptors
6p 21.3–23, 6q25.1, 6p12	Relationship with the inflammatory process and TNF-α. Also associated with bronchial hyperreactivity (HLA-DRB1, HLA-DQB1, IL-17F)
7p14–p15	(AOAH) susceptibility to asthma and IgE
8q21	(RIP2) associated with severe childhood asthma.
9p21–22	Susceptibility-related type I interferon gene for asthma and atopic march
10q 11.2.10q24	(5-LO, PLAU) associated with asthmatic pathogenesis
11q12–13,11p13	Regulates the beta chain of the receptor for IgE. Additionally associated with anti-inflammatory lung proteins (CC16, CC10. CAT and BDNF).
12q13-24,12q14 and 12q22	Genes related to asthmatic development (early onset and exacerbations)
14q11.2, 14q32.3, 14q24–q31	Genes related to childhood asthma. They are also associated with increased bronchial hyperresponsiveness and decreased response to bronchodilator drugs

Table 1. *Cont.*

Chromosome and Region	Genes, Function and/or Association
16p13.13, 16q24.1, 16p11	(SOCS1) related to adult asthma and atopic march. Possible activation of IL-4 and IL-27.
17q12–q21	(ORMDL3) relationship with early onset of asthma
19q13.1–13.3	(PLAUR) increases synthesis of IgE.
20p31, 20q11.2q13.1, 20q12–q13.2	Possible activation of ADAM 33, MMP9 and CD40 associated with childhood asthma, bronchial hyperactivity and IgE.
21q22.3	(RUNX1) relationship with asthma and IgE
Xp21, Xq13.2–21.1 and CySLTR1	Associated with atopic march and asthma induced by NSAIDs

Although asthma affects all ethnic groups, its incidence is more frequent in some economically disadvantaged groups. In addition to genetic factors, some authors consider that socioeconomic status (SES) and access to healthcare generates greater variability in asthmatic prevalence among the different ethnic groups. SES is highly related to ethnicity and it is a risk factor for asthmatic morbidity, especially in poorly developed countries where environmental conditions, stress and psychological/cultural factors play an important role in its incidence [28–30].

Occupational, environmental, and pharmacological agents: Asthma of occupational and environmental origin entertains a close relationship to being caused by exposure to different aeroallergens. Both types of asthma can favor the expression of genes of hypersensitivity, as well as the exacerbation and/or presentation of their symptoms. There are more than 400 aeroallergenic agents, among which are dust (mainly of wood), pollen grains, latex proteins, animal urine and hair, dandruff, mite and fungal proteases, suspended particles [carbon monoxide (CO), nitrogen dioxide (NO_2), sulfur dioxide (SO_2), ozone (O_3) and diesel particles], chemical irritants (acid anhydrides, polyisocyanate polymers, and platinum and persulfate salts), and tobacco smoke, in addition to climate changes, and stress itself. (Table 2) [2,16,22,31–36].

Table 2. Asthma-inducing occupational, environmental, and pharmacological agents.

Agent	Exposure Sites and Individuals	Type of Asthma
Wood dust (cedar, mahogany, ebony, pine and oak)	Carpenters, furniture makers, sawmills	Occupational
Grains (pollen, wheat, barley, coffee, tobacco)	Beekeepers, farmers, bakers, beer industry workers	Occupational
Urine and animal hair	Veterinarians, ranchers, farmers, merchants, daily life (home)	Occupational/environmental
Irritating reagents and/or chemicals (dyes, acid anhydrides, polyisocyanate polymers, and platinum and persulfate salts)	Textile workers, hairdressers, stylists, polyurethane producers, car paint, glue users	Occupational/environmental
Dandruff residue	General employees (offices), daily life (home)	Occupational/environmental
Proteases (mites and fungi)	Field, offices, hospitals, daily life (home)	Occupational/environmental
Suspended particles (CO, NO_2, SO_2, O_3, diesel)	Gas station and refinery employees. Daily life	Occupational/environmental
Tobacco smoke	Employees and workers in general. Daily life	Occupational/environmental
Latex	Health professionals, anyone who uses it	Occupational/environmental
Others (climate changes and stress)	Daily life, employees in general	Occupational/environmental
Medicines (β-lactams and NSAIDs)	Health professionals, daily life (home)	Pharmacological

It is known that exposure to some aeroallergens exacerbates asthma and increases the risk of acute crises in patients with allergy, mainly in children. Therefore, it is important to reduce and to avoid these in order to improve quality of life, thus diminishing the need for employing drugs [2,22]. Relevant data in this context are the following: (a) the exposure of infants to the Great Smog of 1952 (London, UK), in which the rate of this entity increased by approximately 20% [37], and (b) Maciag and Phipatanakul (2019) observed that children who were not breast-fed have a greater incidence of this disease in comparison with those who were breast-fed. Additionally, the authors suggest that vitamin D confers protection against the development of asthma, especially against exposure to the aeroallergens in the traffic-related air contamination of industrialized countries [17].

Antibiotics and non-steroidal anti-inflammatory drugs (NSAIDs) are found among the main drugs that trigger asthmatic crises. In the first case, the β-lactams (such as penicillin, ampicillin, and amoxicillin) have been related to certain allergies and there is evidence that, on their being administered during the first years of an infant's life, can alter the development of intestinal microbiota, generating a greater risk of having asthma [34]. With regard to NSAIDs, practically all of these are potentially capable of precipitating asthma, this due to their capacity to diminish prostaglandins (PGs) and to increase cysteinyl leukotrienes (CysLT) on inhibiting cyclooxygenase (Table 2) [38–40]. Ishitsuka et al., (2020) conducted a review in order to document whether Acetaminophen (N-acetyl-p-aminophenol) presented adverse effects similar to those of NSAIDs. The authors' results indicated that, in high-risk patients such as the elderly, children, and pregnant women, that it can be a drug that cause kidney dysfunction, gastrointestinal injury, asthma and/or bronchospasms [41].

4. Asthma and Its Relationship with Oxidative Stress

As already mentioned, asthma is a chronic inflammatory disease of the respiratory tract whose etiology is multifactorial. Over the past years, the scientific evidence has increased of oxidative stress (reactive oxygen species (ROS), as well as reactive nitrogen species (RNS)) on the induction, activation, and possible treatment of asthma.

Although the generation of both types of free radicals (RONS) form parts of different physiological responses of the organism, on occasion, when an asthmatic crisis presents as a response to diverse stimuli (among these are environmental and occupational allergens), their levels can increase, overcoming the antioxidant mechanisms of the airways and causing structural damage and metabolic alterations that together can favor the pathology of this disease [42,43].

Diverse investigations have produced evidence of and have demonstrated an oxidative process that is generated in the respiratory pathways, a process that is very complex, which it would be difficult to fully describe in this manuscript. Generally, RONS can be produced by different cells, under normal physiological conditions as well as during an asthmatic crisis. In the specific case of ROS, the superoxide anion ($O_2^{\bullet-}$) is importantly generated by the mitochondria and, due to the fact that it is considered a potential microbiocidal agent, its most relevant role is focused on the neutrophils, eosinophils, monocytes, and macrophages. During the respiratory burst of the leukocytes, $O_2^{\bullet-}$ is generated through the activation of the enzyme NADPH oxidase. Later, it is transformed into hydrogen peroxide (H_2O_2) by the action of the Superoxide dismutase enzyme (SOD). This new radical increases its oxidative potential by means of peroxidase enzyme of eosinophils (EPO) and the myeloperoxidase (MPO) of the neutrophils in order to act as a microbiocide. There is evidence that both radicals (superoxide anion and hydrogen peroxide), together with hydroxyl radical ($HO^{\bullet}$), plus the RNS [nitric oxide and ($NO^{\bullet}$) and peroxynitrite ($ONOO^-$)], can produce inflammatory effects and oxidation phenomena in the proteins of the respiratory pathway in patients with asthma [42–44]. On the other hand, $NO^{\bullet}$ is considered a relatively stable radical whose important functions in the lungs comprise regulating the pulmonary vascular tone, stimulating the secretion of mucin, modulating mucociliary clearance, and exercising bactericidal action. There are three nitric oxide synthase isoenzymes in the lungs (iNOS1, iNOS2 and iNOS3), whose main function is to catalyze the conversion of L-arginine into

NO• and L-citrulline. iNOS1 and iNOS2 are always present in the organism at a constant concentration, while iNOS3 is considered inducible when faced of diverse stimuli. iNOS2 is a strong source of NO• in the healthy lung, and there is evidence that certain abnormalities in its genotype and expression favor the increase in this radical and its relation with the incidence of asthma. In addition, it has been suggested that persons with asthma can have three times more NO• in the lower airways and in exhaled air. Therefore, excessive synthesis is related to significant inflammatory processes. Another possible mechanism by which RNS favor asthma is through the processes of nitrosation (a covalent addition between RNS and SH and/or amine groups) and nitration (RNS with aromatic rings) of proteins, which are related to the altered activities of signaling enzymes and molecules [42–46].

In summary, it has been observed that the increase in RONS levels is directly related to the severity of asthma. Higher RONS levels induce respiratory tract inflammation upon activating different transcription factors, highlighting the Nuclear Factor Kappa-Light-Chain-Enhancer of Activated B Cells (NF-κB), mitogen-activated protein kinase (MAPK), and activator protein-1 [43,47–49]. These transcription factors promote the expression of IL-6, IL-8, and TNF-α, inducing an activation of the inflammatory cells that damages and affects the lung tissue [40,50,51].

5. Classification and Diagnosis of Asthma

Initially, this entity was classified considering its causes, intensity, and airway obstruction (frequently estimated by means of maximal expiratory volume at the end of the first second (FEV1) and/or peak expiratory flow (PEF)), a classification that was inappropriate due to the fact that asthma is a disease of multifactorial etiology. Currently, chronic asthma is classified according to GINA 2020 guidelines on controlled, partially controlled, and non-controlled asthma. For investigative purposes, asthma continues to be classified as intermittent, slightly persistent, moderately persistent, and severely persistent (Figure 1). It is noteworthy that these classifications are considered after carrying out a diagnosis, which permits the determining of the scheduling of its pharmacological therapy. In general, the following parameters are taken into account:

(a) Symptom control: good control, partial control, out of control.
(b) Future risk: depends on FEV1 and other factors that increase the risk of exacerbations, irreversible obstruction, or drug-associated adverse effects.
(c) Severity (established based on the clinical history, especially considering the level of medication employed to maintain symptom control): intermittent or slight, moderate, and severe [3–5,52].

The diagnosis is based on an analysis of the clinical history of the patients in which the social and environmental milieu, the familial antecedents, and a physical examination are taken into consideration. In addition, the symptoms of respiratory obstruction (cough, wheezing, thoracic oppression and, in severe cases, respiratory difficulty) are evaluated. For full confirmation of the disease, pulmonary lung function tests are employed.

According to the asthmatic diagnosis algorithm (Figure 1), tests start with a spirometric evaluation to determine the Tiffeneau index (the relationship between FEV1 and forced vital capacity (FVC)), which indicates a possible obstructive pattern when its value is below 70%. Subsequently, the bronchial asthmatic reactivity test is performed by administering a short-acting beta agonist to verify obstruction reversibility and differentiate with chronic obstructive pulmonary disease (COPD).

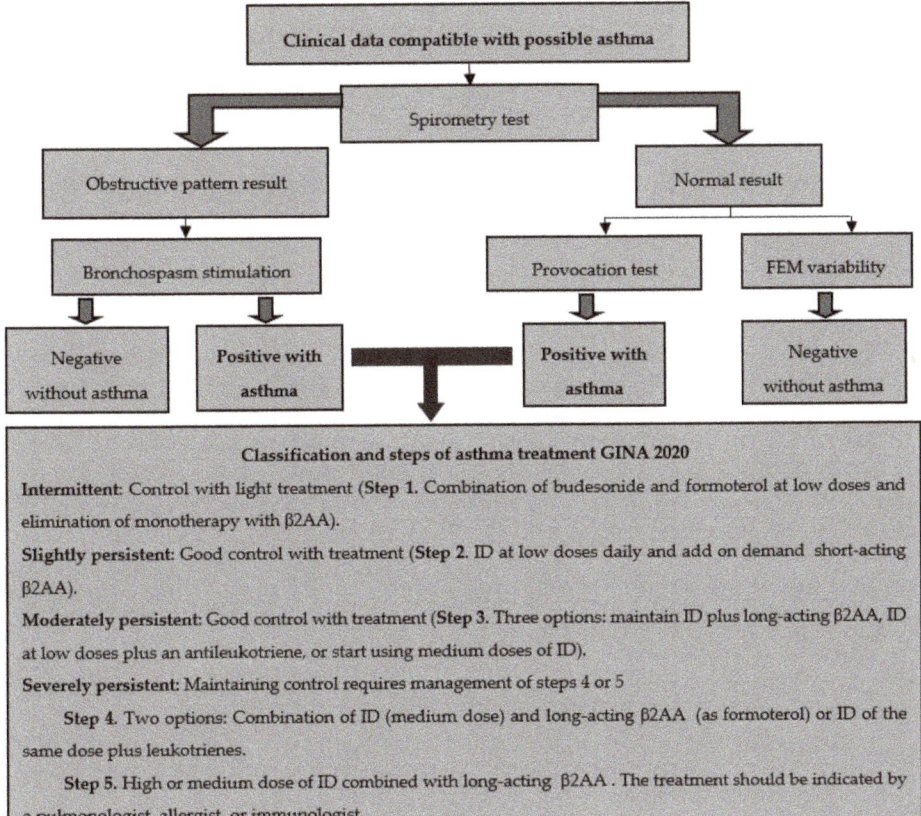

Figure 1. Algorithm of asthmatic diagnosis and steps of its treatment according to GINA 2020.

If the result is normal, two additional tests should be performed with the purpose of discarding the diagnosis of asthma. The primary determination of the variability of the maximal expiratory flow (MEF) is obtained by conducting serial measurements throughout the day and employing the following formula:

$$\text{MEF} = \text{maximal MEF} - \text{minimal MEF} \times 100/\text{maximal MEF}$$

A value of ≥20% over 3 days, across 2 weeks, is highly suggestive of asthma.

The second test comprises the stimulation of a bronchospasm induced pharmacologically with methacholine (cholinergic agonist). If the patient presents a bronchospasm at low doses of the drug, the FEV1 will diminish by 20%; this translates into a positive result and confirms the diagnosis of asthma [3–5,52].

6. Management, Control and the Main Pharmacological Treatments of Asthma

Throughout history, different pharmacological schemas have been used to control and reduce asthma symptoms. The first therapies were unorthodox and absurd since they included "pouring a gallon of ice water on the patient's back from a height of three meters", "applying electric current to the vagus nerve, the accessory, and the sympathetic through an electrode placed on the neck or inserted into the patient's nose". Even smoking was considered as a therapy to avoid bronchospasms. The first antecedent of the 20th century was found in the Orville Brown treatise, where controlling the disease through diet, massages with chest vibrations, breathing exercises and avoiding exposure to allergens, were recommended. Essentially, the pharmacological era of asthma started with Dr. Hirsh (1937) when he prescribed theophylline (methylxanthine alkaloid) suppositories; however, due to their extensive adverse effects, they are no longer used. Later, inhaled treatments were introduced, mainly belladonna, organic nitrites, estramonium, and atropine [53].

During the 1950s, the β_2 adrenergic agonist agents (β2AA) such as albuterol (also called salbutamol) and terbutaline began to be distributed and were considered drugs of first choice at that time. Some years later, the combination of β2AA and corticosteroids was explored to reduce both bronchospasms and inflammation. Corticosteroids were initially prescribed systemically; but they were discontinued due to their high adverse effects. It was not until 1970 that betamethasone and beclomethasone (long-term inhalable corticosteroids (ID)) began to be used and, practically, at the end of the 20th century, the treatment of asthma left its empirical nature behind, and the proper management of asthmatic treatment started under the consensus of national and international guides [53,54].

Currently, the control of chronic asthma seeks five primary goals (Table 3), so the medical guidelines propose a therapeutic scheme in stages; that is, considering that it is a chronic inflammatory entity, the basis of treatment should be early anti-inflammatory therapy, rather than symptomatic treatment. This essentially involves avoiding risk factors to establish a suitable treatment, classifying it by its intensity, increasing the number, frequency and dosage of drugs until possible remission is reached, then carefully reducing the drug dose until it is as small as possible to retain remission; finally, the treatment must be individualized and modified to maintain correct control of the symptoms. In summary, the therapeutic strategy should be divided into: (a) environmental control, (b) patient education, and (c) adequate pharmacological management and immunotherapy [3,52].

Table 3. Main objectives in the control of chronic asthma.

Number	Objectives
1	Absence and/or decrease in chronic symptoms
2	Reduce the frequency of exacerbations
3	Encourage a normal lifestyle without limitations that allows exercise
4	Maintain normal lung function with minimal adverse effects during treatment
5	Decrease the need to use rescue treatments

The Global Initiative for Asthma (GINA) is the most utilized set of guidelines and, in its most recent update (2020), it assembles data derived from the Spanish Guidelines on the Management of Asthma (GEMA 2018) and from the Mexican Asthma Guidelines (GUIMA 2017). This information brings together evidence on the factors associated with asthma, its diagnosis and management in its different stages, and suggestions about the new therapeutic options available in recent decades (especially information related to monoclonal antibodies) [4]. Figure 1 shows the steps of the treatment suggested by GINA 2020.

Clinical efficacy largely depends on adherence to treatment. In general, the drugs used in the management of asthma are divided into two groups, those with bronchodilator potential that achieve symptomatic improvement by relaxing the smooth muscle of the airway (β2AA, anticholinergics, and methylxanthines) and, on the other hand, inflammation-controlling agents (ID and antileukotrienes). Table 4 shows the main characteristics of the drugs used in asthma therapy [2–6].

Table 4. Main drugs used in asthma therapy.

Pharmacological Group	Name(s)	Mechanism of Action	Adverse Effects
Bronchodilator Potential			
β_2 Adrenergic Agonists	First-line drugs. Albuterol, Terbutaline, Pirbuterol and Levalbuterol (Short Action) Formoterol, arformoterol, idacaterol and salmeterol (Long-acting)	They activate adenyl cyclase through the β2AA-receptor and relax smooth muscle, increase mucociliary clearance, and decrease vascular permeability	Uncommon when administered by inhalation. Mainly: Tachycardia, hyperglycemia, hypokalemia, and fine tremors
Anticholinergics	Second-line drugs Ipatropium bromide, and tiotropium bromide. Atropine (prototype agent)	They block the constriction of the smooth muscle of the airways and the secretion of mucus to the muscarinic receptors (M2, M3) of the lung	Atropine: produces thick secretions, blurred vision and cardiac stimulation (all of them limiting its use). Ipatropium bromide: antagonizes both receptors (M3/M2) causing bronchodilation/ bronchoconstriction. Effects related to bronchitis, exacerbation of COPD and headaches
Methylxanthines	Third or fourth line drug Theophylline	Ability to relax the bronchial smooth muscle and pulmonary vessels. Its effect is related to the non-selective inhibition of phosphodiesterase.	According to international guides, its use in children has decreased. Short and long-term effects related to nausea, vomiting, arrhythmias, and gastrointestinal bleeding
Control of inflammation			
Corticosteroids	Beclomethasone Dipropionate Budesonide Fluticasone propionate Ciclesonide Mometasone	Inhalable agents (sometimes administered systemically) that inhibit the inflammatory response by preventing the release of phospholipase A2 and inflammatory cytokines	High and/or accumulated doses can produce suppression of the hypothalamic–pituitary–adrenal glands axis, osteoporosis, cataracts, skin atrophy, weight gain, diabetes, hypertension, psychological disorders and immunosuppression
Antileukotrienes	Zileuton (a) Zafirlukast, montelukast pobilukast and pranlukast (b)	Two mechanisms of action: (a) Inhibition of the enzyme 5-lipooxygenase and (b) antagonistic effect of the cysteinyl leukotriene-1-receptor (CysLT1)	They can cause headache, rash, insomnia, dizziness, tremor, nausea, vomiting, abdominal pain, heartburn, diarrhea, anorexia, constipation, increased liver enzymes, leukopenia, thrombocytopenia, fever, edema, alopecia, and menstrual irregularities
Chromones	Cromolin (Sodium chromoglycate) Nedocromil	They phosphorylate a myosin-like protein in the cell membrane, responsible for the release of mediators from mast cells and prevent the release of histamine	They appear to have a high safety profile, so they can be used in infants and children under the age of two. In general, they cause irritation in the throat and cough when inhaled. While orally they can cause headache and diarrhea

7. Alternative Therapies for Asthma Control

As previously stated, drugs seek to reduce the inflammation of the respiratory tract and alleviate bronchospasms. Unfortunately, symptoms may reappear when administration is discontinued. Despite its existence and the fact that the administration is based on international and national guidelines, controlling asthma continues to be a great challenge. Some studies indicate that more than 50% of asthmatic patients are uncontrolled, even with maintenance treatments (ID combined with a long-acting β2AA). Therefore, new alternatives should be considered:

Immunomodulatory agents: In the past decade, notable advances have been made in biological therapy with monoclonal antibodies (MoAb). Omalizumab was the first and is the only MoAb approved for asthmatic individuals older than 12 years, administered subcutaneously on a monthly basis. Its mechanism of action is based on the protein–protein interaction between its high-affinity receptor and IgE, which prevents binding to mast cells and basophils, decreasing the release of inflammatory mediators [3,55,56]. Due to its interaction with IgE, Omalizumab has shown an important role in atopic or allergic asthma. However, considering that asthma of non-allergic origin presents a similar inflammatory process (increase in TH2 lymphocytes, activation of mast cells and infiltration of eosinophils), this has opened the field of study to other possible MoAbs. Table 5 summarizes the immunomodulatory agents under development and their main characteristics [55,56].

Table 5. Main immunomodulatory agents under development.

Agent	Characteristic and/or Property
MoAb anti IgE	
Quilizumab 8D6	8D6 has an affinity for a conformational epitope in the CH3 domain of IgE. Unlike omalizumab, it can bind to low affinity receptors making it more competitive. The other agent has been studied subcutaneously in three doses (150, 300 and 450 mg) in patients with uncontrolled allergic asthma with ID
MoAb anti IL-5	
Mepolizumab Reslizumab Benralizumab TPI-ASM8	IL-5 is a cytosine modulator of chemotaxis and degranulation of eosinophils. Its receptor is composed of two subunits: (a) specific subunit-α (IL-5Rα) for IL-5 and (b) βc subunit (IL-5Rcβ) responsible for the transduction signal that is shared with specific α subunits of IL-3 receptors and macrophage and granulocyte colony stimulating factor (GM-CSF). Mepolizumab (best known monoclonal antibodies (MoAb) from this group) and together with Reslizumab neutralize IL-5. While Benralizumab acts on IL-5Rα and TPI-ASM8 on IL-5Rβc
IL-4 Antagonists	
Pascolizumab Altrakincept Pitrakinra Dulipumab	Both IL-4 and IL-13 play an important role in TH2 and B lymphocyte responses for IgE synthesis. Despite the fact that both interleukins have different actions in asthma, most of the MoAb are in development or some controlled evaluation studies are being initiated
MoAb IL-13	
Lebrikizumab Anrukinzumab Tralokinumab	All three MoAbs are under evaluation in controlled clinical trials. The main information found corresponds to Anrukinzumab and lebrikizumab. The former has been tested in patients with mild allergic asthma showing a slight reduction in asthmatic responses, while lebrikizumab has been administered subcutaneously to individuals with uncontrolled moderate to severe persistent asthma
Anti-IL-9 monoclonal antibodies	
MEDI-528	IL-9 (produced by TH2 lymphocytes and mast cells) has shown to have an increased expression in the airways of asthmatic individuals. Studies evaluating subjects with mild and moderate asthma suggested that MEDI-528 binds this interleukin and has an acceptable safety profile and a decrease in exacerbations and FEV1 after doing physical exercise.
Anti-TNF-α	
Etanercept Infliximab Adalimumab Golimumab	The four MoAb agents are still under evaluation. Etanercept is a dimeric protein that binds to free TNF-α by neutralizing it; however, it has not shown improvement in any asthmatic parameter so far. While in a single study, golimumab apparently had action on severe asthma. Infliximab (considered for moderate persistent asthma) and adalimumab (tested for severe chronic asthma) have apparently shown reduced exacerbations. Unfortunately, there are no verifying results of its efficacy and safety
MoAb against T cells	
Daclizumab Keliximab Oxelumab KB003	There is little information on these drugs. Inflammation of the airway is known to involve the activation of T lymphocytes, with an increase in T CD25 + cells, in concentrations of IL-2, and a chain receptor of soluble IL-2 (IL-2R). In a single study, daclizumab was confirmed to act on this receptor and appears to have activity against uncontrolled moderate-severe asthma. Apparently, Oxelumab has an effect in patients with controlled mild allergic asthma by blocking OX40. This mechanism is related to the costimulation between the dendritic cell and the T lymphocyte. On the other hand, KB003 has shown changes in FEV1 and lowered the number of exacerbations in individuals with uncontrolled moderate to severe asthma. Keliximab has only been used in the treatment of rheumatoid arthritis

Herbal and/or antioxidant strategies: The WHO estimates that more than 80% of the Earth's inhabitants to trust and have used Traditional Medicine/Complementary and Alternative Medicine (TCAM) for their primary healthcare needs. Among the objectives of this concept are to treat, diagnose and prevent certain diseases such as obesity, diabetes, hypertension, and cancer. Chronic respiratory diseases such as asthma, have also been included [57,58]. Dealing with herbal medicine or herbal interventions for chronic asthma would be a very broad topic difficult to fully address in this review; however, it is possible to highlight their benefits as adjuvant supplementary therapies to the main pharmacological treatment and their possibilities to reduce its doses and potential adverse effects of the latter. In general, this type of intervention is organized into:

(a) Diet, Vitamins and Food Supplements

Various studies have confirmed that food and nutrients can protect the airway from oxidative damage through different mechanisms. For example, some vitamins (soluble (vitamin C) and fat-soluble (vitamin E)) are considered an important defense against RONS. Similarly, carotenoids (α and β), vitamin A, and lycopene have shown significant potential antioxidant effects. Those results also show that asthmatic individuals present lower concentrations of vitamins A, C and E, which may enhance their symptoms. The same happens if selenium levels are low, since this element is essential for the enzyme glutathione peroxidase (GPx) to function properly and to reduce the amount of H_2O_2, preventing the lipid peroxidation of the cell membrane [43,59,60].

Some evidence shows that asthmatic adults with a diet low in antioxidants may have a low FEV1, FVC and more frequent exacerbations. These alterations tend to balance when they ingest a nutritional supplement enriched with antioxidants [43,61]. Research carried out by Hernández et al. (2013) and Peh et al. (2015) with the vitamin E γ-tocotrienol isoform showed that this isoform can inhibit oxidative damage by promoting the production of endogenous antioxidants in the lungs. The process was related to its potential to increase Nrf2 levels by blocking Nuclear Factor Kappa-Light-Chain-Enhancer of Activated B Cells (NF-κB). They also noted that the airway hyperreactivity improved and the lipopolysaccharide-induced neutrophil infiltration decreased [62,63]. All these vitamins and nutrients are essential for humans and are found in different fruits, vegetables, seeds, cereals, seed oils, nuts, shellfish and some red meat [43,59]. Another known and relevant therapy is thiol antioxidants, which induce the conversion of glutathione. N-acetyl cysteine (NAC). NAC treatment is known to reduce the need of bronchodilators and the responsiveness of the airway when irritated by inhaling diesel exhaust. Furthermore, it has also been linked to its potential to significantly inhibit RONS and lipid peroxidation [43,64].

(b) Plants and Natural Extracts

The consumption of medicinal plants to treat different diseases has increased worldwide in recent years. Many asthmatics use plants alone or in combination with prescribed medications to try to reduce and/or control symptoms. Two randomized meta-analysis studies collected different controlled trials to evaluate the effectiveness of herbal medicine in adults with this condition. In the first study (2010), 26 trials on approximately 20 herbal preparations considered in Chinese, Indian and Japanese therapies were analyzed; the evaluation parameters were divided into primary (lung function, number of exacerbations and reduction in the use of corticosteroids) and secondary (symptoms and adverse effects). In summary, their results showed very few relevant data on reductions in exacerbation. Six studies with Chinese therapy indicated changes in FEV1 and a study where 1.8-Cineol (eucalyptol) was used showed evidence of a reduction in the daily dose of oral steroids [65,66]. The second study (2016) consisted of 29 trials that included 3000 participants with an average age of 43 years. Mainly, the anti-asthmatic effect of the plants *Glycyrrhiza uralensis* (licorice root), *Angelica Sinensis*, *Pinellia ternata*, and *Astragalus membraneceus* (the latter two included in traditional Chinese medicine) were evaluated. The diagnosis and treatment of the disease was performed on the basis of parameters of the GINA. The analysis confirmed that almost all plants, as a complement to routine therapy, improved the asthmatic control and lung function. Likewise, the frequency of acute exacerbations and the use of salbutamol decreased [66]. In addition to the examples mentioned above, there are records on the plants "Perpetual" (*Helichrysum stoechas*), "Eucalyptus" (*Eucalyptus globulus*), "Rosemary" (*Rosmarinus officinalis*), "Ginger" (*Zingiber officinale*) and "Elecampane" (*Inula helenium*) that due to their aromas and relaxing effects, they can reduce asthma symptoms [43,67]. It is worth mentioning that the traditional consumption of these medicinal herbs is, in general, orally, on a weekly basis and for one month (mainly as aqueous extracts or tea). According to each area or geographic entity where they are used, their preparation includes the use of the plant alone or a mixture derived from the leaves, stems, roots and/or fruits.

On the other hand, garlic (*Allium sativum* L.), a bulbous perennial plant with a peculiar purgative flavor, has shown antimicrobial, antifungal, analgesic, antihypertensive, anticancer, antioxidant and anti-asthmatic capabilities, attributed to different phytochemicals in its chemical composition, among which organic sulfur compounds (such as diallyl sulfide (DS)) stand out. In the case of its anti-asthmatic potential, studies conducted with DS showed that when it acts on Nrf2 it can reduce ovalbumin-induced infiltrated inflammatory cells and proinflammatory cytokines in BALF mice [57,68].

Finally, research carried out with resveratrol, a phenolic compound found in grapes, indicated that it can decrease ROS production and reverse the high levels of TNF-α and iNOS in the lungs of obese C57BL/6 male mice sensitized with ovalbumin (OVA). This protective effect is probably related to its ability to regulate the decrease in the phosphoinositide 3-kinase-protein kinase B pathway, while regulating or producing an elevation of inositol polyphosphate 4 phosphatase [69,70].

(c) Therapy and Integrative Medicine (IM) for Asthmatic Control

Due to the multifactorial nature of asthma and the fact that the disease has neuromuscular (bronchospasm), immunological (inflammation) and psychological components, another possible alternative for its control and treatment can be through an integrative medicine (IM) approach [this concept was defined by the National Center for Complementary and Integrative Health—NIH (NIH-NCCAM), in other words, approaching all the pathways of its pathophysiology through an integrative medicine that combines the use of complementary evidence-based therapies with conventional medicine. As mentioned already, some studies suggest that more than 50% of asthmatic individuals (children and/or adults) express dissatisfaction with conventional control treatments (β2AA, anticholinergics, methylxanthines, ID and antileukotrienes) and/or unconformity due to the resultant side effects. Among the most common and used IMs are dietary and nutritional therapies, herbal remedies, homeopathy, acupuncture, massage, yoga breathing exercises, relaxation and mind–body therapies (MBSR), and Qigong (a traditional Chinese medicine combining movement, meditation and breathing techniques) [71–73].

Since Arthur Kleinman [74] suggested to the medical field that individuals may have more options to treat their diseases, not just the conventional biomedical approach, research evaluating the combination of traditional practices with conventional therapies have increased. Those that reduce stress and anxiety favor a better attitude towards the disease and therefore asthmatic attacks can also be reduced. One of the first studies (1986) was a prospective, randomized, single-blind controlled trial with 44 adults of both genders. In that study, the use of bronchodilators was reduced and a 70% improvement in their induced airway hyperresponsiveness was evidenced by methacholine after 6-week hypnotherapy [75]. Hypnotherapy has also been successful in the pediatric population; Anbar (2002) confirmed an 80% decrease in asthmatic symptoms (cough, shortness of breath, chest pain and hyperventilation) in children treated with this therapy. This type of therapy has also contributed to reducing school absenteeism [76].

Other studies where different types of yoga programs were analyzed as a treatment therapy showed a progressive improvement in lung function in both children and adults during the course of the treatment. However, the results on the benefits of this type of therapy in asthmatic children were not completely significant and definitive. Thus, is necessary to explore this technique in new clinical trials [77–79].

Mindfulness-based stress reduction (MBSR) is another mind–body approach with some promise of success. This technique has been frequently used for the treatment of anxiety and pain as well as symptoms related to cancer. Pbert et al. (2012) compared a randomized controlled trial of an 8-week MBSR program against an educational program in adult patients with asthma. At the end of the evaluation period, they confirmed clinically significant improvements in their quality of life and stress reduction, which had a favorable impact on their lung function [80].

Finally, research carried out by Cotton et al. (2011) and Shen and Oraka (2012) indicated that approximately 70% of children and adolescents, belonging to poor socioeconomic backgrounds, with poorly controlled asthma, used complementary and alternative medicine for the management of their disease. The most used therapies were relaxation (85%), breathing techniques (58%), and herbal products (12%). The results of both studies conclude that these therapies may be useful to improve asthmatic control [81,82].

8. Perspectives and Conclusions

This review demonstrates the attention that different health professionals have shown to understand more clearly and concisely the pathophysiology of asthma. The data presented confirm that, over the years, the knowledge about the mechanisms involved in the development of this entity, as well as its classification, treatment and control have increased and evolved. The GINA compiled the most outstanding information from GEMA and GUIMA to create the most current version of a catalog or guide for its diagnosis, management and treatment that supports doctors, researchers and scientists.

Currently, GINA 2020 suggests classifying asthma in intermittent cases—slightly persistent, moderately persistent and severely persistent—which allows us to define appropriate guidelines for drug therapy. Given that asthma cannot be completely cured, it is advisable to seek suitable control to decrease severity and possible risks in patients. It is also convenient to encourage people to know more about their disease (patient education) and to reduce or avoid risk factors (occupational/environmental situation), since this is where various allergen agents that activate symptoms are located.

It is of utmost importance that health professionals make an adequate diagnosis based on the patient's medical record considering their social, environmental and family history. When performing a physical examination, evaluating the symptoms of respiratory obstruction (cough, wheezing, chest tightness and possible respiratory distress), is also relevant to fully confirm the disease after analyzing lung function tests established by the asthmatic diagnosis algorithm (Figure 1).

Regarding therapeutic management, which has ceased to have an empirical nature, evolving through the consensus of national and international guidelines, it is convenient to remember that this chronic inflammatory disease should preferably be treated early with an anti-inflammatory therapy. The information shown in this article classifies the drugs used in asthmatic management into two groups, those with bronchodilator potential that achieve symptomatic improvement by relaxing the smooth muscle of the airway (β2AA, anticholinergics and methylxanthines) and, on the other hand, the agents that control inflammation (ID and antileukotrienes).

According to the latest GINA 2020 version, this entity should be managed through five steps. In the first, a combination of budesonide and formoterol should be used at low doses, eliminating monotherapy with β2AA (such as albuterol). During the next step, it would be advisable to start using an ID on a daily basis and include a short-acting β2AA on demand. Subsequently, three possibilities are considered: a) maintaining the IDs combined with long-acting β2AA, b) IDs at low doses plus an antileukotriene, or c) start using a medium-dose of IDs. In the fourth step, two options are considered: a combination of ID (medium dose) and a long-acting β2AA or ID and the same dose plus an antileukotriene. Finally, during the fifth step, it is suggested that a pulmonologist, allergologist or immunologist assesses the use of high or medium doses of ID combined with long-acting β2AA.

However, as with many drugs, IDs can generate different adverse effects when accumulated (mainly in oral and pharyngeal mucous membranes) or used at high doses. These undesirable effects are mainly related to the suppression of the hypothalamic–pituitary–adrenal glands axis and the probability of inducing osteoporosis, cataracts, skin atrophy, weight gain, diabetes, hypertension, psychological disorders and immunosuppression. Unfortunately, if patients interrupt their drug therapy, their symptoms may reappear or increase. Thus, asthmatic control continues to be a great challenge, given that more than 50% of patients are not completely controlled.

Asthmatic treatments continue to evolve in order to reduce symptoms and improve the quality of life of patients. In recent years, notable advances have been made in the biological therapy of monoclonal antibodies (MoAb), among which omalizumab is the only MoAb approved for asthmatic individuals over 12 years of age, administered subcutaneously on a monthly basis and with a mechanism of action based on the protein–protein interaction between its high-affinity receptor and IgE, avoiding binding to mast cells and basophils to decrease the release of inflammatory mediators.

On the other hand, considering that asthma triggers inflammatory processes and that the scientific evidence of its relationship with oxidative stress (ROS/RNS) has increased, herbal strategies and the use of antioxidants might be supportive to traditional pharmacological treatments, probably to reduce doses and adverse effects. Different scientific evidence has suggested that a diet including fruits, vegetables, seeds and cereals, the consumption of vitamins A, C, and E and the use of plants and natural extracts (phytotherapy) contribute to reducing and/or controlling asthmatic symptoms. Different plants, such as *Glycyrrhiza uralensis*, *Angelica Sinensis*, *Pinellia ternata*, *Astragalus membranaceus*, *Helichrysum stoechas*, *Eucalyptus globulus*, *Rosmarinus officinalis*, *Zingiber officinale*, *Inula helenium* and *Allium sativum* L., have shown this benefit and opened up the possibility of analyzing different bioactive compounds, such as diallyl sulfide (extracted from garlic) and resveratrol (obtained from grapes).

It is highly convenient to continue these research studies on other plants and their bioactive compounds (both in preclinical and clinical trials) in order to explore their anti-asthmatic potential, establish their doses and administration intervals and analyze their possible toxic effects in the short, medium and long term. This could contribute to obtaining and preparing new pharmaceutical products for asthma therapy as a relevant goal for the coming decades.

In summary, it is important to consider that, despite the medical progress of asthmatic treatment, its prevalence continues to increase, and its treatment is complicated given the multifactorial nature of the disease. Conventional and newer pharmacotherapies along with integrative herbal and mind–body approaches for asthma may help address symptoms and improve quality of life. A general practitioner and/or specialist must be informed and updated on the subject. They should also be willing to employ different strategies that improve clinical results and are beneficial for quality of life in asthmatic patients.

Author Contributions: E.M.-S., E.M.-B., D.A.A.-B., J.P.-R., J.A.M.-G. designed the concept, conducted the literature search, wrote the majority of the paper and managed the authors; M.S.-G., J.A.I.-V., and Á.M.-G. wrote key sections of the paper; I.Á.-G., N.V.-M., and J.P.-R. wrote sections of the paper and managed the reference list. All authors have read and agreed to the published version of the manuscript.

Funding: This research received no external funding.

Acknowledgments: The authors thank Florencia Ana María Talavera Silva for all her academic support. Her comments and observations in reviewing articles are always valuable and we give her immense recognition for her efforts.

Conflicts of Interest: The authors declare no conflict of interest.

References

1. Beasley, R.; Semprini, A.; Mitchell, E.A. Risk factors for asthma: Is prevention possible? *Lancet* **2015**, *386*, 1075–1085. [CrossRef]
2. The Global Initiative for Asthma. Global Strategy for Asthma Management and Prevention. 2006. Available online: https://ginasthma.org/wp-content/uploads/2019/01/2006-GINA.pdf (accessed on 11 May 2020).
3. Del Río-Navarro, B.E.; Hidalgo-Castro, E.M.; Sienra-Monge, J.J.L. Asthma. *Bol. Med. Hosp. Infant. Mex.* **2009**, *66*, 3–33.
4. Global Strategy for Asthma Management and Prevention. Global Initiative for Asthma (GINA) 2020. Available online: https://ginasthma.org/wp-content/uploads/2020/06/GINA-2020-report_20_06_04-1-wms.pdf (accessed on 11 July 2020).
5. Larenas-Linnemann, D.; Salas-Hernández, J.; Vázquez-García, J.C.; Ortiz-Aldana, I.; Fernández-Vega, M.; Del Río-Navarro, B.E.; Cano-Salas, M.C.; Luna-Pech, J.A.; Ortega-Martell, J.A.; Romero-Lombard, J.; et al. Mexican Asthma Guidelines: GUIMA 2017. *Rev. Alerg. Mex.* **2017**, *64*, s11–s128. [PubMed]
6. Mexican Institute of Social Security (IMSS). Diagnosis, Treatment and Prevention of Exacerbation of Asthma in Adults. Evidence and Recommendations Master Catalog of Clinical Practice Guidelines: IMSS-806-17 Clinical Practice Guide. México. 2017. Available online: http://www.imss.gob.mx/sites/all/statics/guiasclinicas/806GRR.pdf (accessed on 11 May 2020).
7. Plaza-Moral, V.; Alonso-Mostaza, S.; Alvarez-Rodríguez, C.; Gomez-Outes, A.; Gómez-Ruiz, F.; López-Vina, A.; Molina París, J.; Pellegrini-Belinchón, F.J.; Plaza-Zamora, J.; Quintano-Jiménez, J.A.; et al. Spanish guideline on the management of asthma. *J. Investig. Allergol. Clin. Immunol.* **2016**, *1*, 1–92. [CrossRef]
8. Jeffrey, A.Y.; Hubaida, F.; Dawn, C.N. Hormones, Sex, and Asthma. *Ann. Allergy Asthma Immunol.* **2018**, *120*, 488–494.
9. Durán, R. Pathophysiology of asthma: A current view. *Rev. Col. Neumol.* **2015**, *27*, 226–230.
10. Jeffery, P. Inflammation and remodeling in the adult and child with asthma. *Pediatr. Pulmonol.* **2001**, *32*, 3–16. [CrossRef]
11. Rasmussen, F.; Taylor, D.R.; Flannery, E.M.; Cowan, J.O.; Greene, J.M.; Herbison, G.P.; Sears, M.R. Risk factors for airway remodeling in asthma manifested by a low post bronchodilator FEV1/vital capacity ratio. *Am. J. Respir. Crit. Care Med.* **2002**, *165*, 1480–1488. [CrossRef]
12. Holgate, S.T.; Davies, D.E.; Lacke, P.M.; Wilson, S.J.; Puddicombe, S.M.; Lordan, J.L. Epithelial-mesenchymal interactions in the pathogenesis of asthma. *J. Allergy Clin. Immunol.* **2000**, *105*, 193–204. [CrossRef]
13. Joos, G.F. The role of neuroeffector mechanisms in the pathogenesis of asthma. *Curr. Allergy Asthma Rep.* **2001**, *1*, 134–143. [CrossRef]
14. Lemanske, R.F. Inflammatory events in asthma: An expanding equation. *J. Allergy Clin. Immunol.* **2000**, *105*, S633–S636. [CrossRef] [PubMed]
15. Stone, K.D.; Prussin, C.; Metcalfe, D.D. IgE, mast cell, basophils, and eosinophils. *J. Allergy Clin. Immunol.* **2010**, *125*, 73–80 [CrossRef] [PubMed]
16. Martínez-Aguilar, N.E. Aetiopathogenesis, risk factors, and asthma triggers. *NCT* **2009**, *68*, S98–S110.
17. Maciag, M.C.; Phipatanakul, W. Preventing the development of asthma: Stopping the allergic march. *Curr. Opin. Allergy Clin. Immunol.* **2019**, *19*, 161–168. [CrossRef] [PubMed]
18. Mota-Pinto, A.; Todo-Bom, A. The role of the epithelial cell in asthma. *Rev. Port. Pneumol.* **2009**, *15*, 461–472. [PubMed]
19. Huckabee, M.M.; Peebles, R.S., Jr. Novel concepts in virally induced asthma. *Clin. Mol. Allergy* **2009**, *7*, 2. [CrossRef]
20. Kallal, L.; Lukas, N. The Role of Chemokines in virus- associated asthma exacerbations. *Curr. Allergy Asthma Rep.* **2008**, *8*, 443–450. [CrossRef]
21. Reed, C.E.; Kita, H. The role of protease activation of inflammation in allergic respiratory diseases. *J. Allergy Clin. Immunol.* **2004**, *114*, 997–1008. [CrossRef]
22. Abdo, R.A.; Cué, B.M.; Álvarez, C.M. Bronchial asthma: Crisis risk factors and preventive factors. *Rev. Cubana Med. Gen. Integr.* **2007**, *23*, 1561–3038.
23. Furrie, E. Probiotics and allergy. *Proc. Nutr. Soc.* **2005**, *64*, 465–469. [CrossRef]
24. Wood, L.H. Diet, Obesity, and Asthma. *Ann. Am. Thorac. Soc.* **2017**, *14*, S332–S338. [CrossRef] [PubMed]

25. Arias-López, J.C.; Ortíz-Vidal, M.A.; Restrepo, J.C. Asthma in the pediatric population: Risk factors and diagnosis. A current revision. *Salutem Sci. Spiritus* **2018**, *4*, 35–40.
26. Rodrigo, G.J.; Plaza, V. Body mass index and response to emergency department treatment in adults with severe asthma exacerbations: A prospective cohort study. *Chest* **2007**, *132*, 1513–1519. [CrossRef] [PubMed]
27. Shore, S.A. Obesity and asthma: Possible mechanisms. *J. Allergy Clin. Immunol.* **2008**, *121*, 1087–1093. [CrossRef]
28. Forno, E.; Celedón, J.C. Health Disparities in Asthma. *Am. J. Respir. Crit. Care Med.* **2012**, *185*, 1033–1043. [CrossRef]
29. Akinbami, L.J.; Moorman, J.E.; Simon, A.E.; Schoendorf, K.C. Trends in racial disparities for asthma outcomes among children 0–17 years, 2001–2010. *J. Allergy Clin. Immunol.* **2014**, *134*, 547–553. [CrossRef]
30. Brewer, M.; Kimbro, R.T.; Denney, J.T.; Osiecki, K.M.; Moffett, B.; Lopez, K. Does neighborhood social and environmental context impact race/ethnic disparities in childhood asthma? *Health Place* **2017**, *44*, 86–93. [CrossRef]
31. Schwela, D. Air pollution and health in urban areas. *Rev. Environ. Health* **2000**, *15*, 13–42. [CrossRef]
32. Dreborg, S. The implications of nomenclature. *Ann. Allergy Asthma Immunol.* **2002**, *89*, 83–85. [CrossRef]
33. Jindal, S.K.; Gupta, D. The relationship between tobacco smoke & bronchial asthma. *Indian J. Med. Res.* **2004**, *120*, 443–453.
34. Mortimer, K.; Neugebauer, R.; Lurmann, F.; Alcorn, S.; Balmes, J.; Tager, I. Air pollution and pulmonary function in asthmatic children: Effects of prenatal and lifetime exposures. *Epidemiology* **2008**, *19*, 550–557. [CrossRef] [PubMed]
35. Tarlo, S.M. Irritant-induced asthma in the workplace. *Curr. Allergy Asthma Rep.* **2014**, *14*, 406–411. [CrossRef] [PubMed]
36. Rico-Rosillo, G.; Cambray-Gutiérrez, J.C.; Vega-Robledo, G.B. Occupational asthma. *Rev. Aler. Mex.* **2015**, *62*, 48–59.
37. Bharadwaj, P.; Zivin, J.G.; Mullins, J.T.; Neidell, M. Early-Life Exposure to the Great Smog of 1952 and the Development of Asthma. *Am. J. Respir. Crit. Care Med.* **2016**, *194*, 1475–1482. [CrossRef] [PubMed]
38. Rodríguez-Santos, O.; Olea-Zapata, R.; Vite-Juárez, N.E.; Gonzales-Saravia, C.A.; Rojas-Galarza, R.A.; Laurrabaquio-Miranda, A.M.; Díaz-Zúñiga, J.A. Sensitization to penicillin allergens in patients suffering from allergic diseases. *VacciMonitor* **2018**, *27*, 16–21.
39. Duce-Gracia, F.; Sebastián-Ariño, A. Medicines and additives whose use may involve risk in the asthmatic patient. *Med. Respir.* **2013**, *6*, 29–38.
40. Rajan, J.P.; Wineinger, N.E.; Stevenson, D.D.; White, A.A. Prevalence of aspirin-exacerbated respiratory disease among asthmatic patients: A meta-analysis of the literature. *J. Allergy Clin. Immunol.* **2015**, *135*, 676–681. [CrossRef]
41. Ishitsuka, Y.; Kondo, Y.; Kadowaki, D. Toxicological Property of Acetaminophen: The Dark Side of a Safe Antipyretic/Analgesic Drug? *Biol. Pharm. Bull.* **2020**, *43*, 195–206. [CrossRef]
42. Hicks-Gómez, J.J.; Sierra-Vargas, M.P.; Olivares-Corichi, I.M.; Torres-Ramos, Y.D.; Guzmán-Grenfell, A.M. Oxidative stress in asthma. *Rev. Inst. Nac. Enferm. Resp. Mex.* **2005**, *18*, 70–78.
43. Zhu, L.Y.; Ni, Z.H.; Luo, X.M.; Wang, X.B. Advance of antioxidants in asthma treatment. *World J. Respirol.* **2017**, *7*, 17–28. [CrossRef]
44. Dworski, R. Oxidant stress in asthma. *Thorax* **2000**, *2*, 51–53. [CrossRef] [PubMed]
45. Brennan, M.L.; Wu, W.; Fu, X.A. Tale of two controversies: Defining both role of peroxidase in nitrotyrosine formation in vivo using eosinophil peroxidase and myeloperoxidase-deficient mice, and the nature of peroxidase-generated reactive nitrogen species. *J. Biol. Chem.* **2002**, *277*, 17415–17427. [CrossRef] [PubMed]
46. Wu, W.; Chen, Y.; Hazen, S.L. Eosinophil peroxidase nitrates protein tyrosyl residues. Implications for oxidative damage by nitrating intermediates in eosinophilic inflammatory disorders. *J. Biol. Chem.* **1999**, *274*, 25933–25944. [CrossRef] [PubMed]
47. Zuo, L.; Otenbaker, N.P.; Rose, B.A.; Salisbury, K.S. Molecular mechanisms of reactive oxygen species-related pulmonary inflammation and asthma. *Mol. Immunol.* **2013**, *56*, 57–63. [CrossRef]
48. Marwick, J.A.; Tudor, C.; Khorasani, N.; Michaeloudes, C.; Bhavsar, P.K.; Chung, K.F. Oxidants induce a corticosteroid-insensitive phosphorylation of histone 3 at serine 10 in monocytes. *PLoS ONE* **2015**, *10*, e0124961. [CrossRef]

49. Shalaby, K.H.; Allard-Coutu, A.; O'Sullivan, M.J.; Nakada, E.; Qureshi, S.T.; Day, B.J.; Martin, J.G. Inhaled birch pollen extract induces airway hyperresponsiveness via oxidative stress but independently of pollen-intrinsic NADPH oxidase activity, or the TLR4-TRIF pathway. *J. Immunol.* **2013**, *191*, 922–933. [CrossRef]
50. Henricks, P.A.; Nijkamp, F.P. Reactive oxygen species as mediators in asthma. *Pulm. Pharmacol. Ther.* **2001**, *14*, 409–420. [CrossRef]
51. Geraghty, P.; Hardigan, A.A.; Wallace, A.M.; Mirochnitchenko, O.; Thankachen, J.; Arellanos, L.; Thompson, V.; D'Armiento, J.M.; Foronjy, R.F. The glutathione peroxidase 1-protein tyrosine phosphatase 1B-protein phosphatase 2A axis. A key determinant of airway inflammation and alveolar destruction. *Am. J. Respir. Cell Mol. Biol.* **2013**, *49*, 721–730. [CrossRef]
52. Lemanske, R.F.J.; Busse, W.W. Asthma. *J. Allergy Clin. Immunol.* **2003**, *111*, S502–S519. [CrossRef]
53. Gurrola-Silva, A.; Huerta-López, J.G. Asthma history. *Alerg. Asma e Inmunol. Ped.* **2013**, *22*, 77–86.
54. Feldman, A.S.; He, Y.; Moore, M.L.; Hershenson, M.B.; Hartert, T.V. Toward primary prevention of asthma. Reviewing the evidence for early-life respiratory viral infections as modifiable risk factors to prevent childhood asthma. *Am. J. Respir. Crit. Care Med.* **2015**, *191*, 34–44. [CrossRef] [PubMed]
55. Quirce, S.; Bobolea, I.; Domínguez-Ortega, J.; Barranco, P. Future biological therapies in asthma. *Arch. Bronconeumol.* **2014**, *50*, 355–361. [CrossRef] [PubMed]
56. Pelaia, C.; Calabrese, C.; Terracciano, R.; De Blasio, F.; Vatrella, A.; Pelaia, G. Omalizumab, the First Available Antibody for Biological Treatment of Severe Asthma: More Than a Decade of Real-Life Effectiveness. *Ther. Adv. Respir. Dis.* **2018**, *12*, 1–16. [CrossRef] [PubMed]
57. Morales-González, J.A.; Madrigal-Bujaidar, E.; Sánchez-Gutiérrez, M.; Izquierdo-Vega, J.A.; Valadez-Vega, M.D.C.; Álvarez-González, I.; Morales-González, Á.; Madrigal-Santillán, E. Garlic (*Allium sativum* L.): A Brief Review of Its Antigenotoxic Efects. *Foods* **2019**, *8*, 343. [CrossRef] [PubMed]
58. Garcia-Quiala, M.; Díaz-Pita, G. The effectiveness of herbal medicine in patients suffering from bronchial asthma. *Rev. Cienc. Médicas* **2012**, *16*, 118–131.
59. Olivares-Corichi, I.M.; Guzmán-Grenfell, A.M.; Sierra-Vargas, M.P.; Mendoza-Atencio, R.S.; Hicks-Gómez, J.J. Prospects for the use of antioxidants as adjuvants in the treatment of asthma. *Rev. Inst. Nac. Enferm. Resp. Mex.* **2005**, *18*, 154–161.
60. Barrera-Mendoza, C.C.; Ayala-Mata, F.; Cortés-Rojo, C.; García-Pérez, M.E.; Rodríguez-Orozco, A.R. Antioxidant vitamins in asthma. *Rev. Alerg. Mex.* **2018**, *65*, 61–77. [CrossRef]
61. Wood, L.G.; Garg, M.L.; Smart, J.M.; Scott, H.A.; Barker, D.; Gibson, P.G. Manipulating antioxidant intake in asthma: A randomized controlled trial. *Am. J. Clin. Nutr.* **2012**, *96*, 534–543. [CrossRef]
62. Hernandez, M.L.; Wagner, J.G.; Kala, A.; Mills, K.; Wells, H.B.; Alexis, N.E.; Lay, J.C.; Jiang, Q.; Zhang, H.; Zhou, H.; et al. Vitamin E, γ-tocopherol, reduces airway neutrophil recruitment after inhaled endotoxin challenge in rats and in healthy volunteers. *Free Radic. Biol. Med.* **2013**, *60*, 56–62. [CrossRef]
63. Peh, H.Y.; Ho, W.E.; Cheng, C.; Chan, T.K.; Seow, A.C.; Lim, A.Y.; Fong, C.W.; Seng, K.Y.; Ong, C.N.; Wong, W.S. Vitamin E Isoform γ-Tocotrienol Downregulates House Dust Mite-Induced Asthma. *J. Immunol.* **2015**, *195*, 437–444. [CrossRef]
64. Carlsten, C.; MacNutt, M.J.; Zhang, Z.; Sava, F.; Pui, M.M. Anti-oxidant N-acetylcysteine diminishes diesel exhaust-induced increased airway responsiveness in person with airway hyper-reactivity. *Toxicol. Sci.* **2014**, *139*, 479–487. [CrossRef] [PubMed]
65. Clark, C.E.; Arnold, E.; Lasserson, T.J.; Wu, T. Herbal Interventions for Chronic Asthma in Adults and Children: A Systematic Review and Meta-Analysis. *Prim. Care Respir. J.* **2010**, *19*, 307–314. [CrossRef] [PubMed]
66. Shergis, J.L.; Wu, L.; Zhang, A.L.; Guo, X.; Lu, C.; Xue, C.C. Herbal medicine for adults with asthma: A systematic review. *J. Asthma* **2016**, *53*, 650–659. [CrossRef] [PubMed]
67. López-Romero, D.; Izquierdo-Vega, J.A.; Morales-González, J.M.; Madrigal-Bujaidar, E.; Chamorro-Cevallos, G.; Sánchez-Gutiérrez, M.; Betanzos-Cabrera, G.; Alvarez-Gonzalez, I.; Morales-González, A.; Madrigal-Santillán, E. Evidence of Some Natural Products With Antigenotoxic Effects. Part 2: Plants, Vegetables, and Natural Resin. *Nutrients* **2018**, *10*, 1954. [CrossRef] [PubMed]
68. Ho, C.Y.; Lu, C.C.; Weng, C.J.; Yen, G.C. Protective effects of Diallyl Sulfide on ovoalbumin-induced pulmonary inflammation of allergic asthma mice by MicroRNA-144. -34a. and -34b/c-modulated Nrf2 activation. *J. Agric. Food Chem.* **2016**, *64*, 151–160. [CrossRef] [PubMed]

69. André, D.M.; Calixto, M.C.; Sollon, C.; Alexandre, E.C.; Leiria, L.O.; Tobar, N.; Anhê, G.F.; Antunes, E. Therapy with resveratrol attenuates obesity-associated allergic airway inflammation in mice. *Int. Immunopharmacol.* **2016**, *38*, 298–305. [CrossRef]
70. Aich, J.; Mabalirajan, U.; Ahmad, T.; Khanna, K.; Rehman, R.; Agrawal, A.; Ghosh, B. Resveratrol attenuates experimental allergic asthma in mice by restoring inositol polyphosphate 4 phosphatase (INPP4A). *Int. Immunopharmacol.* **2012**, *14*, 438–443. [CrossRef]
71. George, M.; Topaz, M. A systematic review of complementary and alternative medicine for asthma self-management. *Nurs. Clin. N. Am.* **2013**, *48*, 53–149. [CrossRef]
72. McClafferty, H. An overview of integrative therapies in asthma treatment. *Curr. Allergy Asthma Rep.* **2014**, *14*, 464–472. [CrossRef]
73. Yeh, G.Y.; Horwitz, R. Integrative Medicine for Respiratory Conditions: Asthma and Chronic Obstructive Pulmonary Disease. *Med. Clin. N. Am.* **2017**, *101*, 925–941. [CrossRef]
74. Kleinman, A.; Eisenberg, L.; Good, B. Culture, illness, and care: Clinical lessons from anthropologic and cross-cultural research. *Ann. Intern. Med.* **1978**, *88*, 251–258. [CrossRef] [PubMed]
75. Ewer, T.C.; Stewart, D.E. Improvement in bronchial hyper-responsiveness in patients with moderate asthma after treatment with a hypnotic technique: A randomised controlled trial. *Br. Med. J.* **1986**, *293*, 1129–1132. [CrossRef] [PubMed]
76. Anbar, R.D. Hypnosis in pediatrics: Applications at a pediatric pulmonary center. *BMC Pediatr.* **2002**, *2*, 11–17. [CrossRef] [PubMed]
77. Galantino, M.L.; Galbavy, R.; Quinn, L. Therapeutic effects of yoga for children: A systematic review of the literature. *Pediatr. Phys. Ther.* **2008**, *20*, 66–80. [CrossRef] [PubMed]
78. Vempati, R.; Lal Bijlani, R.; Kumar-Deepak, K. The efficacy of a comprehensive lifestyle modification programme based on yoga in the management of bronchial asthma: A randomized controlled trial. *BMC Pulm. Med.* **2009**, *9*, 37–49. [CrossRef]
79. Tahan, F.; Eke Gungor, H.; Bicici, E. Is yoga training beneficial for exercise-induced bronchoconstriction? *Altern. Ther. Health Med.* **2014**, *20*, 18–23.
80. Pbert, L.; Madison, J.M.; Druker, S.; Olendzki, N.; Magner, R.; Reed, G.; Allison, J.; Carmody, J. Effect of mindfulness training on asthma quality of life and lung function: A randomised controlled trial. *Thorax* **2012**, *67*, 769–776. [CrossRef]
81. Cotton, S.; Luberto, C.M.; Yi, M.S.; Tsevat, J. Complementary and alternative medicine behaviors and beliefs in urban adolescents with asthma. *J. Asthma* **2011**, *48*, 531–538. [CrossRef]
82. Shen, J.; Oraka, E. Complementary and alternative medicine (CAM) use among children with current asthma. *Prev. Med.* **2012**, *54*, 27–31. [CrossRef]

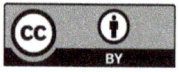

© 2020 by the authors. Licensee MDPI, Basel, Switzerland. This article is an open access article distributed under the terms and conditions of the Creative Commons Attribution (CC BY) license (http://creativecommons.org/licenses/by/4.0/).

MDPI
St. Alban-Anlage 66
4052 Basel
Switzerland
Tel. +41 61 683 77 34
Fax +41 61 302 89 18
www.mdpi.com

Medicina Editorial Office
E-mail: medicina@mdpi.com
www.mdpi.com/journal/medicina

www.ingramcontent.com/pod-product-compliance
Lightning Source LLC
LaVergne TN
LVHW070649100526
838202LV00013B/922